Symposium on the laser in ophthalmology and glaucoma update

TRANSACTIONS OF THE NEW ORLEANS ACADEMY OF OPHTHALMOLOGY

Previously published

Transactions of the New Orleans Academy of Ophthalmology

available from The C.V. Mosby Company are listed below:

Symposium on Glaucoma, 1981

Symposium on Diseases and Surgery
of the Lids, Lacrimal Apparatus,
and Orbit, 1982

Symposium on Medical and Surgical
Diseases of the Retina and
Vitreous, 1983

Symposium on Cataract Surgery, 1984

Symposium on the laser in ophthalmology and glaucoma update

TRANSACTIONS OF THE NEW ORLEANS ACADEMY OF OPHTHALMOLOGY

HUGH BECKMAN, M.D.
DAVID G. CAMPBELL, M.D.
FRANCIS A. L'ESPERANCE, Jr., M.D.
MARTIN A. MAINSTER, M.D., Ph.D.
HARRY A. QUIGLEY, M.D.
ROBERT N. SHAFFER, M.D.
RICHARD J. SIMMONS, M.D.
ROBERT C. WATZKE, M.D.
JAMES WISE, M.D.

with 232 *illustrations*

The C. V. Mosby Company

ST. LOUIS • TORONTO • PRINCETON 1985

MOSBY

A TRADITION OF PUBLISHING EXCELLENCE

Editor: Eugenia A. Klein
Developmental editor: Kathryn H. Falk
Manuscript editor: Roger McWilliams
Design: Staff
Production: Gail Morey Hudson, Mary Stueck, Susan Trail

Printed in the United States of America

The C.V. Mosby Company
11830 Westline Industrial Drive, St. Louis, Missouri 63146

Library of Congress Cataloging in Publication Data

Symposium on the Laser in Ophthalmology and
Glaucoma Update (1984: New Orleans, La.)
Symposium on the Laser in Ophthalmology and
Glaucoma Update.

Thirty-third annual symposium of the New Orleans Academy of Ophthalmology.
Includes bibliographies and index.
1. Glaucoma—Surgery—Congresses. 2. Lasers in surgery—Congresses. 3. Eye—Surgery—Congresses. I. Beckman, Hugh. II. New Orleans Academy of Ophthalmology. III. Title. [DNLM: 1. Lasers—Therapeutic use—Congresses. 2. Glaucoma—Surgery—Congresses. 3. Cataract Extraction—Congresses. WI TR226S]
RE871.S95 1984 617.7′1 84-14813
ISBN 0-8016-3669-8

C/MV/MV 9 8 7 6 5 4 3 2 1 02/D/283

Contributors

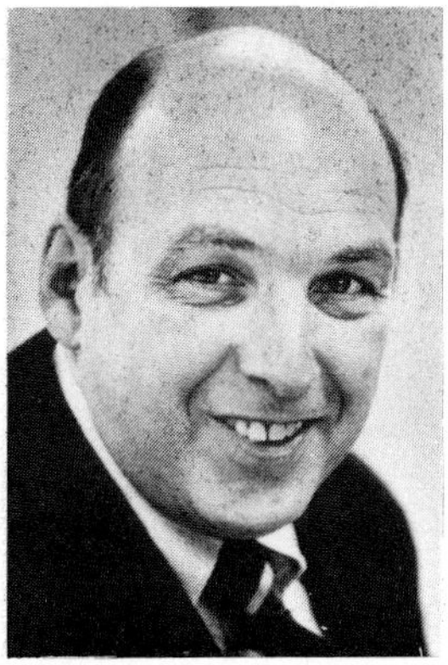

HUGH BECKMAN, M.D.

Chairman, Department of Ophthalmology, Sinai Hospital of Detroit; Associate Professor of Ophthalmology, Wayne State University, Detroit, Michigan

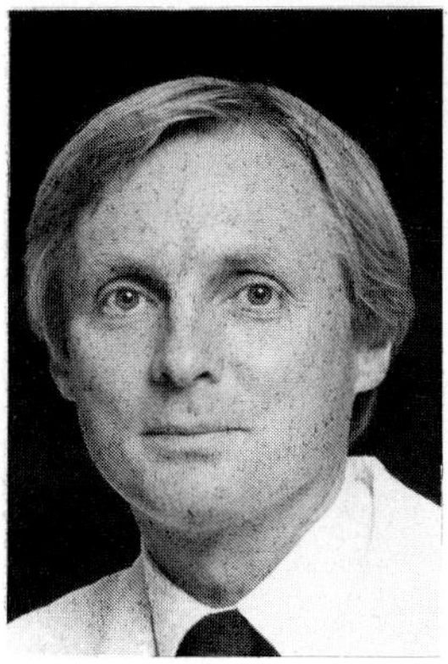

DAVID G. CAMPBELL, M.D.

Associate Professor, Department of Ophthalmology, Emory University School of Medicine; Director of Glaucoma Service, Emory Clinic, Atlanta, Georgia

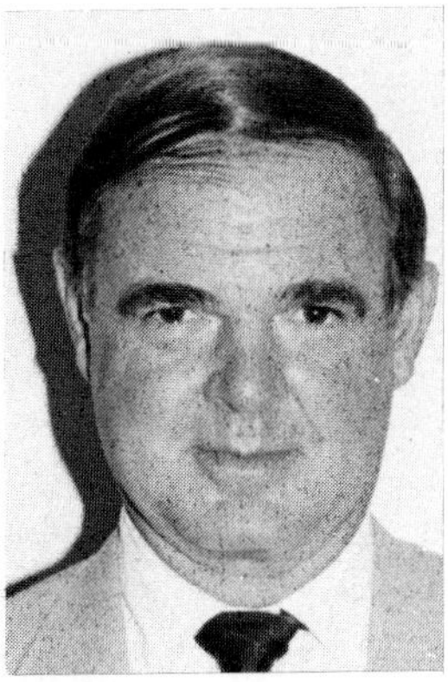

FRANCIS A. L'ESPERANCE, Jr., M.D.

Associate Professor of Clinical Ophthalmology, College of Physicians and Surgeons, Columbia-Presbyterian Medical Center, New York, New York

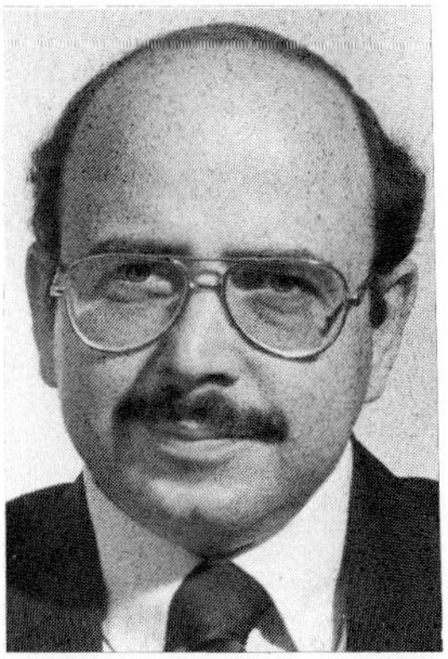

MARTIN A. MAINSTER, M.D., Ph.D.

Retina Associates, Eye Research Institute of Retina Foundation, Harvard Medical School, Boston, Massachusetts

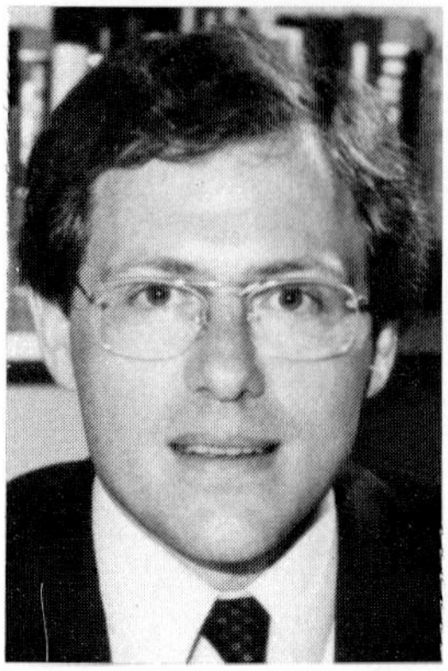

HARRY A. QUIGLEY, M.D.

Associate Professor, Ophthalmology, Director, Glaucoma Service, Wilmer Institute, Johns . Hopkins University School of Medicine, Baltimore, Maryland

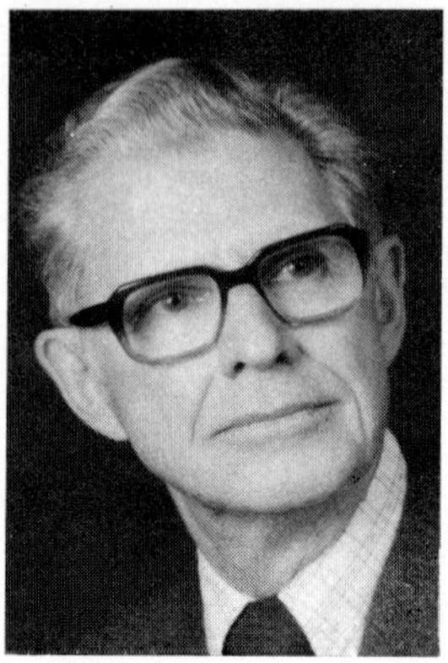

ROBERT N. SHAFFER, M.D.

Clinical Professor Emeritus, University o California San Francisco, San Francisco, California

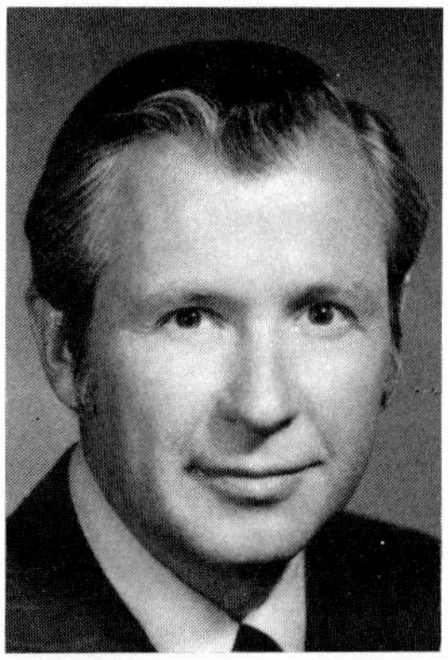

RICHARD J. SIMMONS, M.D.

Associate Clinical Professor of Ophthalmology, Harvard Medical School; Surgeon in Ophthalmology, Massachusetts Eye and Ear Infirmary, Boston, Massachusetts

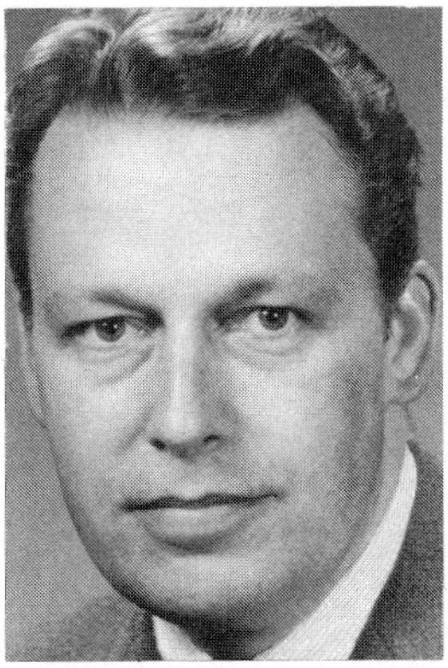

ROBERT C. WATZKE, M.D.

Professor of Ophthalmology, University of Oregon Health Sciences Center, Portland, Oregon; formerly Professor of Ophthalmology, University of Iowa Hospitals and Clinics, Iowa City, Iowa

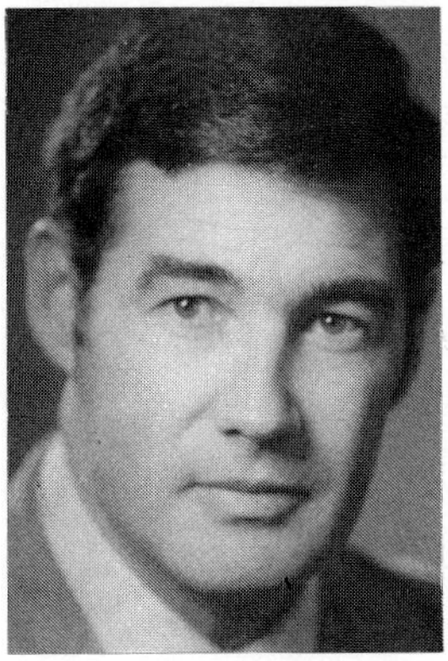

JAMES B. WISE, M.D.

Chairman, Department of Ophthalmology, Baptist Medical Center of Oklahoma, Oklahoma City, Oklahoma

Preface

While ''laser'' is becoming a familiar word to the average American household, ''laser use in medicine'' has been exerting a major force on the direction of future professional health care throughout the world. With the purpose of documenting an up-to-the-minute summary of laser use in the ophthalmic field and providing an in-depth update on a second targeted area of ''glaucoma diagnosis and therapy,'' the New Orleans Academy of Ophthalmology gathered the experts together and convened for its thirty-third annual symposium on March 1st through March 5th, 1984.

We extend our sincere thanks to the guest speakers and to all who participated, for their contributions of technical knowledge to this written record of our Meeting.

We also wish to thank Susan L. Larsen for her assistance with the preparation of this book.

Transactions Committee

Delmar R. Caldwell, M.D., *Chairman*
Walter D. Cockerham, M.D.
H. Frank Boswell, Jr., M.D.
George S. Ellis, M.D.
Robert J. Cangelosi, M.D.

Contents

1

The challenge of when to treat in glaucoma

Harry A. Quigley

In recent years there has been considerable change in the available information about the relationship between abnormal intraocular pressure (IOP) and the damage it can cause to the optic nerve in glaucoma. Whereas some facets of the glaucoma process are now better understood, a number of new questions have arisen about the appropriate time to initiate therapy and even about whether some patients require therapy at all. I will review changing concepts regarding glaucoma management to develop a practical course of action regarding the variety of patients we encounter. Although no single approach can apply to all situations, some general principles can be constructed to guide the individual management plan.

IS IT ELEVATED IOP THAT CAUSES VISION LOSS?

I will propose that most patients with glaucomatous optic disc cupping and visual field loss have or have had elevated IOP. As discussed in Chapter 11, however, the relation between IOP elevation and glaucoma damage remains clouded by discrepancies. Some eyes seem to tolerate short-term elevated IOP without detectable damage.[1,9] The level of IOP that causes visual loss also seems to vary among individuals, and a small number of eyes appear to suffer similar damage with statistically normal IOP (low-tension glaucoma). These inconsistencies continue to challenge our understanding of glaucoma and IOP, although recent clinical research has partly clarified the mystery.

Studies or large groups of patients have shown that elevated IOP is closely linked to glaucoma damage[1,6,9] and that the higher the IOP, the more likely that damage will occur.[3,5] One difficulty with such studies is the infrequency of IOP measurement: at best the IOP level is only checked a few times yearly and in some studies only once. Only a gross estimate of the average IOP over time is thus available. This would be satisfactory if the IOP were stably elevated in glaucoma patients, but it is evident that it is higher than normal on average and also more unstable than normal in these patients. Large swings can occur from hour to hour and day to day.[16] Thus, although the general causal relationship between high IOP level and resulting damage is established, it is not surprising that apparent discrepancies are noted. Our understanding of glaucoma would be greatly enhanced if a continuous monitoring system for IOP could be developed.

Since it is difficult to firmly establish the link between elevated IOP and glaucoma damage, we should question the conclusion that lowering IOP prevents or halts glaucoma damage. During this century some have doubted the efficacy of IOP reduction, although clinical reviews support the role of this action in halting further damage in most eyes, even with advanced optic neuropathy.[8,11] When IOP is lowered in one eye only, the chance of developing field loss is reduced considerably when compared to the untreated eye.[14] However, our ability to accurately monitor the mean IOP in each eye is limited, and data suggest that the susceptibility to damage at a given IOP level might vary from individual to individual. Thus, with no accurate way to assess what IOP level is safe, the ability to determine how much to lower IOP is frustrated.

WHY NOT TREAT EVERYONE WITH ELEVATED IOP?

If high IOP causes the damage and lowering it prevents the damage, why should we not treat anyone with abnormally high IOP? The population studies previously cited provide important data relative to this point. Most patients with abnormal IOP in several studies appeared to suffer no injury without treatment: 90% to 95% of those with IOP above 21 but below 30 mm Hg could be followed for 3 to 5 years untreated without the detection of a first field defect by standard perimetric methods using the Goldmann perimeter. Since therapy may not be benign and to some degree affects the patient's life-style, it would seem important to avoid if nontreatment were safe. One concept suggests that there may be a group of persons with elevated IOP who have no chance of glaucoma damage; the term *ocular hypertension* was applied to those who seemed to qualify.

However, we should also question the idea that most patients with elevated IOP do not merit therapy. First, we do not know if the relatively short-term safety of nontreatment lasts indefinitely. What percentage of the persons followed in the prospective studies would develop field loss 10, 15, or 20 years later? This is clearly an important question for the 40-year-old ''ocular hypertensive.'' If the initial rate of field loss is 1% per year but changes to a higher rate with longer follow-up, then our attitude toward withholding therapy might reverse. I should add that I have no information that the rate of field loss does increase with longer follow-up.

Second, the studies used *visual field loss* as defined by a standard method in the Goldmann perimeter as the criterion for damage—no field defect satisfying a certain definition, no damage. Is it possible that any significant damage occurs before field loss? In the last 5 years I have examined 75 eyes that had a well-documented history of elevated IOP; the group varied from those with normal discs and field tests to those with advanced damage. The number of remaining nerve fibers in the optic nerves was estimated by a histologic counting method and compared to age-matched control eyes similarly prepared. The tissues lead to the confirmation of something previously suspected by many: loss of optic nerve fibers precedes detectable visual field defects by standard methods and criteria with the Goldmann perimeter.[12] At least the first one quarter to one third of the optic nerve can disappear without detection in the field testing carried out during the prospective studies. One half of the nerve was usually gone by the time a reproducible ''early'' paracentral scotoma or nasal step was detected. One can argue that even with a paracentral scotoma the patient usually retains 20/20 vision and normal activity is minimally affected, so it may be acceptable to allow early field loss to occur before treatment. On the other hand, if a lapse in follow-up occurs, major field loss may develop before it is recognized. Compare telling a patient that you will start therapy if any damage is detected and telling him that you are allowing the first stage of damage to go on untreated.

In summary good reasons exist to question the wisdom of treating every eye that has elevated IOP with drops, laser, or surgery, whereas withholding therapy could result in progressive optic nerve damage in patients under our care.

HOW DO WE DECIDE WHOM TO TREAT?

Consider the following typical example: a 46-year-old man comes to your office for reading glasses, and the IOP is 26 mm Hg in each eye. The further information needed to make a management decision comes both from the history and the examination. Two kinds of data must be gathered: (1) risk factors, which do not indicate damage but are associated with greater likelihood that damage will occur; and (2) direct evidence of damage.

Risk factors

The known risk factors associated with glaucoma are older age, family history of glaucoma, higher IOP, large cup/disc ratio, and myopia.[1,6,10] It is important to look at each factor to evaluate its significance and usefulness.

Age

Statistically, the older a patient, the more likely damage will occur, with all other factors being equal. This may simply mean that the older persons are, the more fragile and susceptible they are to injury. An alternate interpretation, however, is that the older patient is more likely to have had elevated IOP longer, having already had time to pass through the silent period of optic nerve damage and being closer to developing detectable damage. For example, we may see two patients with IOP of 28 mm Hg, one 30 and one 70 years of age. If neither had been previously examined, we could not know for how long the IOP had been elevated. However, it is more likely that the younger patient has had elevated IOP for a shorter time and the elderly one for a longer time. Whichever is more correct, the older person is at greater risk to develop detectable damage first.

Family history

Each of us has met a patient who has three brothers and two sisters with glaucoma, with some blind eyes among them. We cannot escape the impression that this patient is at greater risk than another without known affected family members, an impression supported by clinical studies. Yet we must realize that many patients are not aware of eye disease in blood relatives or have no living relatives. I have also had the experience of rechecking with a patient after some follow-up only to find that a relative or two who had not been previously examined had just been found to have glaucoma. The updating of family history is therefore important, and the strong suggestion to each new suspect or glaucoma patient to have family members examined cannot be overemphasized.

IOP level

The level of IOP is also clearly related to the rapidity of damage. As discussed, however, we measure IOP only a few times in each eye, providing a poor estimate of the prevailing IOP over time. To obtain the best estimate of the average IOP in a given patient, it is necessary to measure IOP at various times of the day, or an average IOP level can be constructed from several measurements on different days in a short period. Some of us have taught patients and their families to perform tonometry at home with a Schiøtz tonometer to improve our estimate of prevailing IOP. This has been particularly illuminating in patients with apparent low-tension glaucoma.[7] A number of those thought initially to have normal IOP are shown to have frequent spikes of elevation by this method. An applanation tonometer is now being developed that patients can use themselves to take an accurate IOP at home. In summary the clinical judgment of risk is substantially affected by whether the IOP level is generally in the 20, 30, or 40 mm Hg range.

Cup/disc ratio

The larger the cup/disc ratio, the greater the chance of field loss developing in a suspected glaucoma patient—we know this may result from two possible explanations. First, eyes that have large cups may be more likely to suffer damage at the same IOP level than an eye with a smaller cup. This suggests that the large cup is a reason for greater susceptibility to neural loss. Second, instead of being the reason for faster damage, the large cup may be associated with development of field loss in the cited studies, since the eye with a large cup already has undergone the first phase of damage (cup enlargement) and therefore is closer to the stage of damage characterized by field loss.

In either case the large cup is a warning sign. But how large is large? With the advent of stereoexamination of the disc, cups 0.6 to 0.7 the height of the disc are seen in normal eyes. No single cutoff point exists to separate damaged from normal discs, primarily because the size of the cup is originally determined by the diameter of the scleral canal for the nerve head. The larger the canal, the more leftover space is present after the normal amount of nerve fibers pass through it, and the larger the physiologic cup. Thus, eyes with the normal amount of nerve tissue can have no cup or a 0.8 cup/disc ratio. If an eye starts with a 0.1 cup/disc ratio, the change to 0.6 indicates major loss of tissue. Unless this disc was observed before damage, however, it would not be possible to tell from cup size alone if this were its original size or an acquired enlargement.

Myopia

Recently, accumulating evidence suggests that myopic individuals have a greater chance of developing glaucoma,[10] which confirm the same clinical impressions. However, this finding may be more than a simple relationship. Although myopic eyes may now be considered more likely to develop a first field defect more rapidly than eyes with different refractive errors, they may at the same time be no more or even less likely to undergo further field loss beyond this point. No firm explanation exists for the association between myopia and glaucoma, although several hypotheses can be considered.

Other factors

Other ocular findings are associated with glaucoma in many eyes, but the causal relationship is not fully settled. Two examples are the pigmentary dispersion syndrome and the pseudoexfoliation syndrome. Whereas no population studies have been performed in the United States on the number of patients with these syndromes who develop glaucoma damage, it is probably safe to say that glaucoma occurs more frequently in such eyes.

In conclusion, it is important to use all available information before making therapeutic decisions. The risk factors given are only an indirect expression of the chance of glaucoma damage. By recording and using this information, we can arrive at a higher or lower suspicion of the chance of visual loss, which in turn helps in deciding how frequently a patient should be seen and retested.

Direct evidence of damage

Direct evidence of optic nerve injury is more conclusive in decisions to treat. Two examination areas are important: damage that can be seen in disc and nerve fiber layer and abnormalities in visual function, as indicated primarily by the visual field tests.

It is not the purpose of this chapter to review the disc changes in glaucoma exhaustively—the histologic changes are covered in Chapter 8. The most important sign of damage is progressive cup enlargement. Since the changes observed are often subtle and occur over an extended period, it is essential to establish a system for documentation of disc appearance. A helpful second feature, which can be determined on the first visit, is definite asymmetry of cup size. Cup asymmetry is rare in the normal population, and in early glaucoma it represents tissue loss in the larger-cup eye. One should make certain that no major difference in the disc shape or globe size exists, such as asymmetric myopia. Either of these features can be associated with cup asymmetry that is not representative of glaucoma damage. Splinter hemorrhages at the disc rim are a sign of progressive optic nerve damage in the suspected or established glaucoma patient.[4] Whereas hemorrhages can occur near the disc in other conditions, in glaucoma they must be assumed to represent ongoing damage.

Other signs of disc damage in glaucoma are not as pathognomonic or as clearly indicative of definitive injury but are often helpful. They include loss of all disc rim tissue at the 12 or 6 o'clock position (vertically oval cupping), loss of disc tissue between vessels (hanging vessel or overpass sign), visibility of the laminar pores throughout the cup, and sharply undermined cup edges. As mentioned, the actual size of the cup may be as large as 0.7 the height of the disc in normal eyes. These additional features help to separate the large physiologic cup from those with damage.

We have found that examining the retinal nerve fiber layer is also helpful in directly observing neural damage. In a group of eyes with elevated IOP but no therapy, defects in the nerve fiber layer were visible in almost every eye that developed early field loss before the perimetric defect.[15] In another group an observer looked at photographs of suspected and established glaucoma eyes and recorded the state of the nerve fiber layer. The examinations were done without knowledge of the patient's history and with the disc covered to prevent any bias from the degree of cupping. Eyes with field loss were shown to have detectable nerve fiber layer abnormalities in 84% of cases.[13] This is identical to the accuracy of determining eyes with field loss by examination of the disc. We believe the nerve fiber layer examination will provide additional information about glaucoma damage, and it can be performed with minimal patient cooperation and with available instruments (direct ophthalmoscopy). Our department is now engaged in a study to prove or disprove that nerve fiber layer examination can actually predict which glaucoma suspects will develop field loss. If this study confirms the value of this method, another tool has been added to our diagnostic repertoire.

Perimetry remains a vital clinical measure of glaucoma damage. The typical defects seen in testing with the Goldmann instrument and the representations of similar findings in the newer, computer-assisted machines are well described.[3] It has become evident, however, that the phase of damage in which a field defect is demonstrable is often too late to be taken as the point at which damage is first proved. Patients lose a considerable minority of their optic nerve before perimetric defects are reproducibly shown.[12] Past studies that used field defects as the essential defining characteristic of glaucoma damage were confronted with the paradox that many eyes had elevated IOP but normal field testing. In the opinion of some no damage had occurred until the field was abnormal—hence the ocular hypertension label. Although this is a useful division of different glaucoma phases, some ocular hypertensive patients may have optic nerve damage resulting from cup change, nerve fiber layer defects, afferent pupil defects, and abnormal color vision. The danger in using field loss as the definition of glaucoma and glaucoma damage is creating the mistaken concept that most or all ocular hypertensive persons are free from damage and even immune to glaucoma. There is no harm in using the ocular hypertension label, as long as it is not treated as a diagnosis. It is a *stage* of the glaucoma process, the only stage some patients will reach in their lifetime. Our problem is that we need better tools to identify those whose damage will go further into field and even acuity loss.

PROPOSED GUIDELINES FOR WHEN TO TREAT

A group of experts on glaucoma are not likely to agree about treatment guidelines. The following suggestions are constructed from my experience, from discussions with other glaucomatologists, and from available literature. Each patient must be evaluated individually; these guidelines are an attempt to develop general rules.

Treatment is suggested

Glaucoma should be suspected and treatment is suggested in the following groups of patients.

1. We all agree that the patient with elevated IOP and optic nerve damage requires treatment. Since visual field damage definitely indicates damage, the patient with typical glaucoma field loss should receive therapy.
2. Progressive cup enlargement documented by photographs or drawings should also indicate a need to lower IOP.
3. Therapy is also indicated when major cup asymmetry exists between eyes with no ready alternate explanation.
4. Three other signs of disc damage also suggest acquired damage requiring treatment: loss of disc tissue to the rim (notch), disc rim hemorrhage, and abnormalities of the nerve fiber layer.
5. Each of these patient groups is characterized by visible or detectable damage. However, some patients with elevated IOP have a disc and/or field that cannot be evaluated or have signs of glaucoma damage that may be masked or simulated by concurrent ocular damage. We have lost the ability to judge whether damage has occurred or will occur in such eyes, and therapy is suggested. Included here are eyes with cloudy media (cataract, vitreous hemorrhage), lesions of the disc (optic pit, disc drusen, past anterior ischemic optic neuropathy), retinal disease (macular degeneration, vascular occlusion, diabetic retinopathy), or neurologic field loss. This partial list illustrates the principle that any lesion preventing accurate disc or field evaluation may allow glaucoma damage to occur without our knowledge.
6. The patient who is unable to perform visual field testing after repeated efforts would seem to need therapy. It should be noted, however, that this category is a minority of all patients if appropriate care is exercised. Young children are an obvious example.

7. The patient with functional vision in only one eye should not be allowed to run the risk of damaging the other. There are no one-eyed ocular hypertensive persons.
8. The patient with glaucomatous field loss in the fellow eye should be treated in both eyes. The second eye is at great risk for developing damage.[15] In other words, no person can have glaucoma in one eye and "ocular hypertension" in the other.
9. Some patients worry about withholding therapy. If treatment has few side effects for them, they should be treated. For example, some patients with apparently normal discs and field examinations have used drops for many years. When presented with the option of continuing follow-up without therapy, they become anxious and express dismay at using drops for so long without apparent reason. Although the available alternatives can be presented, the patient's attitude should be respected.
10. The unreliable patient is a no-win situation. There is concern that if no therapy is given and the patient is lost to follow-up, damage could occur. On the other hand, the patient might be just as noncompliant with medical therapy as with returning for tests. It is probably best that they be partly treated and poorly followed than untreated and poorly followed. For some patients the end of the bottle of drops or the expiration of refills may be one of the few successful reminders to return for examination.

Treatment should be strongly considered

This category of patients includes those who are likely to have impending damage or who exhibit signs of damage that are highly suggestive of glaucoma.

1. Patients with high average IOP may be at greater risk for damage than those with lower IOP. No prospective studies are available that show eyes that can or cannot tolerate untreated pressures around 40 mm Hg. Although some discs may tolerate extended IOP in this range, nontreatment of such eyes must be coupled with extremely close and detailed follow-up under optimal conditions.
2. It is best to treat the patient with several risk factors; for example, a 65-year-old with more than one affected family member, an average IOP of 28 mm Hg, and a 0.7 cup/disc ratio in each eye. Since this patient has none of the accepted signs of definite damage, there is no obvious indication for treatment. However, the decision not to treat should again be accompanied by careful observation.

WHAT IS THE END POINT OF THERAPY?

IOP has been lowered to a safe level when no change occurs in the signs of damage being monitored. The theoretically safe IOP may vary from eye to eye; an IOP of 21 mm Hg may be safe for one patient and blinding in another. This stresses the need for disc and field monitoring whether therapy is started or not. Treatment never replaces the need for careful follow-up. If the disc and field cannot be monitored, IOP should be reduced to the normal range for the patient's age, if at all practical.

In some eyes the initial IOP is between 30 and 40 mm Hg and with all available tolerable medications is lowered only to an average of 20 to 24 mm Hg. Although no study can point to the optimal course in this situation, this represents a signficant lowering of IOP. The IOP may now be safe for that eye—at least it deserves a chance at this level. If a substantial lowering is achieved by first-stage treatment, one should continue monitoring optic nerve status before moving on to further steps.

When there is a question of whether treatment is appropriate or not, a therapeutic trial of medication is helpful. This offers the opportunity to determine the patient's tolerance to the therapy and to monitor the IOP-lowering ability of drops. Starting drops in one eye only is most often the best method to judge the effect in a short-run trial, since the eyes often go up or down in IOP together. If both eyes fluctuate down after drops are started in both, a false sense of security is given. With a one-eye trial the difference between eyes shows the true effect. The patient should be told that this is simply a trial; if it does not prove effective or tolerable, it can be terminated. At the same time the patient must understand the importance of complying with the medication regimen during the trial period.

SUMMARY

Several practical approaches to the treatment of glaucoma have been considered. The concept that there are many persons with elevated IOP but few with field loss has led to the proposal that many suspected glaucoma patients do not need treatment. From the concepts developed in this chapter, I would agree that in certain eyes optic nerve function can be monitored without IOP lowering. In general these eyes have the following characteristics: normal fields, no disc rim notch, no history of disc hemorrhage, no nerve fiber layer defect, no major cup/disc asymmetry, stable disc size, no condition that could mask disc or field examination reliability, vision in both eyes, IOP lower than 35 mm Hg, and few associated risk factors. Whether this indicates that many or few persons can be monitored without treatment or not, I do not yet know. This discussion has helped illustrate how data can be gathered to make the best decision.

REFERENCES

1. Armaly, M.F.: Biostatistical analysis of the collaborative glaucoma study. I. Summary report of the risk factors for glaucomatous visual-field defects, Arch. Ophthalmol. **98:**2163, 1980.
2. Drance, S.M., and Lakowski, R.: Early psychophysical disturbances in chronic open-angle glaucoma. In New Orleans Academy of Ophthalmology: Symposium on glaucoma, St. Louis, 1981, The C.V. Mosby Co.
3. Drance, S.M., Wheeler, C., and Patullo, M.: Uniocular open-angle glaucoma, Am. J. Ophthalmol. **65:**891, 1968.
4. Drance, S.M., and others: The importance of disc hemorrhage in the prognosis of chronic open-angle glaucoma, Arch. Ophthalmol. **95:**226, 1977.
5. Harbin, T.S., and others: Visual field progression in open-angle glaucoma patients presenting with monocular field loss, Trans. Am. Acad. Ophthalmol. Otolaryngol. **81:**253, 1976.
6. Hart, W.M., and others: Multivariate analysis of the risk of glaucomatous visual field loss, Arch. Ophthalmol. **97:**1455, 1979.
7. Jensen, A., and Maumenee, A.E.: Home tonometry, Am. J. Ophthalmol. **76:**929, 1973.
8. Kolker, A.E.: Visual prognosis in advanced glaucoma, Trans. Am. Ophthalmol. Soc. **75:**539, 1977.
9. Perkins, E.S.: The Bedford glaucoma survey. I. Long-term follow-up of borderline cases, Br. J. Ophthalmol. **57:**179, 1973.
10. Perkins, E.S., and Phelps, C.D.: Open-angle glaucoma, ocular hypertension, low-tension glaucoma, and refraction, Arch. Ophthalmol. **100:**1464, 1982.
11. Quigley, H.A., and Maumenee, A.E.: Long-term follow-up of treated open-angle glaucoma, Am. J. Ophthalmol. **87:**519, 1979.
12. Quigley, H.A., Addicks, E.A., and Green, W.R.: Optic nerve damage in human glaucoma. III. Quantitative correlation of nerve fiber loss and visual field defect in glaucoma, ischemic neuropathy, papilledema, and toxic neuropathy, Arch. Ophthalmol. **100:**135, 1982.

13. Quigley, H.A., Miller, N.R., and George, T.: Clinical evaluation of nerve fiber layer atrophy as an indicator of glaucomatous optic nerve damage, Arch. Ophthalmol. **98:**1564, 1980.
14. Shin, D., and others: Long-term epinephrine therapy of ocular hypertension, Arch. Ophthalmol. **94:**2059, 1976.
15. Sommer, A., and others: The nerve fiber layer in the diagnosis of glaucoma, Arch. Ophthalmol. **95:**2149, 1977.
16. Worthen, D.M.: Effect of pilocarpine drops on the diurnal intraocular pressure variation in patients with glaucoma, Invest. Ophthalmol. **15:**784, 1976.

2

Problems and prognosis of the developmental glaucomas

Robert N. Shaffer

It often seems foolish to present information on the congenital glaucomas to a general ophthalmologic audience. The averagely busy ophthalmologist may see a new congenital glaucoma patient once every 10 years; even the general pediatric ophthalmologist may see no more than one a year. However, the impact on the life of that child and the cost to society if vision is impaired or lost can hardly be overstated. It is important to be occasionally reminded of the signs and symptoms that should alert us to this danger and lead to prompt diagnosis. The ophthalmologist who recognizes the glaucoma and can institute appropriate treatment before severe optic nerve damage occurs has taken a significant step toward preserving vision and promoting a more useful and happy future for the young patient and his family.

CLASSIFICATION, SIGNS, AND SYMPTOMS

In 1980, at the Glaucoma Symposium of the New Orleans Academy of Ophthalmology, my partner, Dunbar Hoskins, presented a new morphologic classification of the developmental glaucomas.[1] This is based on the appearance of the tissues during slit-lamp and gonioscopic examination of the iris, the trabecular meshwork, and the cornea. Its use facilitates generalizations about appropriate therapy and prognosis, avoiding the need to diagnose from among the multitude of potentially confusing syndromes.

Isolated trabeculodysgenesis

This group makes up more than 50% of the developmental glaucomas and has been termed *primary* or *infantile* congenital glaucoma. It is characterized by epiphora, photophobia, corneal enlargement and hazing, pressure elevation, rapid cupping of the optic disc, and an anterior flat insertion of iris into a thickened trabecular meshwork.[2,4,5] The ophthalmologist who mistakenly treats these early cases of epiphora as a tear duct obstruction can be in serious legal difficulties when the true nature of the condition becomes apparent. The glaucoma should be treated promptly by goniotomy or, if corneal haze prevents accurate trabecular surgery, by trabeculotomy.

Almost 20% of these patients have hazy corneas and increased intraocular pressure at birth. Their prognosis is considerably poorer than those diagnosed after the age of 1 month. The prognosis is still poorer if an iris anomaly is also noted, changing the diagnosis to "iridotrabecular dysgenesis."

Iridotrabecular dysgenesis

In addition to the flat iris insertion into the trabecular meshwork, these patients may have iris stromal hypoplasia, absent collarette, and frequently tiny blood vessels crossing irregularly over the iris surface. The prognosis is poor but may be slightly better if immediate surgery is performed.

Included in iridotrabecular dysgenesis are familial hypoplasias of the iris and aniridia. Both should be treated medically as long as possible because surgical success is low.

Iridocorneal trabeculodysgenesis

This group includes Rieger's, Axenfeld's, and Peter's anomalies. As in iris hypoplasia, aniridia, and Sturge-Weber syndrome, pressure tends to become elevated much later than in trabeculodysgenesis. Also, there are usually no symptoms or signs, and glaucomatous damage can be extensive before it is diagnosed. Therefore, the alert clinician must note these anomalies of iris, cornea, and skin and carefully monitor pressure and discs indefinitely.

Since surgical success in these patients is low, medical treatment is advisable as long as optic disc integrity can be maintained.

TREATMENT

Trabeculodysgenesis

By using Hoskins' classification, valid generalizations on treatment can be made. Patients with isolated trabeculodysgenesis are usually candidates for prompt trabecular surgery. The exception is trabeculodysgenesis with increased episcleral venous pressure—the Sturge-Weber syndrome—which should be treated medically as long as possible.

Trabeculodysgenesis and iridotrabecular dysgenesis present at birth have a poorer prognosis, but these eyes should undergo one or two trabecular surgeries before resorting to medical therapy or filtering procedures.

The best opportunity to cure isolated trabeculodysgenesis is in the first trabecular surgery. The inexperienced surgeon should not attempt either goniotomy or trabeculotomy, since both require precise technique to avoid complications and to achieve success. Goniotomy is preferred unless the cornea is too hazy to permit accurate surgery.

Iridotrabecular dysgenesis and iridocorneal trabeculodysgenesis

Since surgical results in these forms of developmental glaucoma are poor, medical therapy is usually advisable if pressure can be kept low enough to avoid disc damage. The carbonic anhydrase inhibitors should be used with care in pediatric patients. Timoptic should also be used with some caution in babies. It must be remembered that almost half of the eyedrop dose ends up in the nose, where it is rapidly absorbed. This seldom causes symptoms in adults, but the dose per body weight in the infant is almost 10 times that of the adult. In addition to the obvious precipitation of asthma in predisposed children, some develop chronic upper respiratory ailments. Always ask the parents about respiratory complaints when using Timoptic in children. If possible, block the tear duct for a few moments after instilling the Timoptic.

GONIOTOMY

Safety

Complications of goniotomy are almost nonexistent when skillfully performed. Analysis of 695 goniotomies performed in our office revealed only one complication resulting in severe visual loss.[3] This was an eight-ball hemorrhage in a child with Lowe's syndrome. Minor complications have included small hyphemas and a rare shallow anterior chamber lasting 1 or 2 days. Small iridodialyses and cyclodialyses noted in the past have not been seen in recent years when trabeculotomy has been used in patients with cloudy corneas. There have been six cases of cardiopulmonary arrest during anesthesia which were frightening, although all recovered. These anesthetic-induced complications have resulted in our custom of performing bilateral goniotomy in bilateral cases rather than risking two anesthesias in these infants. (See Table 2-1.)

Effectiveness

When the signs and symptoms of glaucoma from trabeculodysgenesis occur in the first to 24 month of life, surgical control of intraocular pressure (IOP) is almost 100%. Patients were considered to be cured if pressures were less than 20 mm Hg without medications and if optic disc cupping was the same or better than at the first examination at least 6 months after the surgery. Adequate follow-up examinations were possible in 205 patients between the ages of 1 and 24 months. One hundred twenty-nine (75%) were cured with one goniotomy, and 66 more (19%) with a second goniotomy—a total of 94%. The remaining 10 (5%) were controlled either by goniotomy or trabeculotomy. None was using medications.

In contrast, there were 50 cases diagnosed at birth. Most of them were bilateral and usually had considerable clouding of the cornea. These represent a more severe arrest in fetal development. In addition to trabeculodysgenesis, iridodysgenesis was often present, with hypoplasia of the iris, imperfectly formed collarette, and occasionally with small superficial blood vessels coursing irregularly over the iris surface. The prognosis of these eyes was poor. One or two goniotomies controlled only 13 of these 50 eyes (26). Even with multiple operations, the remaining 37 eyes were controlled, if at all, by intense medical therapy. Pressures tended to remain borderline, often with slow progression of optic nerve damage.

Over the age of 24 months, eyes with trabeculodysgenesis, typical flat iris insertion into the trabeculum, and increased IOP also had a poor prognosis. Thirty-two eyes in this category were surgically treated; only 12 (38%) were controlled by one or two goniotomies. The remainder required maximal medical therapy and often filtering surgery. (See Table 2-2.)

Even in cases that require multiple operations and intensive medical therapy, it is usually possible to obtain at least partial control. Various setons, such as the Molteno valve, may increase the success rate in the future. Meanwhile, it is of great importance to maintain the child's visual life as long as possible. The longer that the child can be kept in visual contact with the environment, the better the adaptation to the world if vision is eventually lost.

Short-term prognosis

It must be remembered that IOP is reduced by anesthesia, so one must not depend on pressure measurements alone as a sign of surgical success. The corneal haze, other than Haab's striae, should promptly clear. Most important, the cupping of the optic nerve should not increase and usually decreases if a cure has been accomplished. If the pressure under anesthesia is still 20 to 24 mm Hg, one remains concerned that a cure has not been effected. However, in the absence of symptoms or disc change and if tensions remain below 20 mm Hg without medication 6 months after surgery, one can be quite certain of a cure. One is usually sure after 6 weeks.

There have been some disappointing visual results. Visual acuity was determined in only 52 eyes. Twenty-eight had a vision of 20/20 to 20/40; 11, 20/50 to 20/200; and 13, less than 20/200. The decreased vision was largely caused by deprivation amblyopia resulting from anisometropia, marked astigmatism, and breaks in Descemet's membrane in the visual axis. Visual fields remained intact unless there had been severe damage before surgery.

Long-term prognosis

In general patients who are not well controlled were usually returned by the referring physicians. Those with a favorable surgical result are often not seen after the initial follow-up examination. Frequently when letters of enquiry are sent, the family has moved and left no fowarding address. The mobility of a young population makes accurate long-term follow-up extremely difficult.

Satisfactory follow-up examinations were obtained in 82 eyes that had had goniotomies at least 5 years before. (See Table 2-3.) Fifty-two of the eyes had been followed

Table 2-1. Complications in 695 consecutive goniotomies

Complication	*Number*
Hemorrhage	2; severe, one lost vision
Iridodialysis	4; small, without sequellae
Cyclodialysis	2; small, without sequellae
Shallow chamber	5; 1 to 2 days' duration
Lens injury, infection	None
Cardiopulmonary arrest	6; all recovered

Table 2-2. Efficacy of 287 goniotomies by age

	Birth-1 month	*1-24 months*	*Over 24 months*
Number of cases	50	205	32
1 goniotomy	8 (16%)	129 (75%)	11 (35%)
2 goniotomies	5 (10%)	66 (19%)	1 (3%)
Total %	26%	94%	38%
Multiple operations	37 (74%)	10 (6%)	20 (64%)

Table 2-3. Fifty-two successful goniotomies (IOP: 10-20 mm Hg)—complications noted after 15-25 years

Complication	*Number*
Amblyopia (vision 20/50 or less)	20 (46%)
Tension 24 to 32 mm Hg after 18 years	3
Endothelial dystrophy after 17 years	2
Retinal detachment after 20 years	2
Visual loss from trauma after 20 years	2

between 15 and 25 years. All had pressures ranging between 10 and 20 mm Hg without medical therapy. There had been no change in disc cupping or in fields when these findings were available. No complications had appeared under 15 years; between 15 and 25 years seven had developed complications (14%). Three had an increase in IOP into the 25 to 35 mm Hg range, and two had developed a mild endothelial dystrophy with some corneal edema. Two retinal detachments occurred, and two had a neovascular glaucoma following blunt trauma. No change in disc cupping was noted. Most of the eyes had full visual fields unless there was already severe damage to the optic nerve at the time of the goniotomy.

For 15 years none of these eyes had any problem. However, it has been disturbing to find a complication rate of 14% in these presumably cured eyes 15 to 25 years after successful goniotomies. Very few patients have reached the third or fourth decade of life after goniotomy, so we cannot be at all sure what the complications will be in the latter half of their lives. There is no doubt that periodic follow-up of all cases of developmental glaucoma is necessary if unsuspected loss of sight is to be avoided.

SUMMARY

Goniotomy is a safe and highly successful operation in developmental glaucoma with trabeculodysgenesis (primary infantile glaucoma). Trabeculotomy should be reserved for patients with marked corneal edema or for those in which two goniotomies have failed. The prognosis varies markedly with the age of onset of signs and symptoms. When present at birth or after age 2 years, two goniotomies will only cure some 30% of cases. Between ages 1 and 24 months, 94% of cases will be cured by two goniotomies.

Eyes with successful goniotomies have now been followed for over 25 years with maintenance of pressure control without medication. A deprivation amblyopia has been the most marked complication, as caused by marked astigmatism, anisometropia, and tears of Descemet's membrane involving the visual axis. Between 15 and 25 years two cases developed an endothelial dystrophy, two had retinal detachments, and three had pressure elevation. One fears added complications in the next 25 years. Obviously periodic ophthalmic examinations are indicated the rest of these patients' lives.

REFERENCES

1. Hoskins, D., and others: Developmental glaucoma: diagnosis and classification. In New Orleans Academy of Ophthalmology: Symposium on glaucoma, St. Louis, 1981, The C.V. Mosby Co.
2. Kolker, A., and Hetherington, J.: Becker-Shaffer's diagnosis and therapy of the glaucomas, ed. 5, St. Louis, 1983, The C.V. Mosby Co.
3. Litinsky, S., and others: Operative complications of goniotomy, Trans. Am. Acad. Ophthalmol. **83:**78, 1977.
4. Maumenee, A.E.: The pathogenesis of congenital glaucoma: a new theory, Trans. Am. Ophthalmol. Soc. **56:**507, 1958.
5. Maumenee, A.E.: Further observations of the pathogenesis of congenital glaucoma, Trans. Am. Ophthalmol. Soc. **60:**140, 1962.

3

New concepts in angle-closure glaucoma

David G. Campbell
Angela Vela*

MODERN GONIOSYNECHIALYSIS

The development of severe synechial angle-closure glaucoma can present a severe problem for both patient and clinician. Grant[10] made the initial observation that long-standing synechial closure can damage the underlying trabecular meshwork (TM), rendering it unable to function normally even if the synechiae are lysed and the TM is reexposed. However, Grant did show that function could return in perfused enucleated eyes if the synechiae were not long-standing.

Recently we have had success in surgically opening the TM in four eyes with severe synechial angle-closure glaucoma (more than 9 hours of closure) of 1 year's duration or less, with a return to normal intraocular pressure (IOP) without medication in all four cases and a follow-up of 7 to 15 months.[8,36] One patient with synechiae of at least 6 years' duration showed no improvement in function.

Four recent advances

In the past attempts to perform goniosynechialysis have been difficult and hazardous. Attempts to sweep open a synechially closed angle with a cyclodialysis spatula have often failed because of imprecise surgical technique and unwanted and occasionally uncontrollable hemorrhage. Modern advances in four different areas now enable modern goniosynechialysis to be performed safely with rewarding results if patient selection has been appropriate (Fig. 3-1).

The first advance was the introduction of the chamber-deepening procedure. This procedure, first introduced by Chandler and Simmons[11] to evaluate the degree of synechial angle closure following the development of angle-closure glaucoma, surgically pushes the lens and iris—including the peripheral iris—posteriorly, making obvious any synechial closure and creating a large and safe entrance to the angle region. Surgical instruments can then be placed across the anterior chamber into the angle without danger to the endothelium, iris, or lens. Thus, an anterior chamber converted to the chamber-deepened configuration provides a safe entrance for angle manipulation.

The second advance was the development of the sodium hyaluronate[26,27] for ocular surgery. This clear, sterile viscous gel holds the anterior chamber in the deepened con-

*Assistant Professor, Department of Ophthalmology, University of Texas School of Medicine, Galveston, Tex.

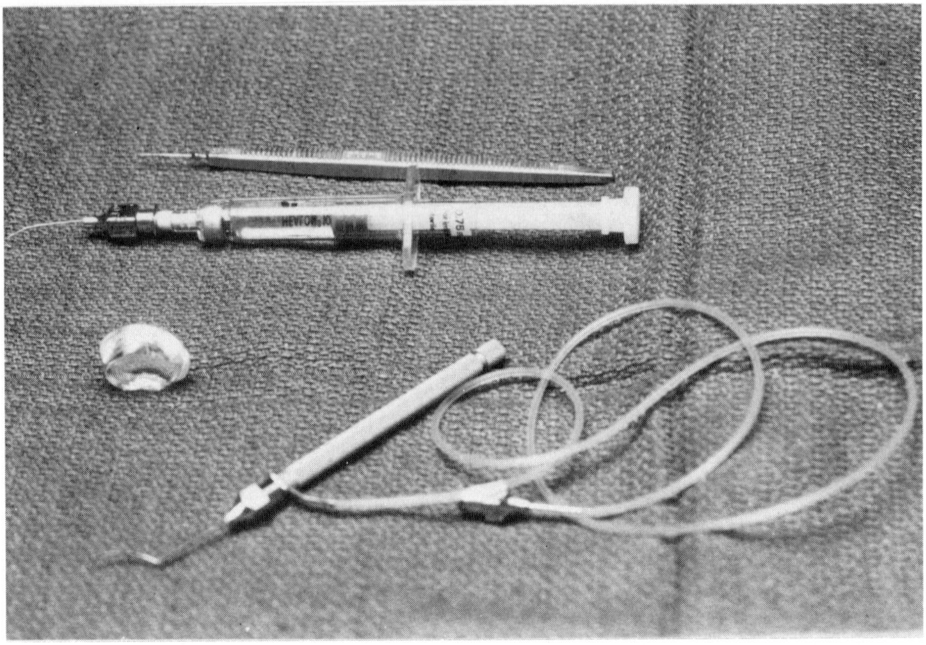

Fig. 3-1. Equipment needed to perform goniosynechialysis. Top to bottom, Ziegler knife, sodium hyaluronate, Barkan gonioscopy lens—pediatric size, and cyclodialysis spatula.

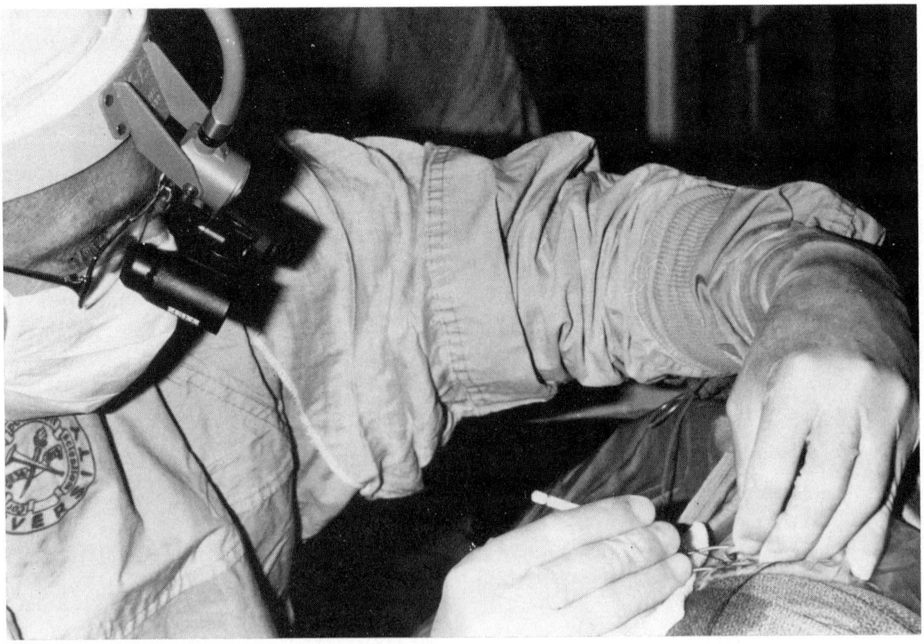

Fig. 3-2. Additional equipment needed includes a bright fiber optic headlight and ocular loupes.

figuration much more reliably than balanced salt solution, since it cannot escape quickly out of the entrance incisions and thus prevents rapid and unwanted flattening of the anterior chamber. This allows angle surgery to be performed safely. In addition, if unwanted hemorrhage develops in the area of lysis, the hyaluronate helps to quickly coagulate bleeding that might otherwise obscure the surgical view. The hyaluronate also localizes the bleeding, generally in a droplet adjacent to the hemorrhage site, thereby avoiding dispersion of blood that again might obscure the surgical view.

The third advance was the development of a curved irrigating cyclodialysis spatula.[2] Although not created specifically for goniosynechialysis, this curved spatula fits into the angle well and can gently lyse the adhesions. The irrigation from within the spatula is indispensable, since it can be used to help hold the chamber deep during the procedure and can stop bleeding instantly by elevating the IOP.

The final advance was the use of direct visualization of the angle with high magnification. The development of reliable operative loupes with 4× to 6× enlargement provides the necessary magnification when used with a Barkan goniotomy lens and illuminating fiberoptic headlight (Fig. 3-2). Research is currently underway to see if a reliable cutaway indirect gonioscopy lens can be developed for use with the operating microscope, but for the present the direct Barkan system is advised. The use of direct visualization of the angle for this procedure is very important, since attempts to sweep the angle without it generally do more harm than good.

Simmons[33] has described successful goniosynechialysis using direct visualization and chamber deepening in a patient with recent synechial angle closure secondary to retinal detachment surgery. Our technique expands on this work by adding the use of sodium hyaluronate and an irrigating cyclodialysis spatula and broadens the indication for surgery in regard to the duration of known synechial closure.

Surgical technique

The technique used is as follows. The patient is supine, and local anesthesia is generally used. A paracentesis incision is made in the inferior cornea (Fig. 3-3, *A*), and a chamber-deepening procedure is performed as originally described by Chandler and Simmons.[11] Fluid is evacuated from the anterior chamber and is then pushed from the posterior chamber into the anterior chamber by depression at the limbus for 360 degrees with a muscle hook (Fig. 3-3, *B*).[5] Fluid is evacuated once again from the anterior chamber, and the chamber is shallowed to a depth of approximately two corneal thicknesses (Fig. 3-3, *C*). The chamber is then deepened with sodium hyaluronate to a depth of approximately six to eight corneal thicknesses centrally (3 to 4 mm) (Fig. 3-3, *D*). Then, using either a sterile Koeppe lens system or a sterile indirect gonioscopy lens and an operating microscope, the angle is examined and significant synechial angle closure (generally 9 hours or greater) is confirmed. An incision is then made at the temporal limbus, and the irrigating cyclodialysis spatula is passed through the deepened anterior chamber to the opposite angle (Fig. 3-4). Using a headlight for illumination and 4× to 6× ocular loupes combined with a Barkan surgical goniotomy lens, the synechiae over the opposite 180 degrees are lysed by gentle anterior to posterior movements of the spatula (Fig. 3-5).

If bleeding is encountered, as is more likely with long-standing synechiae, the IOP is quickly increased by elevation of the irrigation bottle to a level sufficient to stop the bleeding. The bottle is elevated for 30 to 60 seconds and generally lowered again. The hemorrhage usually localizes as a drop within the hyaluronate, and the operation may

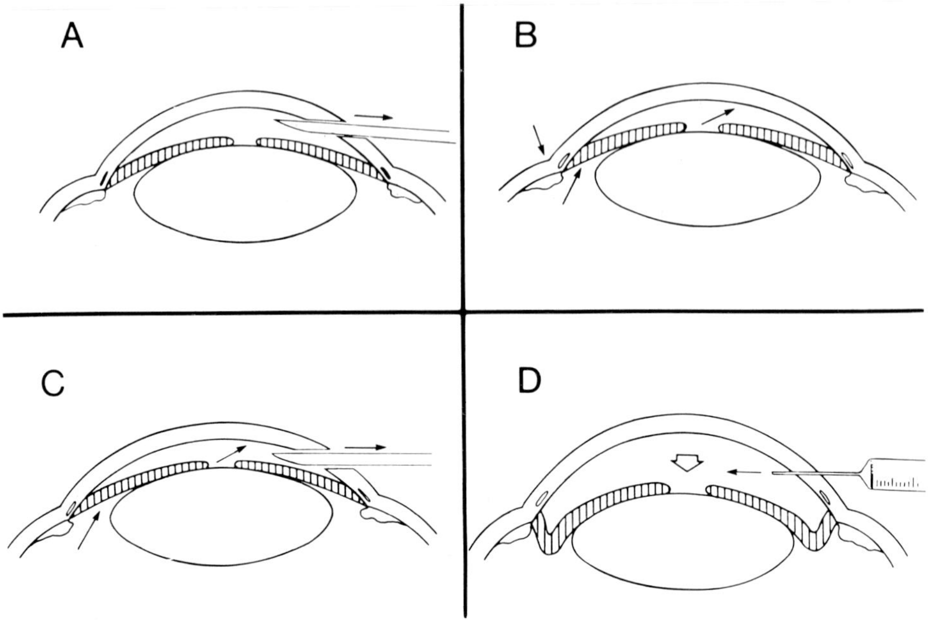

Fig. 3-3. The surgical goniosynechialysis procedure (see text). (Published with permission from The American Journal of Ophthalmology **88**(2):199, 1979. Copyright by The Ophthalmic Publishing Co.)

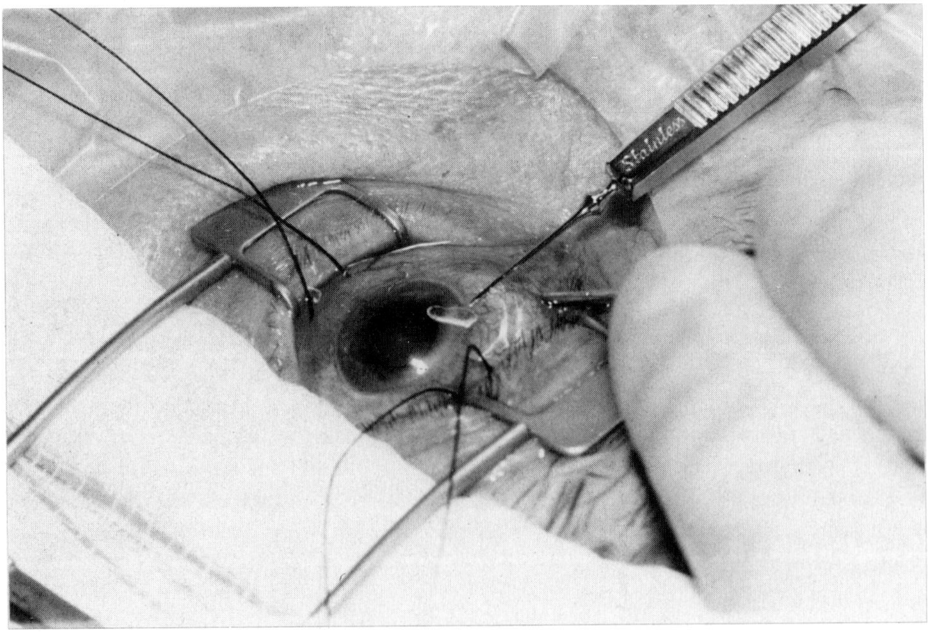

Fig. 3-4. Limbal incision to allow future passage of cyclodialysis spatula.

continue. If a sheet of blood develops within the hyaluronate, obscuring the surgical view, this can be aspirated, and the anterior chamber can be refilled with clear hyaluronate.

When the first half of the operation is complete, a similar incision is made on the nasal side, and the temporal 180 degrees of the angle is surgically treated. The sodium hyaluronate is then evacuated from the anterior chamber and replaced with balanced salt solution to avoid a prolonged postoperative pressure rise caused by the hyaluronate. The two surgical incisions are closed with individual 10-0 nylon sutures. Postoperatively patients are generally placed on topical antibiotics, steroids, and a pupillary constricting agent to hold the peripheral iris away from the surgical area.

Other considerations

Aside from intraoperative hemorrhage, which has been controlled, there have been no complications to date. Damage to the endothelium or lens or the creation of an inadvertent cyclodialysis cleft have also been avoided.

Good candidates for this procedure should be those with significant (generally 9 hours or greater) and definite synechial angle closure, generally 1 year or less in duration. In general candidates should also have a severe pressure elevation uncontrolled by maximum medical therapy. Further studies and experience with the procedure may change the parameter in regard to the length of known synechial closure.

Obviously the cause of the initial angle closure must also be treated so that the closure will not recur. If the cause was relative pupillary block, then laser iridotomy or

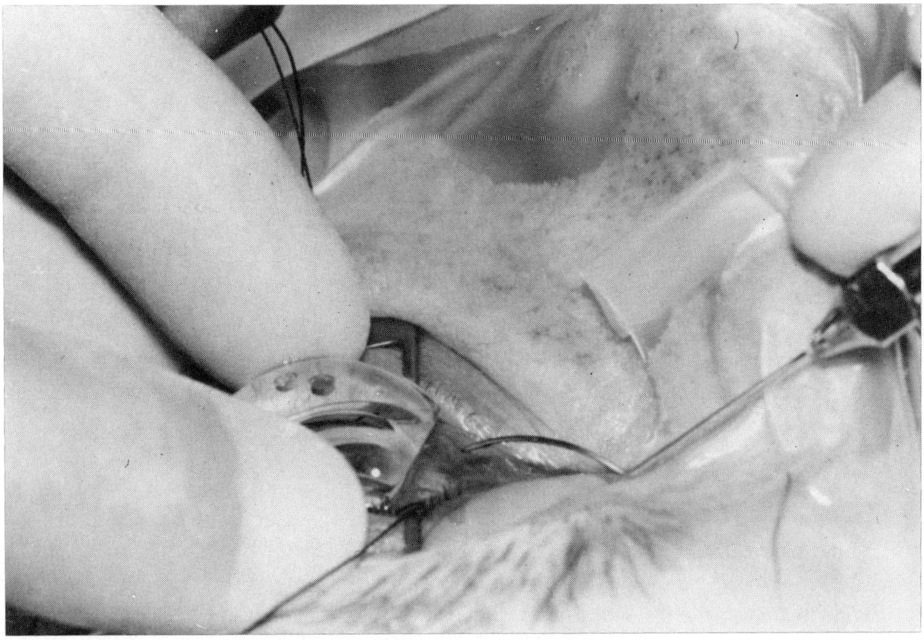

Fig. 3-5. Barkan gonioscopy lens and irrigating cyclodialysis spatula about to be placed into anterior chamber.

surgical iridectomy should be performed. If the cause was plateau iris configuration or syndrome,[38] then peripheral iridotomy and chronic miotic therapy should be used, possibly combined with a laser peripheral iridoplasty. If the cause was forward movement of the lens or angle closure precipitated by pilocarpine, postoperative mydriatic-cycloplegic therapy may be effective in moving the lens posteriorly and helping to hold the angle open. If peripheral iris and ciliary body cysts[37] caused the closure, they must be ruptured by argon or YAG laser treatment; if this is impossible, intentional mild recession of the angle in addition to lysis should be considered.

The surgical technique is new and still somewhat difficult and should be performed by surgeons familiar with the chamber-deepening procedure, operative gonioscopy, and operative surgical angle techniques such as goniotomy. Further long-term studies will delineate the procedure's usefulness, but the short-term (7 to 15 months) results have been encouraging.

IRIS RETRACTION SYNDROME

One of the interesting aspects of a rhegmatogenous retinal detachment is that the IOP generally drops a few mm Hg in the detached eye.[14] Also, in some cases the pressure can drop to hypotonous levels,[3,17,18,22] that is, to pressures close to 0 and well below the normal episcleral venous pressure of 9 to 10 mm Hg. These very low pressures indicate either that aqueous production is drastically reduced or that fluid is leaving the eye via an unconventional outflow pathway, one which bypasses the TM and Schlemm's canal. The development of a most peculiar anterior chamber configuration can be associated with this precipitous drop in pressure, one that I call the *iris retraction configuration.*[6,7] In this configuration the peripheral iris drops back posteriorly and then returns forward, hugging the anterior surface of the lens (Fig. 3-6, *A*). The appearance is much as if someone had placed a syringe in the vitreous cavity and created suction in that space that pulled the iris posteriorly (Fig. 3-6, *B*). In the past the term used to describe the syndrome was the *vitreous traction syndrome,*[15] since it was generally assumed that the iris was pulled posteriorly by the force of vitreous retraction. Also of interest is that many of these patients[4,20] went on to develop inoperable retinal detachments because of the development of advanced proliferative vitreoretinopathy.[24]

Etiology of low pressure in retinal detachment

The cause of reduced IOP accompanying retinal detachment has been believed to be either posterior fluid flow out of the eye from the subretinal space[3,22,30] (generally assumed to be through the retinal pigment epithelium to the choroid[16,25]) or decreased aqueous production[21,28,31,32,34] caused by the retinal detachment in a manner not clearly defined. Arguments and proofs have been forwarded to support both contentions. It is clear, however, that a functioning fluid pump does exist in the subretinal space. Both the rapid removal of fluid from this space following reattachment and closure of a detached retinal hole[13,23] and the rapid removal of inflammatory subretinal fluid following institution of steroid therapy prove the existence of an active pump, one to which ocular fluid obviously has access in the presence of a rhegmatogenous retinal detachment. It seems likely, therefore, that fluid is constantly leaving the eye via this pathway in the presence of a rhegmatogenous retinal detachment. Corroborative laboratory proof has been provided by Pederson,[29] Marmor,[25] and others,[1,9,19,35] although definite clinical proof has been lacking until recently.

Clinical observations

Intriguingly, clinical proof has come from the observation of patients with the iris retraction syndrome. I have introduced the term *iris retraction syndrome* to include those patients who present with a rhegmatogenous retinal detachment, hypotony, and a posteriorly displaced iris—an iris in the iris retraction configuration, often associated with a secondary inflammation and in some instances with a secondary ciliochoroidal detachment. Particular insight into the syndrome was obtained from observing those patients who initially presented with angle closure caused by iris bombe and who were then converted to the iris retraction syndrome. Careful observations indicated that this

A

B

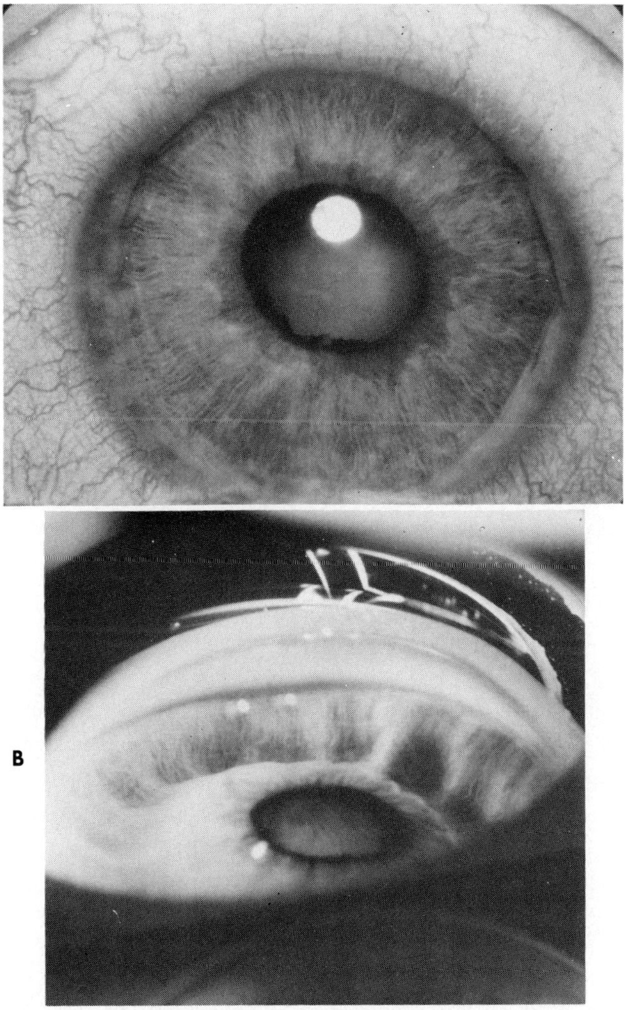

Fig. 3-6. A, Anterior view of eye in iris retraction configuration. Note peripheral iris step off as peripheral iris falls posteriorly. Note also synechiae to lens. **B,** Gonioscopic view of eye in iris retraction configuration showing marked peripheral posterior displacement of iris and adherence of central iris to anterior lens contour.

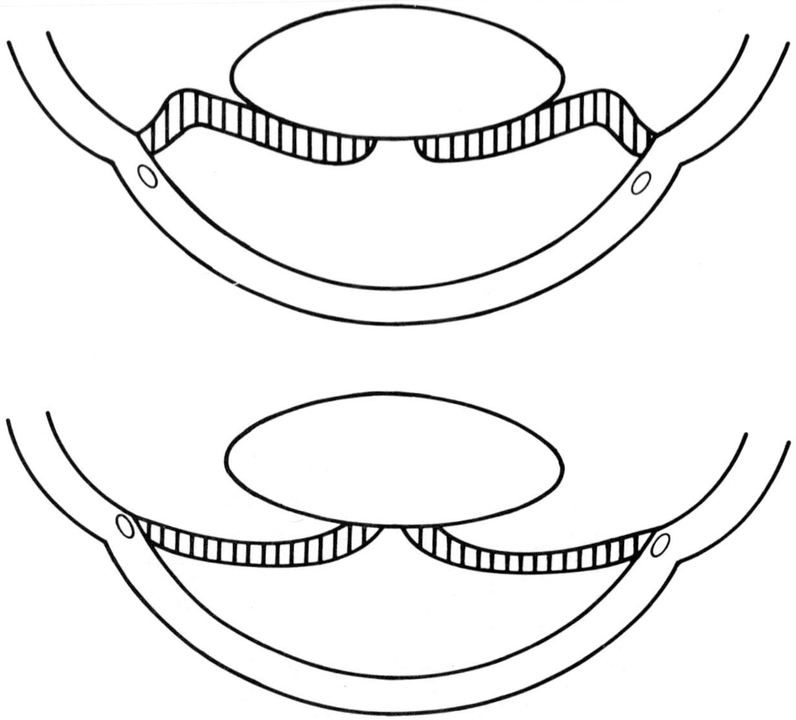

Fig. 3-7. Demonstration that an eye can present in iris bombe configuration with angle closure *(top),* and configuration of eye following administration of carbonic anhydrase inhibitor showing change to iris retraction configuration.

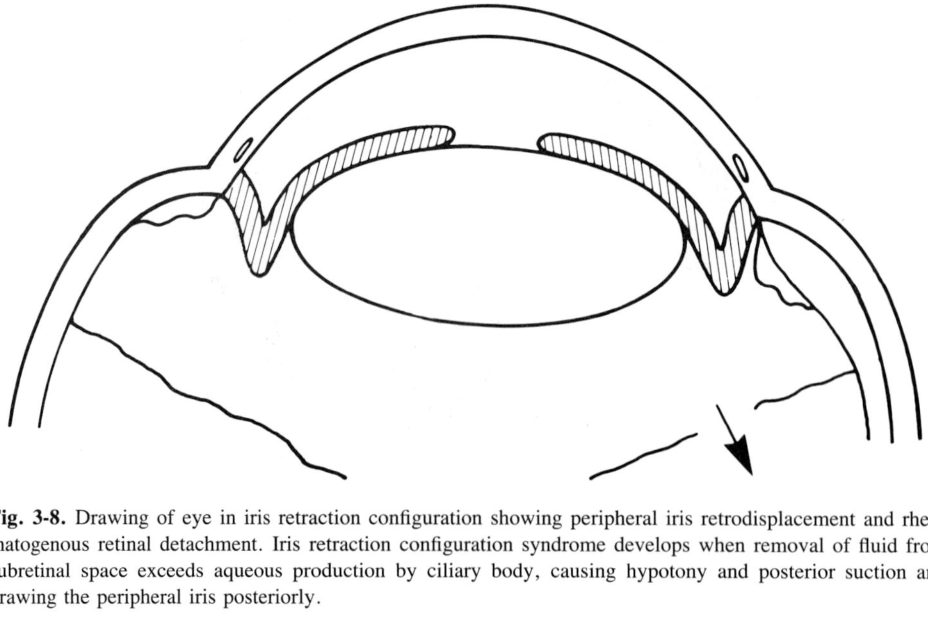

Fig. 3-8. Drawing of eye in iris retraction configuration showing peripheral iris retrodisplacement and rhegmatogenous retinal detachment. Iris retraction configuration syndrome develops when removal of fluid from subretinal space exceeds aqueous production by ciliary body, causing hypotony and posterior suction and drawing the peripheral iris posteriorly.

syndrome was not a result of vitreous retraction but was instead caused by hydrodynamic changes in the eye that rendered the pressure behind the iris so low that it was sucked posteriorly. Studies showed that whenever a patient presented with the iris retraction syndrome, the pupil was always sequestered, or totally bound down to the lens, preventing fluid flow between the anterior and posterior chambers. Thus, the iris served as a pressure-sensitive diaphragm, indicating regions of higher and lower pressure. In addition, disruption of the barrier by a peripheral iridectomy or pharmacologic pupillary dilation to disrupt posterior synechiae to the lens caused the iris to flatten slowly. Such action indicated that the pressure had been lower posteriorly than anteriorly in the retraction configuration and that it had now become equalized.

Finally and most importantly, study of two patients with angle closure and iris bombe confirmed the hydrodynamic nature of this configuration. These patients, who presented with rhegmatogenous retinal detachment and angle closure secondary to iris bombe and resultant elevation of IOP, converted to the iris retraction configuration under the influence of the carbonic anhydrase inhibitor, acetazolamide. Following the decrease in aqueous production caused by this medication, the iris flattened slowly and converted to the retraction configuration (Fig. 3-7). This was associated with a concomitant decrease in pressure from a high level to a hypotonous level. When the carbonic anhydrase inhibitor was discontinued, the eye returned to the iris bombe configuration, with angle closure and elevated IOP. These clinical observations indicated that when the eye was in the bombe configuration, aqueous production behind the sequestered iris-lens diaphragm exceeded aqueous removal, causing the iris to bulge forward in the bombe configuration, closing the angle and elevating the IOP. When carbonic anhydrase inhibitors were administered, aqueous production was reduced to a level that allowed aqueous removal to overcome production, causing hypotony and a suction that drew the iris posteriorly (Fig. 3-8). These observations proved that constant activity of the subretinal pump contributes to the decrease in IOP typically seen with a rhegmatogenous retinal detachment.

Relationship between the subretinal pump and proliferative vitreoretinopathy

The importance of a functional subretinal pump in rhegmatogenous retinal detachment cannot be overemphasized if one considers its possible relationship to the development of proliferative vitreoretinopathy, the most serious complication of retinal detachment. If one accepts this reasoning, it would not be surprising that the incidence of proliferative vitreoretinopathy increases dramatically in hypotonous eyes with rhegmatogenous retinal detachment. It is not difficult to reason that cells drawn into the eye by the hypotony would be drawn posteriorly by the diverted fluid flow and would tend to line the retina, to proliferate there, and to cause proliferative vitreoretinopathy.

Although most studies have indicated that subretinal fluid flow occurs toward the choroid and thus that the pump resides in this region, four clinical and/or pathologic observations make us wonder if the retina might not also play a role in fluid removal. First, pathologists have long known that a chronically detached retina will develop large cysts on its posterior surface, as seen following gross section of the eye and easily documented microscopically (Fig. 3-9, *A*). Specifically, chronic detachment and deterioration may cause the retina to lose its ability to remove accumulated fluid, thus accounting for the cyst formation.

Second, ophthalmologists have long known that the outpouring of fatty exudate from peripheral arteriovenous fistulas associated with Von Hippel-Landau disease can be associated with an accumulation of this material not only in the immediate area, but also in the distantly located macula (Fig. 3-9, *B*). This phenomenon constitutes part of what Wise[39] has called the "exaggerated macular response." It appears that the exudate travels in the subretinal space to the macular region and is then carried into the retina, where it accumulates in a star pattern in Henle's fiber layer. The material does not accumulate in the retinal pigment epithelium or in the choroid, again suggesting a fluid flow toward the retina and retinal removal of fluid.

Third, in patients with retinal degenerations such as retinitis pigmentosa, pigment released from the retinal pigment epithelial layer does not collect and find its way back into the choroid, as one might suspect if the choroid were removing large amounts of fluid. Instead it is carried forward singly or in macrophages to the retina, generally perivascularly, again suggesting a flow toward the retina (Fig. 3-9, *C*).

Finally, in the development of proliferative vitreoretinopathy following rhegmatogenous retinal detachment (Fig. 3-9, *D*), cells shown by Machemer[24] to originate from the pigment epithelium and elsewhere find their way to both surfaces of the retina. It is intriguing to speculate that they may be drawn there by fluid flow.

If fluid flow to the subretinal space—and possibly to the retina—plays an important role in the development of proliferative vitreoretinopathy, this would explain the vastly increased incidence of this complication in hypotonous eyes, since these eyes would have almost all fluid flow in the eye directed posteriorly. In contrast, a much smaller portion of the total fluid flow in the eye would be diverted posteriorly in a routine rhegmatogenous retinal detachment without hypotony.

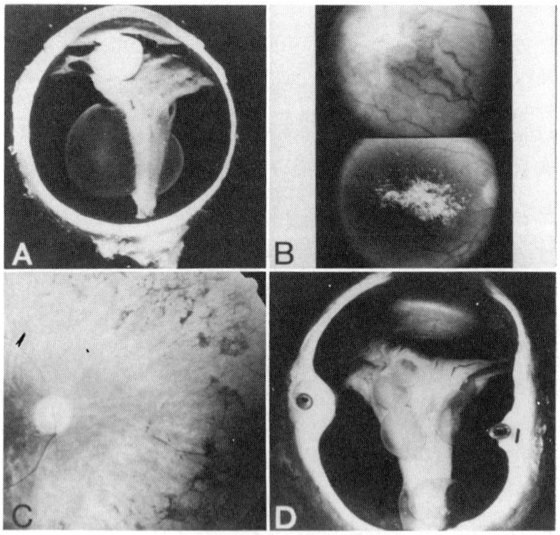

Fig. 3-9. Pathologic events that may suggest role for retina in subretinal fluid removal. **A,** Large retinal cysts associated with long-standing retinal detachment may indicate failure of chronically detached retina to remove fluid. **B,** Peripheral arteriovenous malformation *(top)* and distant secondary macular lipid deposit in von Hippel-Lindau disease *(bottom)* indicates that fluid from fistula is drawn to macular region, where it deposits within retina. **C,** Typical pigmentation pattern of retinitis pigmentosa, which indicates that pigment released from retinal pigment epithelium is drawn forward into retina, generally perivascularly. **D,** Massive proliferative vitreoretinopathy associated with rhegmatogenous retinal detachment. Cells that cause this disease line retina, and some may be drawn there by fluid flow.

Summary

The study of the relationship between angle closure and the iris retraction syndrome has clarified the pathophysiology of this syndrome, and this elucidation has led to possible further insight into the etiology of proliferative vitreoretinopathy. Further laboratory studies are certainly needed to delineate more exactly the direction and quantification of posterior fluid flow in the presence of rhegmatogenous retinal detachment in general and in the fascinating and rare iris retraction syndrome.

REFERENCES

1. Arruga, H.: Ueber die ruhigstellung des angapfels in der behandlung der netzhautablosung, Klin. Monatsbl. Augenheilkunde **93:**52, 1934.
2. Barraquer, J.: Separation of synechiae. In Surgery of the iris and the ciliary body, Adv. Ophthalmol. **30:**201, 1975.
3. Beigelman, M.N.: Acute hypotony in retinal detachment, Arch. Ophthalmol. **1:**463, 1929.
4. Boke, W., and Hubner, H.: Acute retinal detachment with severe uveitis and hypotony of the eyeball, Mod. Probl. Ophthalmol. **10:**245, 1972.
5. Campbell, D.G.: A comparison of diagnostic techniques in angle closure glaucoma, Am. J. Ophthalmol. **88:**197, 1979.
6. Campbell, D.G.: Iris retraction associated with the syndrome of rhegmatogenous retinal detachment and hypotony: a new explanation, Arch. Ophthalmol. (In press.)
7. Campbell, D.G., and Bell, F.C.: On the cause of hypotension in retinal detachment, Invest. Ophthalmol. Vis. Sci. **18**(suppl.):65, 1979.
8. Campbell, D.G., and Vela, A.: Modern goniosynechialysis for the treatment of synechial angle closure glaucoma. (Submitted to Ophthalmology.)
9. Cantrill, H.L., and Pederson, J.E.: Experimental retinal detachment. III. Vitreous fluorophotometry, Arch. Ophthalmol. **100:**1810, 1982.
10. Chandler, P.A., and Grant, W.M., editors: Glaucoma, ed. 2, Philadelphia, 1979, Lea & Febiger.
11. Chandler, P.A., and Simmons, R.J.: Anterior chamber deepening for gonioscopy at the time of surgery, Arch. Ophthalmol. **74:**177, 1965.
12. Cogan, D.G.: Symposium: primary chorioretinal aberrations with night blindness. Pathology, Trans. Am. Acad. Ophthalmol. Otolaryngol. **54:**629, 1949.
13. Custodis, E.: Bedeutet die plombenaufreihung auf der sklera einen fortschritt in der operativen behandlung der netzhautablosung? Ber Deutsch Ophth. Gesellsch. **58:**102, 1953.
14. Dobbie, J.G.: A study of the intraocular fluid dynamics in retinal detachment, Arch. Ophthalmol. **69:**159, 1963.
15. Donaldson, D.D.: Atlas of external diseases of the eye. Vol. 4. Anterior chamber, iris, and ciliary body, St. Louis, 1973, The C.V. Mosby Co.
16. Frambach, D.A., and Marmor, M.F.: The rate and route of fluid resorption from the subretinal space of the rabbit, Invest. Ophthalmol. Vis. Sci. **22:**292, 1982.
17. Gonin, J.: L'hypotonie oculaire dans ses relations avec le decollement retinien, Arch. d'Ophtalmol. **51:**426, 1934.
18. Gonin, J.: La pathogenie du decollement spontane de la retine, Ann. d'Oculiste **132:**30, 1904.
19. Heath, H., Beck, T.G., and Foulds, W.S.: Chemical composition of subretinal fluid, Br. J. Ophthalmol. **46:**385, 1962.
20. Jarett, W.H.: Rhegmatogenous retinal detachment complicated by severe intraocular inflammation, hypotony and choroidal detachment, Trans. Am. Ophthalmol. Soc. **79:**664, 1981.
21. Langham, M.E., and Regan, C.D.J.: Circulatory changes associated with onset of primary retinal detachment, Arch. Ophthalmol. **81:**820, 1969.
22. Leber, T.H.: Die krankheiten der netzhaut. In Graefe, F.W.E., and Saemisch, E.T.: Handbuch der gesamten Augenheilkunde **7:**1422, 1916.
23. Lincoff, H.A., Baras, I., and McLean, J.: Modifications to the Custodis procedure for retinal detachment, Arch. Ophthalmol. **73:**160, 1965.
24. Machemer, R.: Pathogenesis and classification of massive periretinal proliferation, Br. J. Ophthalmol. **62:**737, 1978.

25. Marmor, M.F., Abdul-Rahim, A.S., and Cohen, D.S.: The effect of metabolic inhibitors on retinal adhesion and subretinal fluid resorption, Invest. Ophthalmol. Vis. Sci. **19:**893, 1980.
26. Miller, D., and Stegmann, R.: Use of sodium hyaluronate in anterior segment eye surgery, Am. Intraocular Implant Soc. J. **6:**13, 1980.
27. Miller, D., O'Conner, P., and Williams, J.: Use of sodium hyaluronate during intraocular lens implantation in rabbits, Ophthalmic Surg. **8:**58, 1977.
28. Pederson, J.E.: Experimental retinal detachment. IV. Aqueous humor dynamics in rhegmatogenous retinal detachments, Arch. Ophthalmol. **100:**1814, 1982.
29. Pederson, J.E., Gaasterland, D.E., and MacLellan, H.M.: Experimental ciliochoroidal detachment—effect on intraocular pressure and aqueous humor flow, Arch. Ophthalmol. **97:**536, 1979.
30. Poos, F.: Die amotio retinae als krankheitsprozess. 2. Mitteilung. Uber die vorgange bei ablosung und weideranlegung der netzhaut nach foramenbildung, Graefes Arch. Augenheilkunde **156:**191, 1955.
31. Regan, C.D.J., and Rousseau, A.P.: The intraocular dynamics of eyes with retinal detachment. Am. J. Ophthalmol. **61:**696, 1966.
32. Seelenfreund, M.H., and others: Choroidal detachment associated with primary retinal detachment, Arch. Ophthalmol. **91:**254, 1974.
33. Simmons, R.J.: Angle closure glaucoma after scleral buckling operations for separated retina. In Chandler, P.A., and Grant, W.M., editors: Glaucoma, ed. 2, Philadelphia, 1979, Lea & Febiger.
34. Syrdalen, P.: Intraocular pressure and ocular rigidity in patients with retinal detachments. I. Preoperative study. Acta Ophthalmol. **48:**1024, 1970.
35. Van Heuven, W.A., Lam, K.W., and Ray, G.S.: Source of subretinal fluid on the basis of ascorbate analyses, Arch. Ophthalmol. **100:**976, 1982.
36. Vela, A., and Campbell, D.G.: Modern goniosynechialysis, Invest. Ophthalmol. **25**(suppl.): 194, 1984.
37. Vela, A., Rieser, J.C., and Campbell, D.G.: The heredity and treatment of angle closure glaucoma secondary to iris and ciliary body cysts, Ophthalmology **91:**332, 1984.
38. Wand, M., and others: Plateau iris syndrome, Trans. Am. Acad. Ophthalmol. Otolaryngol. **83:**122, 1977.
39. Wise, G.N., and Wangvivat, Y.: The exaggerated macular response to retinal disease. Part II. Am. J. Ophthalmol. **61:**1359, 1966.

4

The glaucomas and extracapsular cataract surgery with posterior chamber lens implantation

Richard J. Simmons
James A. Savage*
John V. Thomas*
C. Davis Belcher III*

Cataract and glaucoma commonly coexist. Both are seen with increased incidence in elderly age-groups. In addition, miotic medication and surgery for glaucoma both carry with them the possibility of increasing the likelihood of significant lens opacity.[41,49,51] Surgery for the cataract frequently needs to be considered in such cases. One must also consider the indications for cataract surgery and for glaucoma therapy in each individual. Mere coexistence of the two entities is not enough to indicate intervention for the glaucoma or the cataract.[43-45]

In regard to the glaucoma, the indications for and type of therapy should be carefully evaluated. To treat the glaucoma, medical therapy in progressive increments up to maximum tolerated level should be employed as needed. If additional control of glaucoma is required, laser trabeculoplasty should be considered in the case of open-angle glaucoma. If medication or laser therapy controls the glaucoma, there is generally no indication for glaucoma surgery; surgery for the cataract should be done without combined glaucoma procedure. On the other hand, if medical and laser therapy do not sufficiently control the glaucoma, then one should consider either (1) glaucoma surgery, combined with the cataract surgery; or (2) a glaucoma filtration procedure before cataract surgery followed months later by cataract removal.[16,25,26,42-45,48] Evaluation of the glaucoma in such cases is therefore important, since appropriate glaucoma therapy must be determined and carried out before or in combination with cataract surgery.

As noted, the simple existence of a cataract in the presence of glaucoma does not mandate intervention. One should consider the visual needs of the patient, the status of the fellow eye, the amount of disability caused by the cataract, and the fact that any surgery, including cataract surgery, can carry risks to normal eyes as well as glaucomatous ones. In addition, when removal of the cataract is indicated, one must decide on

*Glaucoma Consultation Service, Massachusetts Eye and Ear Infirmary, Harvard Medical School and the New England Glaucoma Research Foundation, Boston, Mass.

the surgical technique. For years intracapsular cataract extraction (ICCE) surgery was the standard, but recently extracapsular cataract extraction (ECCE) techniques have been shown to possess several theoretic and real advantages for many patients.[29] The choice of the technique of cataract surgery should be considered in conjunction with the relative safety of each procedure, the skills of the surgeon, and the procedure with which he or she is most familiar.

One must also decide whether to use an intraocular lens (IOL). For years many glaucoma specialists have believed that in no circumstance is an IOL indicated for a glaucomatous eye.[2,13,20,36] Some experienced surgeons, however, have suggested that implanting IOLs in glaucomatous eyes is a possibility to consider and can be done, at least in some eyes, without disadvantage.[10,13,14,21-24,46,47]

In eyes without glaucoma, what are the risks of ECCE and what is the risk of adding a posterior chamber IOL? In glaucomatous eyes how do these risks of ECCE with and without posterior chamber lens implantation compare?[30,31] Also, all glaucomatous patients are not the same: some have mild glaucoma, others are controlled with medical

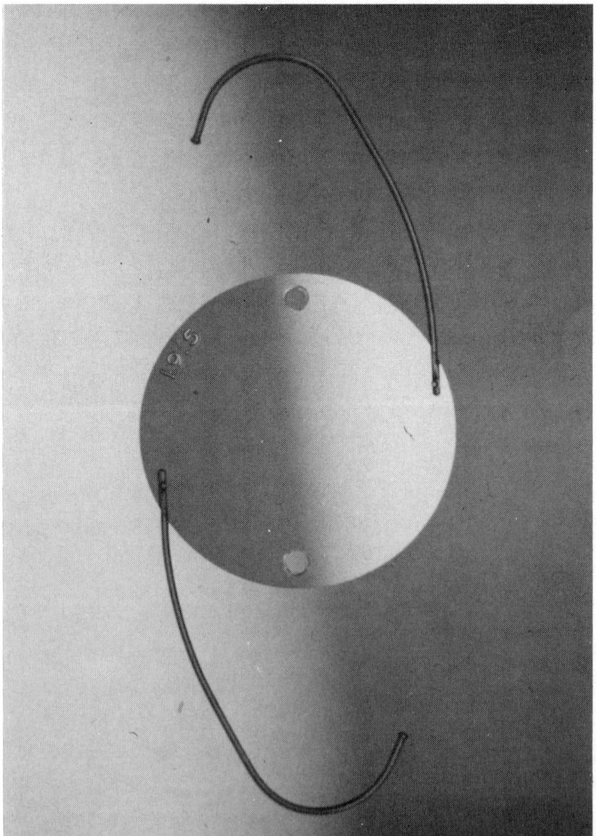

Fig. 4-1. Photograph of Sinskey-style posterior chamber lens implant. Haptic configuration is helpful for lens insertion, particularly in glaucomatous eyes with miotic and less mobile pupils.

or laser therapy, and still others require one of the surgical procedures already mentioned. What is the risk of ECCE and posterior chamber lens implantation in each of these different groups of glaucomatous eyes? Finally, what is the risk of these cataract procedures in glaucomatous patients who have had previous angle-closure glaucoma?

We have attempted an ongoing analysis of our experience with these various groups to determine the risks involved and to answer these questions. Following long experience with ICCE, we have found a minimal but variable influence of ICCE used alone on glaucoma.[3,10,14,15,32,50] On the average, ICCE from below in the presence of a filtration bleb above has produced minimal but definite worsening of intraocular pressure (IOP) in our patients.[44] The addition of anterior chamber lenses to ICCE appears to be potentially damaging to the trabecular meshwork and in our experience can aggravate glaucoma. ECCE, with the advantage of intact zonules and posterior capsule to keep vitreous out of the anterior chamber, seems to offer theoretic advantages for the glaucomatous eye. Also, the use of a posterior chamber IOL, which keeps vitreous posteriorly in its normal position even after capsulotomy and does not allow contact of haptics or the lens with the corneal endothelium or the trabecular meshwork when properly placed, would seem to be the ideal site for a pseudophakos, especially in a glaucomatous eye (see Fig. 4-1). It also seems logical that the placement of an anterior chamber pseudophakos near the trabecular meshwork would carry entirely different and worse implications for a patient with open-angle glaucoma than posterior placement in the capsular bag, ciliary sulcus, or both.[6,7,12,17,27,30,33,35,37,39] Although we have come to favor ECCE with posterior chamber lens implantation for visual reasons and the theoretic benefits in glaucomatous eyes mentioned, we have been concerned not only with whether this operation can cause glaucoma, but with whether it aggravates existing glaucoma.

Since cataract is frequently found in elderly patients, the present population is living longer than ever before, and IOLs allow theoretic and practical advantages over contact lenses or spectacles, we believe it is important to consider these questions. The use of contact lenses over filtering blebs presents a risk of infection and damage to the bleb from insertion. The administration of glaucoma drops to patients with contact lenses or aphakic spectacles can be difficult, especially when the patient attempts to administer the drops to himself. Using an IOL that permits better peripheral vision and better use of a central island of vision can help such patients. For this reason the following study has been conducted to determine what the results have been in a series of glaucomatous and normal eyes. What is the risk of this procedure? Does the procedure aggravate glaucoma? If so, how significant is the aggravation and what can be done about it? What is the place of ECCE with or without a posterior chamber intraocular lens in glaucomatous eyes? This chapter attempts to answer these questions.

MATERIALS AND METHODS

Patient population

In 233 eyes of 200 patients ECCE was performed and ongoing follow-up was conducted by members of our group, including Stephen R. Deppermann, Thomas M. Richardson, and Omah S. Singh. Preexisting glaucoma of varying severity was present in 116 eyes, 87 with and 29 without the implantation of a posterior chamber IOL. Fifty-eight eyes, 39 of the pseudophakic and 19 of the aphakic eyes, had at least a 6-month follow-up (Table 4-1). The pseudophakic and aphakic groups were each further subdivided into five categories, based on the methods of IOP control employed before the cataract surgery (see boxed material). The decision of whether or not to employ an IOL in a particular eye was based on such considerations as myopia, aphakia in the other eye, and associated pathologic conditions in the eye; the presence or status of glaucoma was not used as a criteria for employing or omitting lens implantation.

In addition to the glaucomatous eyes, two groups of nonglaucomatous "control" eyes—healthy except for the presence of a cataract—were studied. Of these 117 eyes, 100 had ECCE with the implantation of a posterior chamber IOL and 17 had ECCE alone. Forty-two of the pseudophakic and nine of the aphakic eyes had a minimum of 6 months' follow-up. Eyes of patients with diabetes were eliminated from these groups, as were eyes with a history of trauma, known senile macular degeneration, retinal detachment, uveitis, amblyopia, corneal disease, or other known ocular disease. The preoperative and postoperative examination strategies were identical to those employed in

Table 4-1. Patient groups in ECCE study

	ECCE with posterior chamber IOL		*ECCE alone*		*Total*	
Patient groups	*Total eyes*	*Eyes with 6-mo follow-up*	*Total eyes*	*Eyes with 6-mo follow-up*	*Total eyes*	*Eyes with 6-mo follow-up*
Group A	25	14	6	4	31	18
Group B	33	14	9	7	42	21
Group C	13	8	9	6	22	14
Group D	6	1	2	1	8	2
Group E	10	2	3	1	13	3
Total glaucoma groups	87	39	29	19	116	58
Group F (nonglaucoma)	100	42	17	9	117	51

Patient groups in ECCE study

Group A Open-angle glaucoma with IOP controlled before cataract surgery with medications alone

Group B Open-angle glaucoma controlled preoperatively with argon laser trabeculoplasty (LTP) and medications

Group C Open-angle glaucoma controlled preoperatively with glaucoma filtration surgery; ECCE done from below because of a filtering bleb above

Group D Open-angle glaucoma inadequately controlled before ECCE; cataract surgery combined with glaucoma surgery

Group E Previous primary angle-closure glaucoma successfully treated with surgical or argon laser iridectomy without residual open-angle glaucoma component and no more than 1 clock hour of peripheral anterior synechiae

Group F Nonglaucomatous eyes without preexisting glaucoma or other ocular pathology; also excluded: eyes of patients with diabetes and of those under age 50

the glaucoma groups. The operative techniques were also the same, except for various modifications employed in the glaucoma eyes, such as posterior synechialysis, sphincterotomy, sector iridectomy, cataract extraction combined with glaucoma filtration surgery or cyclodialysis, and cataract extraction from below because of a filtering bleb above.

Preoperative assessment

The preoperative evaluation of all eyes included corrected Snellen visual acuity, applanation tonometry, and when possible, examination of the disc. Gonioscopy, Chandler-Harrington visual fields, and in some cases tonography were done in the eyes with preexisting glaucoma. If more than one preoperative measurement of IOP existed during the 2 months before cataract surgery, we averaged the values—as long as all measurements were taken when glaucoma medications were the same and at least 2 months had passed since prior laser or surgical glaucoma procedures.

We also recorded the preoperative medicines required for glaucoma control. To quantitate these medical requirements, we devised a point system, assigning values to various medication concentrations to enable comparisons and quantitation of changes in the requirements for control of the glaucoma (Table 4-2). For instance, a change from timolol 0.25% b.i.d. (2 points) to timolol 0.5% b.i.d. (4 points) would be a net increase of 2 points.

Postoperatively we gave particular attention to those eyes with severe preoperative glaucomatous visual field loss. Those eyes with arcuate scotomata involving fixation and those with double arcuate scotomata producing central islands were closely followed postoperatively for changes in visual acuity and visual field status.

Surgical procedure

All cases were performed by a member of one glaucoma surgical group consisting of five surgeons. The choice of technique was by the individual surgeon, but the same

Table 4-2. Glaucoma medication point values

Medication	*Strength*	*Frequency*	*Weighted value (units)*
Timolol	0.25%	b.i.d.	2
	0.5%		4
Epinephrine	1.0%	b.i.d.	2
Dipivalyl epinephrine	0.1%	b.i.d.	2
Pilocarpine	1.0%	q.i.d.	1
	2.0%		2
	3.0%		3
	4.0%		4
Carbachol	0.75%	t.i.d.	1
	1.5%		2
	3.0%		4
Phospholine	0.25%	b.i.d.	4
Acetazolamide	250 mg	q.i.d.	4
	500 mg (seq.)	b.i.d.	4
Methazolamide	50 mg	t.i.d.	2
	100 mg	t.i.d.	4

basic technique was employed in all. The surgical procedure employed was microscopic ECCE. Some surgeons preferred a mechanized method of cortical removal, while others preferred a manual technique. In 134 cases the cortical cleanup was accomplished manually by the technique advocated by Gills.[18] In the remaining 99 eyes a mechanized irrigation/aspiration method was used. The preoperative preparation of the eye was found to be critical; preoperative injections and the application of a compression device were timed to obtain an exceedingly soft eye (Fig. 4-2, *A*). When this was achieved, ECCE was much easier, without troublesome and potentially dangerous posterior pressure. Following sedation with diazepam and fentanyl in suitable doses, we administered retrobulbar and lid blocks (0.75% Bupivocaine with epinephrine, 2% Xylocaine, hyaluronidase). For mydriasis, a combination of 0.8% tropicamide and 5% phenylephrine was given topically. An orbital vascular compression device was then applied to obtain a suitably soft eye for the procedure, which was particularly important when the "open eye" manual technique was employed. The goal was to apply the compression device 20 to 45 minutes before surgery.

Before commencing with the operation, we tested the IOP with a Schiøtz tonometer. For scale readings less than 12 (5.5 g weight), concentrated digital pressure was applied to the eye and orbit until the eye was suitably soft (Fig. 4-2, *B*). In many such situations we administered a 50 cc bolus of intravenous 25% mannitol to further soften the eye.

Except in cases of combined ECCE and glaucoma filtration surgery, a fornix-based conjunctival flap was used. For the limbal incision and anterior capsulotomy, hyaluronic acid was injected into the anterior chamber for endothelial protection. A two-plane corneoscleral incision was employed, with beveling of the inner cut. This permitted entrance to the anterior chamber in front of the trabecular meshwork to minimize any effect on outflow from subsequent wound closure with sutures.[8,15,38]

For hemostasis during the conjunctival and limbal incisions, we used a monopolar coaxial microdiathermy. This instrument has a 0.2 mm diameter tip, and we found it to be the safest, most precise method of microsurgical hemostasis.[40] In particular, the delicate size of the tip is ideally suited to the elimination of bleeding vessels within the cataract wound, where the excessive tissue shrinkage produced by several of the larger, currently popular bipolar instruments may result in faulty wound apposition and closure. Also, when combined cataract/glaucoma filtration surgery was done, the pinpoint hemostasis provided by the diathermy was particularly desirable during the conjunctival flap dissection and for any bleeding in the depths of the sclerostomy, since it minimizes excessive charring and shrinkage of adjacent tissue.

A square anterior capsulotomy was made using microscissors with hyaluronic acid in the anterior chamber. The nucleus was gently expressed using an irrigating vectis with its tip beneath the superior pole of the nucleus and its shaft pressing on the posterior lip of the wound. Occasionally counterpressure inferiorly was required for the nucleus removal. During this maneuver care was taken not to rupture the zonules or posterior capsule, especially in highly myopic eyes and in those with extremely large nuclei.

Cortical removal was then performed using the manual technique advocated by Gills. Since this is an open-eye technique, the meticulous attention paid to obtaining a soft eye with preinjection and ocular compression emerged as a critical determinant in making the surgery easier.

Sinskey-style posterior chamber IOLs were used in all 187 cases of implantation in

A

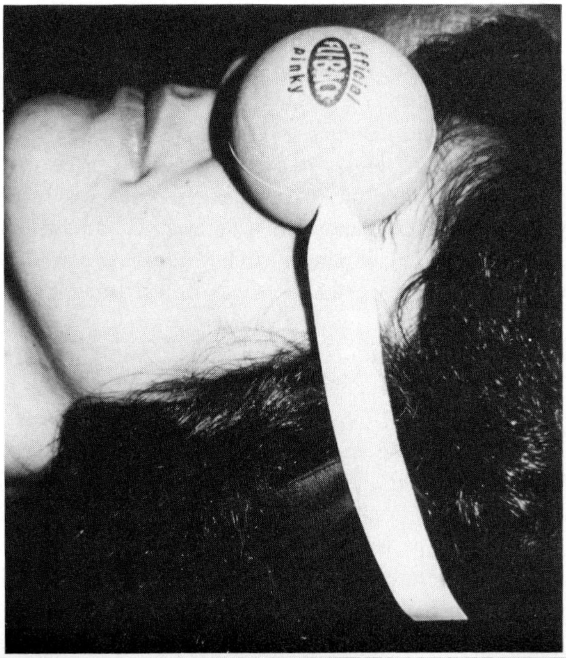

B

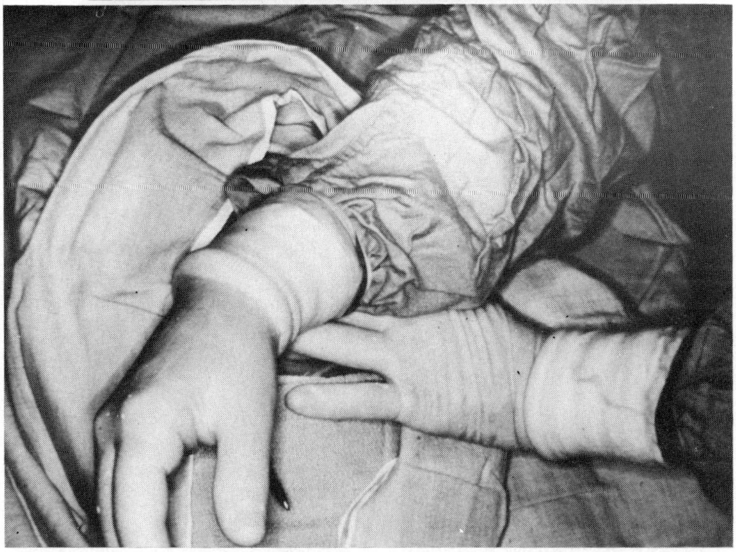

Fig. 4-2. A, Orbital vascular compression device that we prefer. This appliance is inexpensive, well tolerated, and valuable in producing a soft eye for surgery. **B,** Method of digital ocular compression, as taught by Paul A. Chandler. We use it, when necessary, for additional softening.

the series; 181 (96.8%) had posterior angulation of the haptics to avoid pupillary capture. Balanced salt solution followed by acetylcholine was generally injected into the anterior chamber following lens implantation. This resulted in little or no residual hyaluronic acid in the anterior chamber at the conclusion of the procedure. The corneoscleral incision was closed with interrupted 10-0 nylon sutures. In cases of combined ECCE and glaucoma filtration, the conjunctival incision was closed using a running, intermittently locked, subcuticular 10-0 nylon suture. This avoided stiff, exposed nylon sutures that might redden the eye postoperatively.

In some eyes, where chronic miosis had resulted from prior glaucoma therapy, a sphincterotomy (Fig. 4-3) or sector or keyhole iridectomy was required for adequate pupil size to safely complete the maneuvers required for controlled ECCE.[10] These sector or keyhole iridectomies were left open and were not repaired with monofilament suture, as some have advocated.[10,11] This step was omitted to minimize the number of intraocular maneuvers done in these eyes. Optical complaints by the patients were an infrequent occurrence.

Several techniques of combined cataract/glaucoma surgery were employed in cases where inadequate glaucoma control existed preoperatively. Combined cataract/trabeculectomy was done by extending the trabeculectomy incision to permit the cataract extraction. Combined cataract/cyclodialysis was done in either of two ways. In one case the cyclodialysis was performed with a rectangular trabeculectomy-like dissection superiorly.[18] The inner scleral layer was then disinserted anteriorly and reflected into the suprachoroidal space. The other combined cataract/cyclodialysis procedures were done from an external approach through an inferotemporal sclerotomy.

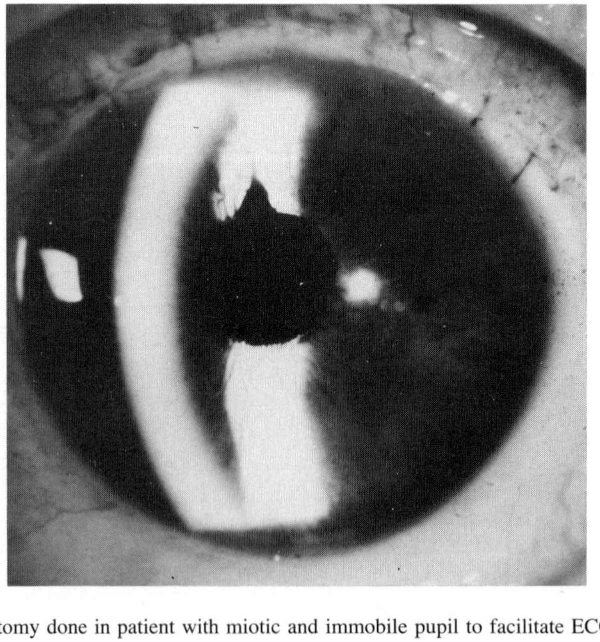

Fig. 4-3. Sphincterotomy done in patient with miotic and immobile pupil to facilitate ECCE with insertion of posterior chamber IOL.

Postoperative care

We performed postoperative examinations with frequent IOP determinations. Biomicroscopy, ophthalmoscopy, keratometry, and refraction were done when indicated. Comparison of preoperative and postoperative visual acuity was represented as the number of Snellen lines improved. In the eyes with preexisting glaucoma, gonioscopy, visual field testing, and in some cases tonography were done at appropriate times.

We divided postoperative pressure rises into "early" and "lasting" groups. Early rises were those occurring during the first 8 weeks following surgery. Lasting rises were those pressure rises found later than 8 weeks postoperatively that required additional glaucoma therapy. Only those eyes with at least a 6-month follow-up were considered in determinations of average changes in pressure, changes in medical requirements for pressure control, visual field changes following surgery, improvement in visual acuity, and postoperative complications. All eyes with at least 8 weeks of follow-up were considered in calculations of frequency of early pressure rises. Pressure rises were divided into those 5 mm or greater, greater than 10 mm, and greater than 15 mm Hg above the preoperative IOP value.

RESULTS (Tables 4-3 and 4-4)

Groups of eyes in which an IOL was implanted were referred to as "pseudophakic"; if no implant was used, the eyes were termed "aphakic." For instance, "pseudophakic/glaucoma" would denote those eyes with preexisting glaucoma that underwent ECCE with the implantation of a posterior chamber IOL; "aphakic/control" would denote nonglaucomatous eyes that underwent ECCE without lens implantation; and so on.

Group A (see previous box)

ECCE with posterior chamber IOL. In the medically controlled group 25 eyes had a posterior chamber lens implanted, and six eyes had ECCE alone. In the pseudophakic group, for those 14 eyes with at least 6 months of follow-up, the average change in IOP was −5.5% (average preoperative tension: 18.7 mm Hg; average postoperative tension: 16.7). In the 25 eyes of the pseudophakic group, 16 (64%) had an early tension rise of 5 mm Hg or more, 12 (48%) of greater than 10 mm Hg, and 4 (16%) of greater than 15 mm Hg. In the 14 eyes with at least 6 months of follow-up, two (14.2%) had a lasting pressure elevation of 5 mm Hg or greater, and one (7.1%) had a lasting rise of greater than 10 mm Hg. There were no lasting pressure elevations greater than 15 mm Hg (see Fig. 4-4).

For these eyes the medication requirements for glaucoma control increased by an average of 0.5 units. The average improvement in visual acuity following cataract surgery was +6.1 Snellen lines.

ECCE alone. For those four medically controlled eyes with ECCE alone with a minimum of 6 months of follow-up, the average change in IOP was −14.8% (average preoperative tension: 18.2 mm Hg; average post-operative tension: 15.4 mm Hg). Of five eyes with at least 8 weeks of follow-up, three (60%) had early pressure rises of 5 mm Hg or greater, one (20%) of greater than 10 mm Hg, and none greater than 15 mm Hg. There were no lasting pressure rises as high as 5 mm Hg in the four eyes with at least 6 months of follow-up (see Fig. 4-4).

The postoperative glaucoma medication requirements were decreased by an average of 0.5 units. The average improvement in visual acuity was +8.3 Snellen lines.

Table 4-3. Average results for patients after ECCE with at least 6 months of follow-up*

	Group A		*Group B*		*Group C*		*Group D*		*Group E*		*Group F*	
Parameters	*PC-IOL*	*No IOL*	*PC-IOL*	*No IOL*	*PC-IOL*	*No IOL*	*PC-IOL*	*No IOL*	*PC-IOL*	*No IOL*	*PC-IOL*	*No IOL*
Total eyes	25	6	33	9	13	9	6	2	10	3	100	17
Eyes with 6-mo follow-up	14	4	14	7	8	6	1	1	2	1	42	9
Follow-up (weeks)	47.4	51.8	42.4	52.3	41.3	55.2	40	71	47.5	32	50.1	42.8
Age (years)	73.9	67.3	75.2	74.4	71.6	70.8	73	75	69.0	81	69.6	68.7
Sex (male/female)	6:8	4:0	6:8	2:5	4:4	2:4	0:1	0:1	0:2	0:1	21:21	5:4
Race	White	White	White	White	One Black	White	White	White	White	White	White	White
Tn before previous LTP or filter op	—	—	21.4	21.0	33.8	24.0	—	—	—	—	—	—
Interval before ECCE (months)	—	—	11.3	10.4	52.8	48.7	—	—	—	—	—	—
Preop IOP	18.7	18.2	17.3	13.7	12.7	10.5	15	22	17.5	22	15.7	15.4
Postop IOP	16.7	15.4	16.5	13.6	12.4	12.4	9	13	15.5	20	15.0	13.7
% change Tn IOP	−5.5	−14.8	−3.6	+1.2	−4.1	+27.1	−40	−40.9	−12.5	−9.1	−3.8	−11.2
Change in Meds	+0.5	−0.5	+0.9	−3.1	+2.4	+2.3	+4	−16	−0.5	−4	—	—
Snellen lines improved	+6.1	+8.3	+6.6	+4.4	+5.8	+6.0	+1	+9	+5.5	+8	+6.8	+5.6

*Abbreviations: IOP, intraocular pressure in mm Hg; PC-IOL, Sinskey-style posterior chamber intraocular lens; Meds, weighted medication values (Table 4-2); LTP, laser trabeculoplasty; filter-op, glaucoma filtration surgery.

Table 4-4. Early vs. lasting tension rises following ECCE in eyes with preexisting glaucoma and in control eyes

	Early rise (0-8 weeks postop)			*Lasting rise (eyes with 6-mo follow-up)*		
Groups	*≥5 mm Hg*	*≥11 mm Hg*	*≥16 mm Hg*	*≥5 mm Hg*	*≥11 mm Hg*	*≥16 mm Hg*
Group A						
PC-IOL*	16/25 (64%)	12/25 (48%)	4/25 (16%)	2/14 (14.2%)	1/14 (7.1%)	0/14 (0%)
No IOL	3/5 (60%)	1/5 (20%)	0/5 (0%)	0/4 (0%)	0/4 (0%)	0/4 (0%)
Group B						
PC-IOL	28/30 (93.3%)	17/30 (56.7%)	12/30 (40.0%)	1/14 (7.1%)	0/14 (0%)	0/14 (0%)
No IOL	8/9 (88.9%)	4/9 (44.4%)	2/9 (22.2%)	0/7 (0%)	0/7 (0%)	0/7 (0%)
Group C						
PC-IOL	11/12 (91.7%)	8/12 (66.7%)	1/12 (8.3%)	3/8 (37.5%)	1/8 (12.5%)	0/8 (0%)
No IOL	8/9 (88.9%)	4/9 (44.4%)	2/9 (22.2%)	2/6 (33.3%)	1/6 (16.7%)	0/6 (0%)
Group D						
PC-IOL	0/4 (0%)	0/4 (0%)	0/4 (0%)	1/1 (100%)	0/1 (0%)	0/1 (0%)
No IOL	0/2 (0%)	0/2 (0%)	0/2 (0%)	0/1 (0%)	0/1 (0%)	0/1 (0%)
Group E						
PC-IOL	2/8 (25%)	1/8 (12.5%)	0/8 (0%)	0/2 (0%)	0/2 (0%)	0/2 (0%)
No IOL	0/2 (0%)	0/2 (0%)	0/2 (0%)	0/1 (0%)	0/1 (0%)	0/1 (0%)
Group F						
PC-IOL	19/91 (20.9%)	9/91 (9.9%)	4/91 (4.4%)	3/42 (7.2%)	1/42 (2.4%)	0/42 (0%)
No IOL	4/13 (30.8%)	2/13 (15.4%)	1/13 (7.7%)	0/9 (0%)	0/9 (0%)	0/9 (0%)

*PC-IOL, posterior chamber intraocular lens.

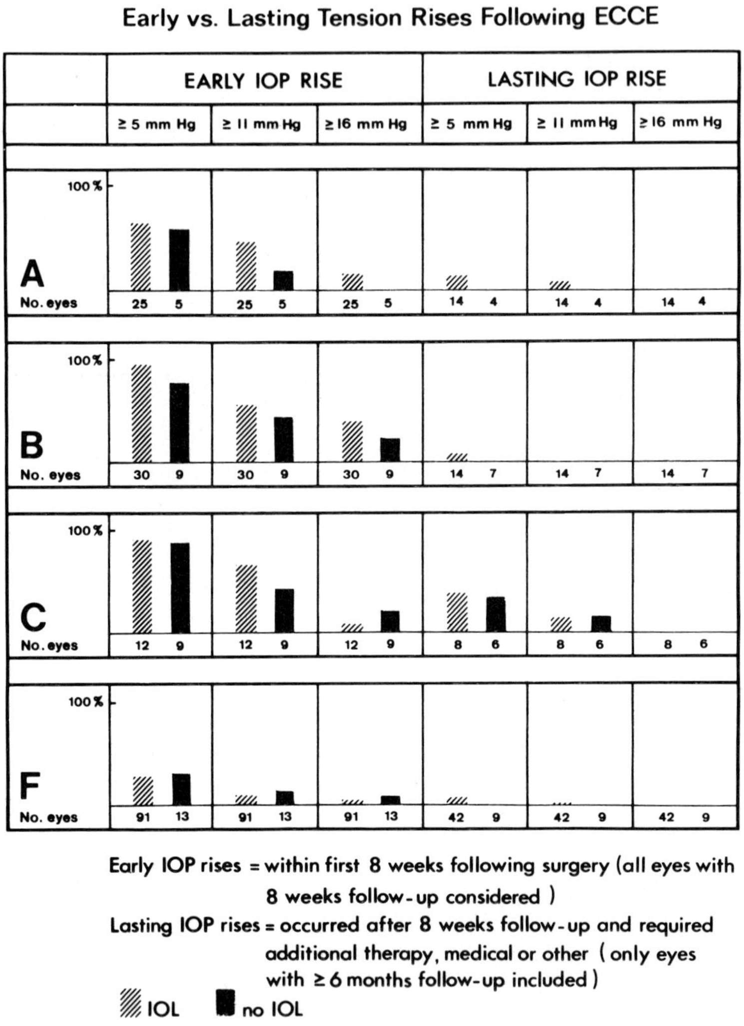

Fig. 4-4. Graph showing early and lasting rises in IOP following ECCE with and without posterior chamber lens insertion in glaucomatous eyes controlled preoperatively with medications (group A), with argon laser trabeculoplasty (group B), and with glaucoma filtration surgery (group C). Control eyes (group F) are shown for comparison *(bottom)*.

Group B

ECCE with posterior chamber IOL. In the group that underwent argon laser trabeculoplasty before cataract surgery, 33 had a posterior chamber lens implanted and nine had ECCE alone. For those 14 eyes in the pseudophakic group with at least 6 months of follow-up, the average change in IOP was −3.6% (average preoperative tension: 17.3 mm Hg; average postoperative tension: 16.5 mm Hg). The average time from completion of laser to cataract surgery was 11.3 months. An average of 10.7 clock hours of trabecular meshwork had been treated with laser therapy. The change in tension achieved with laser surgery was from 21.4 mm Hg to 17.3 mm Hg just before cataract surgery, or an average improvement after 11.3 months of 4.1 mm Hg (19.2%) (Fig. 4-5).

Early tension rises of 5 mm Hg or greater in the 30 pseudophakic eyes with at least 8 weeks of follow-up occurred in 28 (93.3%), greater than 10 mm Hg in 17 (56.7%), and greater than 15 mm Hg in 12 (40%). In the 14 eyes with at least 6 months of follow-up, a lasting tension rise of 5 mm Hg or gretaer was seen in one (7.1%). None of these eyes had lasting elevations of greater than 10 mm Hg (see Fig. 4-4).

The average change in glaucoma medication requirements between prelaser and precataract surgery was −2.4 units; from precataract surgery to postoperatively, +0.9 units. Therefore, the net change in medication requirements from prelaser to postcataract surgery was −1.5 units. The average improvement in visual acuity following cataract surgery was +6.6 Snellen lines.

ECCE alone. The seven aphakic eyes with at least 6 months of follow-up had an average change in IOP of +1.2%, although the average preoperative tension was 13.7 mm Hg and the average postoperative tension was 13.6 mm Hg. The average time from completion of laser to cataract surgery was 10.4 months. Twelve clock hours of angle were treated with laser therapy in all cases. The change in IOP achieved with laser surgery was from an average tension of 21.0 mm Hg to 13.7 mm Hg after laser inter-

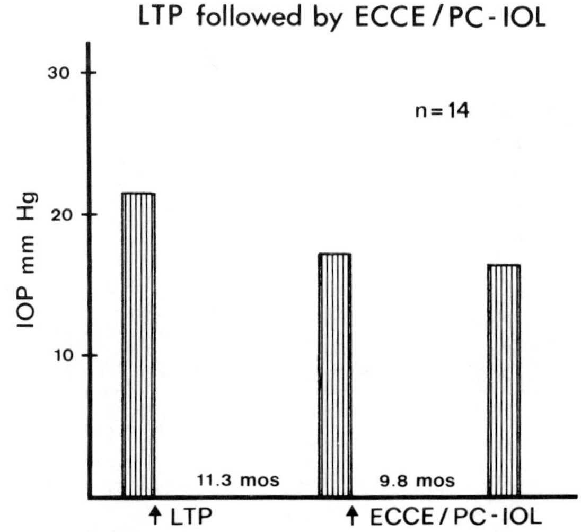

Fig. 4-5. Graph showing IOP before and after argon laser trabeculoplasty and following subsequent ECCE with posterior chamber lens implantation.

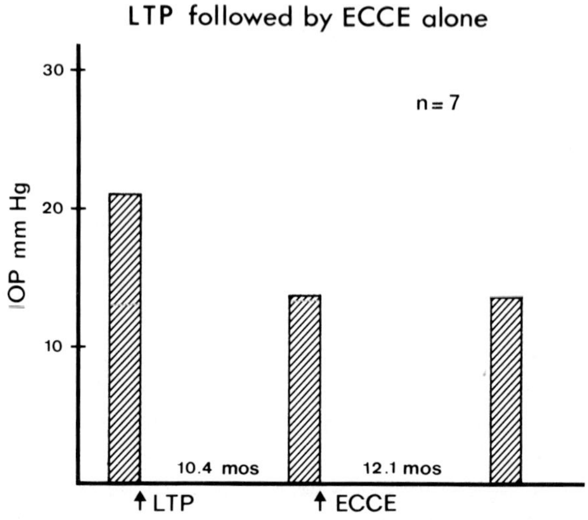

Fig. 4-6. Graph showing IOP before and after argon laser trabeculoplasty and following subsequent ECCE with no lens implant.

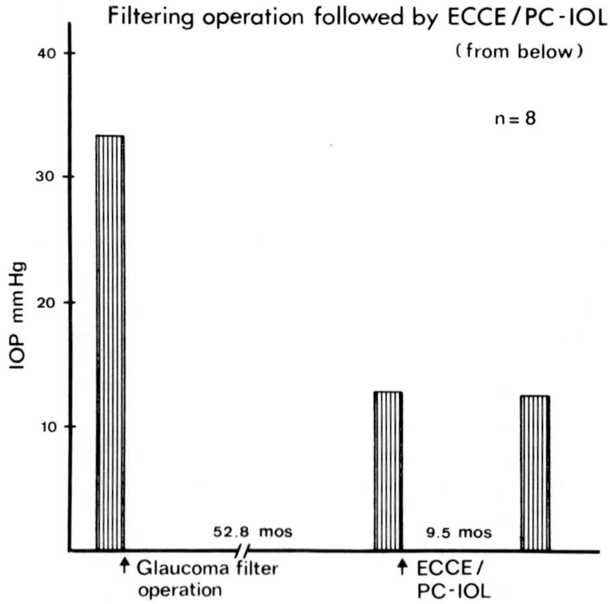

Fig. 4-7. Graph showing IOP before and after glaucoma filtration surgery and following subsequent ECCE with posterior chamber lens implantation.

vention, or an average improvement of −7.3 mm Hg (34.8%) after 10.4 months (Fig. 4-6).

Early tension rises of 5 mm Hg or greater in those nine aphakic eyes with at least 8 weeks of follow-up were seen in eight (88.9%), of greater than 10 mm Hg in four (44.4%), and of greater than 15 mm Hg in two (22.2%). No lasting tension rises of 5 mm Hg or greater were seen in the seven aphakic eyes with at least 6 months of follow-up (see Fig. 4-4).

The average change in glaucoma medication requirements from prelaser to precataract surgery was −0.1 units; from precataract surgery to postoperatively, −3.1 units—a net decrease of −3.2 units. The average improvement in visual acuity was +4.4 Snellen lines.

Group C

ECCE from below with posterior chamber IOL. In the eyes with previously successful glaucoma filtration surgery, 13 had ECCE done from below with a posterior chamber IOL, and nine had ECCE done from below alone. Of those eight pseudophakic eyes with at least 6 months of follow-up, the average change in IOP was −4.1% (average preoperative tension: 12.7 mm Hg; average postoperative tension: 12.4 mm Hg). The previous filtration surgery in these eyes (four trabeculectomies and four full-thickness operations) had been done an average of 52.8 months before the cataract extraction. The average prefilter tension was 33.8 mm Hg for these eyes, so the change in tension from prefilter to precataract surgery, 52.8 months later, was −21.1 mm Hg (62.4%) (Fig. 4-7).

Early tension rises in the 12 pseudophakic eyes with at least 8 weeks of follow-up included 11 (91.7%) with rises 5 mm Hg or more, eight (66.7%) greater than 10 mm Hg, and one (8.3%) greater than 15 mm Hg. In the eight pseudophakic eyes with at least 6 months of follow-up, three eyes (37.5%) had a lasting pressure elevation of 5 mm Hg or greater, and one (12.5%) had a lasting elevation of 10 mm Hg or greater. None of these eyes had lasting elevations of greater than 15 mm Hg (see Fig. 4-4).

The average change in glaucoma medication requirements from prefilter to precataract surgery was −7.7 units; the change from precataract surgery to postoperatively, +2.4 units—a net change of −5.3 units. The average improvement in visual acuity following cataract surgery was +5.8 Snellen lines.

ECCE alone from below. Of the six aphakic eyes with previously successful filter surgery with at least 6 months of follow-up, the average change in IOP was +27.1% (average preoperative tension: 10.5 mm Hg; average postoperative tension: 12.4 mm Hg). The average change in glaucoma medication requirements was +2.3 units. The previously successful glaucoma filtration surgery in these eyes (two trabeculectomies and four full-thickness operations) had been done an average of 48.7 months before ECCE from below. The average prefilter tension was 24.0 mm Hg, for an average net change in tension of −11.6 mm Hg (Fig. 4-8). The average improvement in visual acuity following cataract surgery was +6.0 Snellen lines.

Of the nine aphakic eyes, eight (88.9%) had early tension rises of 5 mm Hg or more, four (44.4%) of greater than 10 mm Hg, and two (22.2%) of greater than 15 mm Hg. Of the six aphakic eyes with at least 6 months of follow-up, two (33.3%) had a lasting elevation in pressure of 5 mm or greater and one (16.7%) of greater than 10 mm Hg. No lasting elevations of tension greater than 15 mm Hg were seen in this aphakic group (see Fig. 4-4).

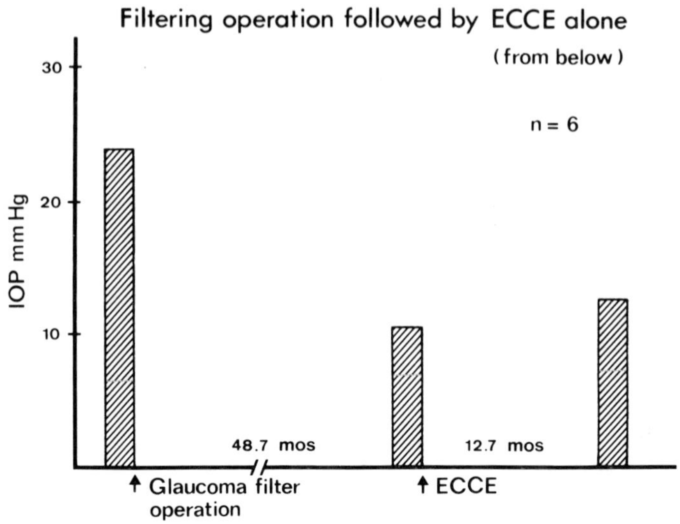

Fig. 4-8. Graph showing IOP before and after glaucoma filtration surgery and following subsequent ECCE with no lens implant.

Group D

ECCE/posterior chamber IOL/glaucoma operation. The eyes with inadequately controlled open-angle glaucoma that underwent combined ECCE and glaucoma surgery were less in number than the other groups and were thus less easily compared to them. Of the six pseudophakic eyes, one had follow-up of at least 6 months. That patient was a 73-year-old white woman who had combined ECCE/posterior chamber lens implantation/cyclodialysis (the cyclodialysis was done by internal eversion of a partial-thickness scleral flap, as advocated by Gills[18,34]). The preoperative tension was 15 mm Hg with a nearly totally cupped disc and a small central island on visual field testing. The glaucoma medication requirement preoperatively was 12 units. The postoperative tension fluctuated widely, from 0 to the middle teens until the 35th postoperative week, when it was found to be 22 mm Hg. A repeat cyclodialysis (external) was done, and 2 weeks later the tension was 9 mm Hg, with a medical requirement of 16 for a net increase in medications of 4 units.

In the other five pseudophakic eyes (four ECCE/posterior chamber lens implantation/trabeculectomy; one ECCE/posterior chamber lens implantation/external cyclodialysis), insufficient follow-up exists to make long-term comparisons. Three of these eyes had at least 8 weeks of follow-up, and none had early tension rises of 5 mm Hg or greater.

ECCE and glaucoma operation. Of the two aphakic eyes, only one had at least 6 months of follow-up. This was in a 71-year-old white woman who had combined ECCE and posterior lip sclerectomy. The preoperative tension was 22 mm Hg, and medical requirement for glaucoma control was 16 units. No view of the disc was possible, but a large Bjerrum scotoma had split fixation. Seventy-one weeks postoperatively, the IOP was 13 mm Hg and she was taking no glaucoma medications. The visual field had not progressed, and visual acuity was corrected to 20/30. No early tension rise occurred.

The other aphakic eye—in a 75-year-old white woman who had ECCE and external cyclodialysis—had shorter follow-up. No early postoperative tension rise occurred, and at 18 weeks the tension was 15 mm Hg, down from 21 mm Hg preoperatively. The visual acuity was corrected to 20/40. Glaucoma medical requirements were up from 4 to 8 units. A central island present preoperatively on visual field testing had not worsened.

Group E

ECCE with posterior chamber IOL. Of the 10 pseudophakic eyes, two had at least 6 months of follow-up. In these two the average change in IOP was −12.5% (average preoperative tension: 17.5 mm Hg; average postoperative tension: 15.5 mm Hg). Of the eight pseudophakic eyes with at least 8 weeks of follow-up, two (25%) had an early tension rise of 5 mm Hg or greater, one (12.5%) of greater than 10 mm Hg, and none of greater than 15 mm Hg. Neither of the two eyes with at least 6 months of follow-up had lasting elevations of 5 mm Hg or greater.

The average change in glaucoma medication requirements was −0.5 units, and neither patient was on glaucoma medication at the most recent postoperative visit (average: 47.5 weeks of follow-up). The average improvement in visual acuity following cataract surgery was +5.5 Snellen lines.

ECCE alone. Of the three aphakic eyes, one had at least 6 months of follow-up. This eye was that of an 81-year-old white woman whose preoperative IOP was 22 mm Hg and whose postoperative tension was 20 mm Hg (32 weeks of follow-up). Her glaucoma medication requirement had decreased from 4 to 0 units. She improved from 20/100 to 20/20. None of the aphakic eyes had early tension rises of 5 mm Hg or greater.

Group F

ECCE with posterior chamber IOL. In this control group of 117 eyes, 100 had ECCE with the implantation of a posterior chamber IOL. In the pseudophakic group, of the 42 eyes with at least 6 months of follow-up, the average change in IOP was −3.8% (average preoperative tension: 15.7 mm Hg; average postoperative tension: 15.0 mm Hg). In this group, of the 91 eyes with at least 8 weeks of follow-up, 19 (20.9%) had early tension rises of 5 mm Hg or more, nine (9.9%) of greater than 10 mm Hg, and four (4.4%) of greater than 15 mm Hg. Of the 42 eyes with at least 6 months of follow-up, three (7.2%) had a persistent tension rise of 5 mm Hg or more, and one (2.4%) of greater than 10 mm Hg. No lasting tension rises of greater than 15 mm Hg were found in this group. The average improvement in visual acuity following cataract surgery was +6.8 Snellen lines.

ECCE alone. In the control group 17 eyes had cataract extraction alone. Of the nine eyes that had at least 6 months of follow-up, the average change in IOP was −11.2% (average preoperative tension: 15.4 mm Hg; average postoperative tension: 13.7 mm Hg). Of the 13 eyes with at least 8 weeks of follow-up, four (30.8%) had early tension rises of 5 mm Hg or more, two (15.4%) of greater than 10 mm Hg, and one (7.7%) of greater than 15 mm Hg. None of the nine eyes in which there was at least 6 months of follow-up had lasting rises in tension of 5 mm Hg or greater. The average improvement in visual acuity following cataract surgery was +5.6 Snellen lines.

COMPLICATIONS

Intraoperative (Table 4-5)

ECCE, with or without posterior chamber IOL, in eyes with preexisting glaucoma. Of the 87 eyes glaucomatous eyes to have ECCE with the implantation of a posterior chamber pseudophakos, two (2.3%) had significant intraoperative hyphema, one of which was associated with a sector iridectomy. Two (2.3%) also had small central capsular holes, but there were no instances of vitreous loss.

Of the 29 glaucomatous eyes to have ECCE without the implantation of an IOL, one (3.4%) had hyphema, and in this case a sector iridectomy had been done. Two (6.9%) had small central capsular tears, and one (3.4%) had vitreous loss.

ECCE, with or without a posterior chamber IOL, in control eyes. In the 100 control eyes to have ECCE with the implantation of a posterior chamber lens, one (1%) had a central capsular tear, but there were no instances of vitreous loss. No intraoperative hyphemas were noted in these groups.

In the 17 aphakic control eyes, 2 (11.8%) had capsular tears and two (11.8%) had vitreous loss. There were no instances of hyphema. In one case a suprachoroidal hemorrhage occurred when the patient coughed following insertion of a posterior chamber lens implant. The implant was extruded, and the eye was immediately closed and sclerostomies performed. Corrected visual acuity was 20/70 12 weeks postoperatively, and the tension was 12 mm Hg.

Postoperative (Table 4-6)

Postoperative complications were noted and reported for those eyes with at least 6 months of follow-up in all groups. The number of eyes with sufficient follow-up to be considered were pseudophakic/glaucoma, 39 eyes; aphakic/glaucoma, 19 eyes; pseudophakic/control, 42 eyes; and aphakic/control, 9 eyes.

Hyphema. Postoperative hyphemas were observed in four (10.3%) of the pseudophakic/glaucoma eyes and in one (5.3%) of the aphakic/glaucoma eyes. These were not observed in any of the control eyes.

Iritis. Significant iritis was not noted in any of the pseudophakic or aphakic eyes with preexisting glaucoma. In three (7.1%) of the pseudophakic/control eyes, iritis required additional treatment, such as with intensive topical steroids. No significant episodes of iritis were noted in the aphakic/control eyes.

Transient corneal edema. Transient corneal edema was noted in none of the pseudophakic/glaucoma eyes but was seen in one (5.3%) of the aphakic/glaucoma eyes. Corneal edema that subsequently resolved was noted in two (4.8%) of the pseudophakic/control eyes and in one (11.1%) of the aphakic/control eyes.

Posterior synechiae. Posterior synechiae to the posterior capsule or intraocular lens were seen in one (2.6%) of the pseudophakic/glaucoma eyes and in one (5.3%) of the aphakic/glaucoma eyes. No posterior synechiae were observed in control eyes.

Decreased filtration bleb. In the eight pseudophakic eyes with preexisting glaucoma filtration blebs, two (25%) were observed to have less diffuse and desirable-appearing filtration blebs in the months following ECCE. This was not observed in any of the six aphakic eyes with preexisting filtration blebs.

Subsequent glaucoma operation or laser procedure for glaucoma. In two (5.1%) of the pseudophakic/glaucoma eyes, subsequent laser or operative procedures were required to adequately control glaucoma. None of the aphakic/glaucoma eyes or control eyes subsequently required glaucoma surgery.

Cystoid macular edema. Clinically significant cystoid macular edema was noted in two (5.1%) of the pseudophakic/glaucoma eyes and one (5.3%) of the aphakic/glaucoma eyes. In the control groups this edema was seen in two (4.8%) of the pseudophakic and none of the aphakic eyes.

Posterior capsule opacity. Posterior capsule opacity was noted in seven (17.9%) of the pseudophakic/glaucoma eyes and four (21.1%) of the aphakic/glaucoma eyes. In the control groups nine (21.4%) of the pseudophakic and two (22.2%) of the aphakic eyes had this complication. Nd:YAG posterior capsulotomy was performed in six (15.4%) of the pseudophakic/glaucoma eyes and one (5.3%) of the aphakic/glaucoma eyes. Cap-

Table 4-5. Intraoperative complications of ECCE

	Preexisting glaucoma		*Control eyes*	
Complication	*PC-IOL (87 eyes)*	*No IOL (29 eyes)*	*PC-IOL (100 eyes)*	*No IOL (17 eyes)*
Torn posterior capsule	2 (2.3%)	2 (6.9%)	1 (1.0%)	2 (11.8%)
Vitreous loss	0	1 (3.4%)	0	2 (11.8%)
Hyphema	2* (2.3%)	1† (3.4%)	0	0
Suprachoroidal hemorrhage	0	0	0	1 (5.9%)

*One of the two following sector iridectomy.
†Following sector iridectomy.

Table 4-6. Postoperative complications of ECCE (eyes with at least 6 months of follow-up)

	Preexisting glaucoma		*Control eyes*	
Complication	*PC-IOL (39 eyes)*	*No IOL (19 eyes)*	*PC-IOL (42 eyes)*	*No IOL (9 eyes)*
Hyphema	4 (10.3%)	1 (5.3%)	0	0
Iritis	0	0	3 (7.1%)	0
Transient corneal edema	0	1 (5.3%)	2 (4.8%)	1 (11.1%)
Posterior synechiae	1 (2.6%)	1 (5.3%)	0	0
Decreased filtration bleb	2/8 (25%)	0/6	— —	— —
Subsequent operative or laser procedure for glaucoma	2 (5.1%)	0	0	0
Cystoid macular edema	2 (5.1%)	1 (5.3%)	2 (4.8%)	0
Nd:YAG capsulotomy	6 (15.4%)	1 (5.3%)	0	1 (11.1%)
Posterior capsule opacity	7 (17.9%)	4 (21.1%)	9 (21.4%)	2 (22.2%)
Postop diagnosis of glaucoma in control eye	— —	— —	1 (2.4%)	0

sulotomy was done in none of the pseudophakic/control eyes and in one (11.1%) of the aphakic/control eyes.

Postoperative diagnosis of glaucoma in control eyes. Of the 42 pseudophakic/control eyes with at least 6 months of follow-up, only one (2.4%) required medication for IOP control. This was a 71-year-old white male whose preoperative IOP was 19.5 mm Hg; this slowly rose to 25 mm Hg 52 weeks following ECCE with posterior chamber lens implantation. Sixty-one weeks postoperatively, he was using timolol, 0.5% b.i.d., in the operated eye only for an IOP of 18. None of the aphakic/control eyes developed postoperative glaucoma.

Effect of ECCE, with and without posterior chamber IOL, on eyes with severe glaucomatous visual field loss (Table 4-7)

Preoperative scotomas with split fixation. Of the 39 pseudophakic/glaucoma eyes, five (12.8%) had preoperative arcuate scotomas splitting fixation. The postoperative visual fields were better or unchanged in all five (100%); none worsened. In the 19 aphakic/glaucoma eyes, five (26.3%) had split fixation preoperatively and all (100%) had improvement or no change in visual field status postoperatively.

Preoperative double arcuate scotomas with central islands. Two (5.1%) of the pseudophakic/glaucoma eyes had central islands preoperatively; neither worsened. Of the aphakic/glaucoma eyes, three (15.8%) had central islands preoperatively, two of which had postoperative improvement or no change in visual field status. The one that worsened was that of a 72-year-old white female who had ECCE from below 13 years after a successful filtering operation. The preoperative tension was 11 mm Hg, and the postoperative tension was 14 mm Hg 33 weeks postoperatively. The highest recorded postoperative tension was 16 mm Hg.

Table 4-7. Eyes with severe preoperative glaucomatous visual field loss following ECCE (at least 6 months of follow-up)

Field loss	*ECCE with IOL (39 eyes)*	*ECCE with no IOL (19 eyes)*
Preoperative arcuate scotoma with split fixation	5 (12.8%)	5 (26.3%)
Field better or same postoperatively	5 (100%)	5 (100%)
Field worse postoperatively	0	0
Preoperative double arcuate scotomas with central island 10 degrees or less	2 (5.1%)	3 (15.8%)
Field better or same postoperatively	2 (100%)	2 (66.6%)
Field worse postoperatively	0	1 (33.3%) (6.7% of all eyes with severe loss)

DISCUSSION

Risk of elevated IOP and glaucoma in nonglaucomatous eyes following ECCE with or without posterior chamber lens implantation

Of 117 previously nonglaucomatous eyes, only one developed postoperative elevation of pressure requiring treatment. That was in a 71-year-old man who had uncomplicated ECCE with posterior chamber lens implantation. The preoperative tension was 19.5 mm Hg, and the maximum postoperative tension was 25 mm Hg 52 weeks following surgery. The angle was open, and no excess inflammation had been noted. No other cause for increased pressure, such as peripheral anterior synechiae or steroid response, was present. The pressure in the operated eye was 18 mm Hg 61 weeks postoperatively on timolol, 0.5% b.i.d.

Therefore, the risk of open-angle glaucoma following ECCE with or without posterior chamber lens implantation in previously nonglaucomatous eyes is low. In the one instance when it did occur in this series, it was readily controlled.

Table 4-8. Eyes with preexisting glaucoma and early tension rises of ≥16 mm Hg following ECCE*

Group	*Preop tension*	*Postop tension*	*Peak tension*	*Medication change*	*Visual fields*
Group A					
Pseudophakic					
PA7	21.3	15.5	44	+1	
PA10	11	21	30	+2	Split fixation
PA11	16.7	12	42	0	Central island
PA18	24	25	48	−7	
Group B					
Pseudophakic					
PB4	12.5	12	35	0	
PB5	11.3	10	40	−3	
PB8	17.8	24.5	40	−4	
PB10	19.5	15.5	36	+2	
PB13	21	15	45	+4	
PB14	19.7	14	42	+3	
PB15	16.7	14	38	+4	
PB18	12	11	35	0	
PB22	13.5	17	48	0	
PB28	12	11	35	−2	
PB30	22	16	42	+3	
PB33	17	11	44	0	
Aphakic					
AB1	15.3	16	34	0	Split fixation
AB7	12	16	40	0	
Group C					
Pseudophakic					
PC11	8	3	25	+8	Split fixation
Aphakic					
AC4	10.8	11	29	0	Split fixation
AC9	7	8	35	0	

*All tensions in mm Hg; medication values in units as given in Table 4-2.

Risk to glaucomatous eyes of exacerbation of glaucoma following ECCE with or without posterior chamber lens implantation

Early elevations in tension following ECCE, with or without lens implantation, were much more frequent in the glaucoma groups than in the nonglaucomatous eyes (see Fig. 4-4). The elevations were usually transient.

In eyes with early pressure elevations of 16 mm Hg or greater, the peak tension averaged 39.4 mm Hg in 17 pseudophakic/glaucoma eyes and 34.5 mm Hg in four aphakic/glaucoma eyes (Table 4-8). In control eyes with similar early elevations in pressure, the peak tensions averaged 40.8 mm Hg in the four pseudophakic eyes and 33 mm Hg in one aphakic eye. Such pressure elevations represent a definite potential danger to severely damaged glaucomatous eyes and merit prompt recognition and treatment.

Groups A and B, the medical- and laser-controlled groups, represent the most commonly encountered glaucomatous eyes in clinical practice. For these groups during the early postoperative period, pressure elevations were much more frequent than in the nonglaucomatous eyes, group F. Considering these two common groups together, there was a 26% incidence of an early pressure rise greater than 15 mm Hg during the 8 weeks following surgery and an 8% incidence of a lasting elevation in pressure of 5 mm Hg or greater (Tables 4-8 and 4-9). None of the eyes in these groups required subsequent laser or surgery for glaucoma within the period of follow-up. In the entire study only two of the glaucomatous eyes did require subsequent glaucoma procedures, one laser and one operative.

Table 4-9. Eyes with preexisting glaucoma and lasting tension rises of ≥5 mm Hg following ECCE* (at least 6 months of follow-up)

Group	*Weeks of follow-up*	*Preop tension*	*Postop tension*	*Peak tension*	*Medication change*	*Visual fields*
Group A						
Pseudophakic						
PA10	53	11	21	23	+12	Split fixation
PA13	30	17.3	25	25	−2	
Group B						
Pseudophakic						
PB11	53	27.7	32	33	−2	
Group C						
Pseudophakic						
PC6	40	16.5	18	23	0	
PC8	64	14.8	20	27	+8	Split fixation†
PC12	28	7.5	16	16	+4	
Aphakic						
AC3	87	6.5	12	20.5	+4	
AC4	52	10.8	11	17	0	Split fixation
Group D						
Pseudophakic						
PD1	41	15	6	22	+7	Central island‡

*All tensions in mm Hg; medication values in units as given in Table 4-2.
†Laser trabeculoplasty (3 clock hours/session) required 54 and 63 weeks postoperatively.
‡Cyclodialysis required 39 weeks postoperatively.

Certain operative and postoperative complications such as hyphemas and posterior synechiae were found in more of the glaucomatous eyes than in the nonglaucomatous eyes. This is not surprising, since the pupils in these eyes are frequently miotic and immobile from chronic medical therapy. To adequately visualize the anterior segment structures for controlled ECCE, synechialysis, iridectomy, or sphincterotomy may be required in these difficult cases (Fig. 4-9). Such iris surgery can result in bleeding into the anterior chamber. In the nonglaucomatous eyes, which usually had easily dilated pupils, no hyphemas or posterior synechiae were noted (Fig. 4-10). It is possible that discontinuing epinephrine products and strong miotics, if possible, several days before surgery may help decrease anterior segment congestion and the likelihood of hyphema.[28,51]

Therefore, there is some risk of pressure elevation with these procedures in glaucomatous eyes. However, especially in eyes previously controlled with medications or laser therapy, postoperative IOP elevations are almost always temporary. When lasting pressure elevation does occur, it is usually manageable by increased medical therapy, by laser trabeculoplasty when it has not been previously performed, or rarely by conventional glaucoma surgery when needed.

ECCE with posterior chamber lens implantation vs. ECCE with no implantation: Does the posterior chamber implant make a difference to the risk of pressure elevation?

Whether posterior chamber lens implantation following ECCE subjects glaucomatous eyes to increased risk is a critical question. Table 4-5 shows the early and lasting pressure elevations for the eyes in the glaucomatous and nonglaucomatous groups. In nonglaucomatous eyes no statistically significant difference was found for the incidence of early elevations in IOP when comparing ECCE with lens implantation to ECCE with no implant. In addition, in the glaucomatous eyes controlled preoperatively with medications, with laser trabeculoplasty, or with filtration surgery (see Figs. 4-11 and 4-12), there was no statistically significant difference in early pressure elevation, whether a posterior chamber implant or no implant was used. The presence of the posterior chamber lens, therefore, made no difference to glaucoma control.

Risk to severely damaged glaucomatous eyes following ECCE with or without posterior chamber lens implantation

Senile macular degeneration has been an accepted indication for IOL implantation because of the distortion-free peripheral and midperipheral visual field that a pseudophakos provides. Such patients depend on these portions of the visual field for ambulation and day-to-day tasks. In the case of a patient with severe glaucomatous visual field loss, the opposite situation exists; that is, the peripheral visual field is severely affected and the central visual field is relatively spared, such as with double arcuate scotomas leaving a central island.

Following removal of the crystalline lens, as the correcting lens is moved posteriorly, progressively less image magnification occurs. Typical magnification with aphakic spectacles at a vertex distance of 12 mm is 25%, compared to 7% with a contact lens and even less with an IOL. This may be important in the case of severe glaucomatous visual field loss, since in such a patient with a small central island of vision, a fixed area of retina is capable of receiving visual stimuli. With a magnified image, such as results from aphakic spectacle correction, less information would be reflected on the

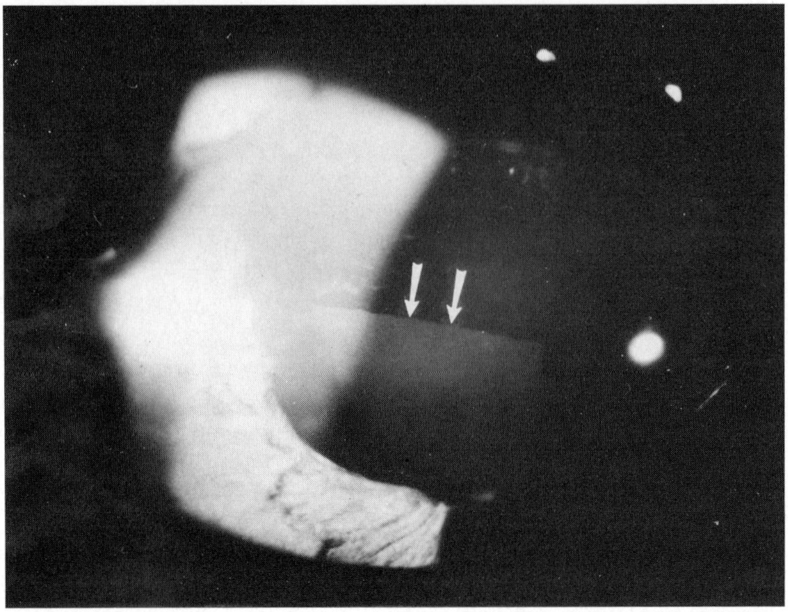

Fig. 4-9. Sector iridectomy for immobile pupil. Note hyphema *(arrows)* between the posterior capsule and posterior chamber lens implant, a rare complication. Patient required subsequent neodymium:YAG laser capsulotomy for posterior capsule opacity.

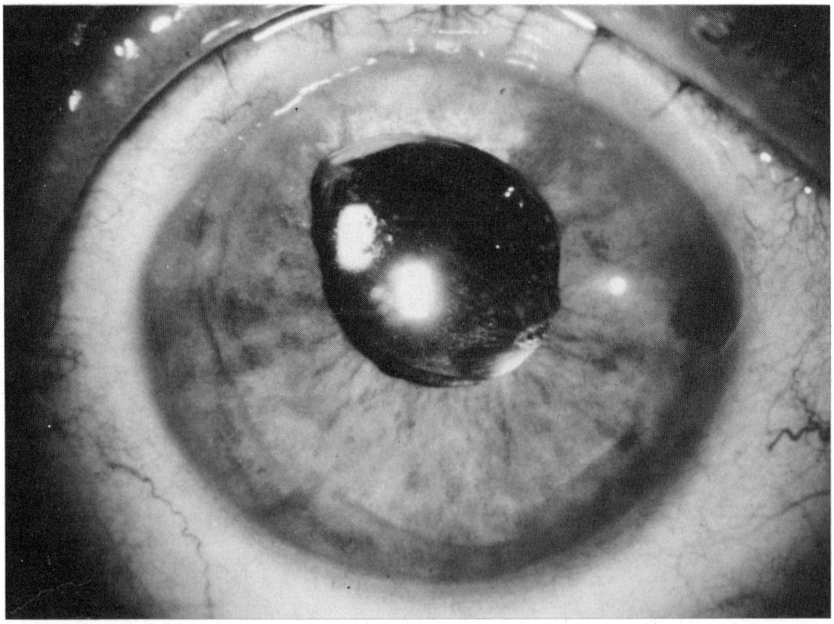

Fig. 4-10. Postoperative appearance of eye with immobile pupil preoperatively. Note iris trauma and posterior synechiae to implant, which usually can be avoided.

A

B

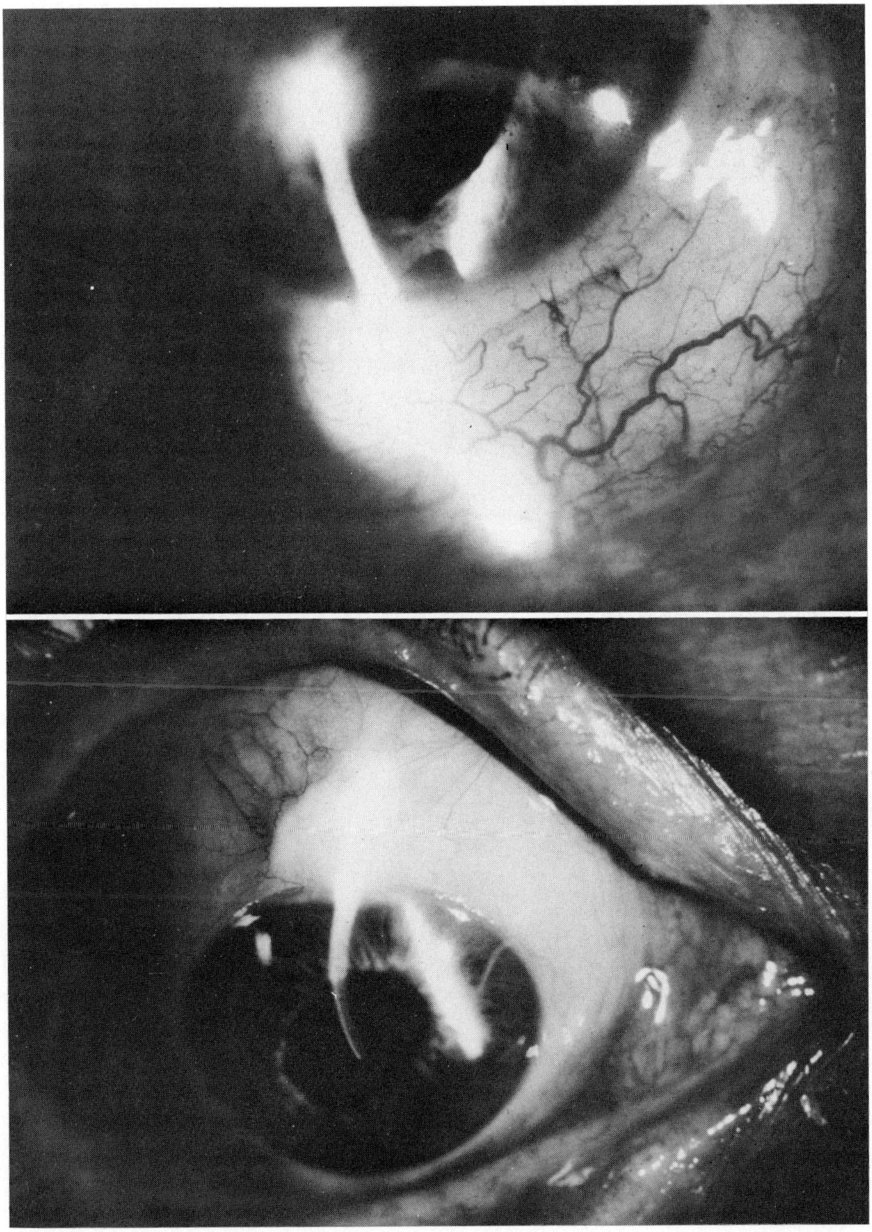

Fig. 4-11. A, Filtration bleb below following ECCE combined with trabeculectomy and posterior chamber lens implantation from below in presence of filtration above. **B,** Preservation of filtration bleb above.

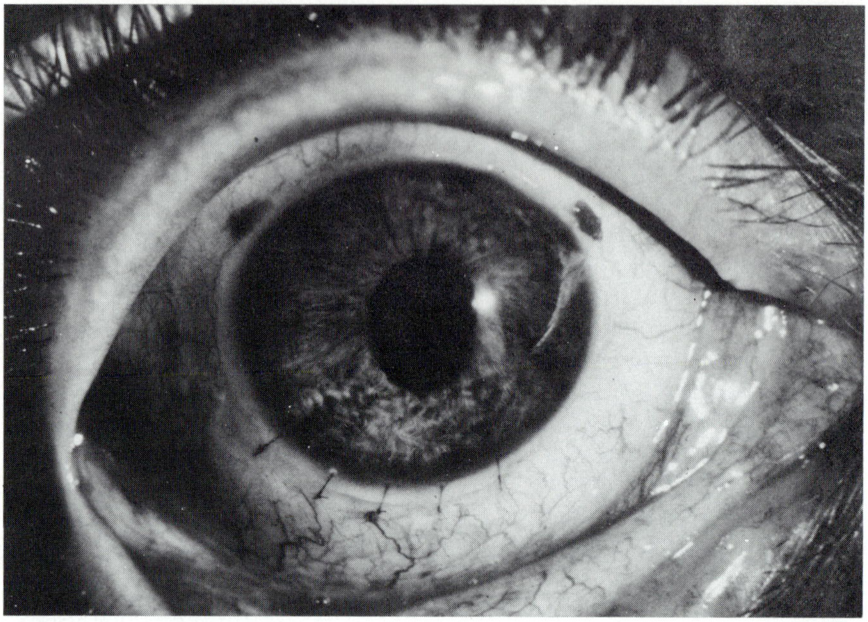

Fig. 4-12. ECCE with posterior chamber lens implantation from below. Note preservation of filtration above.

limited area of functional retina in the posterior pole. With the minimal magnification of posterior chamber pseudophakia, more of the visual panorama would fit into this retinal area. Whether this theoretic optical advantage with pseudophakia in eyes with small central visual islands is sufficient to make a difference in practical terms deserves investigation.[4,5]

Severely damaged glaucomatous eyes with split fixation or central island on visual field testing may be especially susceptible to fluctuations in pressure, and the early elevations shown in the graphs could conceivably contribute to loss of fixation and precipitous decrease in acuity.[1,9,19] In Kolker's series 21 of 23 such eyes had ICCE, and 8.7% lost central island fixation during the immediate postoperative period.[28] Of the 15 similarly damaged eyes in our series, none lost fixation (see Table 4-8), but one (6.7%) did go from a preoperative central island to split fixation—the 70-year-old white woman who had undergone a successful full-thickness glaucoma filtration operation 13 years before ECCE from below without IOL implantation. She had also had argon laser trabeculoplasty 3 months before cataract surgery. Preoperative tension was 11 mm Hg, and the maximum postoperative tension was 16 mm Hg; 33 weeks postoperatively her tension was 14 mm Hg. A tiny central island that was present preoperatively has progressed to split fixation. Her macula appears to be normal.

Meticulous attention for prompt recognition and treatment of postoperative pressure elevations may minimize the problem of visual field progression in these damaged and vulnerable eyes. In the present series of 15 severely damaged eyes with central islands or split fixation, 6.7% had postoperative visual field progression following ECCE extraction with or without posterior chamber lens implantation, a result that compares favorably with ICCE.[28]

SUMMARY

We have examined the preoperative status, results, and complications in 233 eyes having ECCE with or without the implantation of a posterior chamber IOL. One hundred and sixteen eyes with preexisting glaucoma of varying severity were compared with 117 nonglaucomatous eyes having this surgery. The results show that the major risk is elevation of IOP, usually transient, in glaucomatous eyes having ECCE. This risk was not enhanced with the implantation of a posterior chamber IOL. The elevation of IOP was successfully managed with a temporary increase in medical therapy in almost all cases, but one eye required laser therapy and one required subsequent glaucoma surgery. We have presented several theoretic and practical advantages of ECCE and posterior chamber lens implantation in glaucomatous eyes compared to other methods of cataract surgery.

REFERENCES

1. Abedin, S., Simmons, R.J., and Grant, W.M.: Progressive low-tension glaucoma: treatment to stop glaucomatous cupping and field loss when these progress despite normal intraocular pressure, Ophthalmology **89:**1, 1982.
2. Arnott, E.J.: Consideration for lens implantation in patients with glaucoma, Glaucoma **4:**56, 1982.
3. Bigger, J.F., and Becker, B.: The effect of uncomplicated cataract extraction on glaucoma control, Trans. Am. Acad. Ophthalmol. **75:**260, 1971.
4. Binkhorst, R.: Personal communication.
5. Boeder, P.: Personal communication.
6. Bresnick, G.H.: Eyes containing anterior chamber acrylic implants, Arch. Ophthalmol. **82:**726, 1969.
7. Byron, H.M.: Anterior segment complications of implant surgery, Ophthalmology **86:**621, 1979.
8. Campbell, D.G., and Grant, W.M.: Trabecular deformation and reduction of outflow facility due to cataract and penetrating keratoplasty sutures, Invest. Ophthalmol. **16:**126, 1977.
9. Chandler, P.A., Grant, W.M., editors: Glaucoma, Philadelphia, 1979, Lea & Febiger.
10. Clayman, H.M., and others: Lens implantation, miosis, and glaucoma, Am. J. Ophthalmol. **87:**121, 1979.
11. Cohan, B.E., and others: Broken nylon iris fixation sutures, Am. J. Ophthalmol. **88**982, 1979.
12. Crawford, J.B.: A histopathologic study of the position of the Shearing intraocular lens in the posterior chamber, Am. J. Ophthalmol. **91:**458, 1981.
13. Drews, R.C.: Case selection in the use of intraocular lenses, Int. Ophthalmol. Clin. **19:**33, 1979.
14. Drews, R.C.: Lens implantation in patients with glaucoma, Ophthalmology **87:**665, 1980.
15. Galin, M.A., and others: Cataract surgery and intraocular pressure, Trans. Ophthalmol. Soc. U.K. **98:**124, 1978.
16. Galin, M.A., and others: Cataract extraction in glaucoma, Am. J. Ophthalmol. **87:**124, 1979.
17. Galin, M.A., and others: Experimental cataract surgery-electron microscopy, Ophthalmology **86:**608, 1979.
18. Gills, J.P.: Personal communication.
19. Haik, K.G.: Personal communication.
20. Herschler, J.: Editorial: glaucoma and the intraocular lens, Ann. Ophthalmol., July 1979, p. 1057.
21. Jaffe, N.S.: Symposium: IOLs . . . . indications and contraindications, Trans. Am. Acad. Ophthalmol. **81:**93, 1976.
22. Jaffe, N.S.: Suggested guidelines for intraocular lens implant surgery, Arch. Ophthalmol. **94:**214, 1976.
23. Jaffe, N.S.: Changing guidelines for intraocular lens implantation: an opinion, Glaucoma **9:**309, 1983.
24. Jaffe, N.S.: The way things were and are: changing indications for IOL implantation, Ophthalmology **90:**318, 1983.
25. Johns, G.E., and Layden, W.E.: Combined trabeculectomy and cataract extraction, Am. J. Ophthalmol. **88:**973, 1979.
26. Kass, M.A.: Cataract extraction in an eye with a filtering bleb, Ophthalmology **89:**871, 1982.
27. Keates, R.H., and Ehrlich, D.R.: "Lenses of chance"—complications of anterior chamber implants, Trans. Am. Acad. Ophthalmol. **85:**408, 1978.
28. Kolker, A.E.: Visual prognosis in advanced glaucoma: a comparison of medical and surgical therapy for retention of vision in 101 eyes with advanced glaucoma, Trans. Am. Ophthalmol. Soc. **75:**539, 1977.

29. Kratz, R.P.: Intracapsular versus extracapsular cataract extraction for intraocular lens implantation, Int. Ophthalmol. Clin. **19:**179, 1979.
30. Kratz, R.P.: Complications associated with posterior chamber lenses, Ophthalmology **86:**659, 1979.
31. Layden, W.E.: Pseudophakia and glaucoma, Ophthalmology **89:**875, 1982.
32. Linn, J.G.: Cataract extraction in management of glaucoma, Trans. Am. Acad. Ophthalmol. **75:**273, 1971.
33. McDonnell, P.J., and others: Pathology of IOLs in 33 eyes examined post mortem, Ophthalmology **90:**386, 1983.
34. Montgomery, D., and Gills, J.P.: Extracapsular cataract extraction, lens implantation and cyclodialysis, Ophthalmic Surg. **11:**343, 1980.
35. Obstbaum, S.A., and Galin M.A.: Glaucoma, cataract surgery and the intraocular lens, Int. Ophthalmol. Clin. **19:**139, 1979.
36. Podolsky, M.M., and Ritch, R.: Secondary glaucoma in aphakia. In Ritch, R., and Shields, M.B., editors: The secondary glaucomas, St. Louis, 1982, The C.V. Mosby Co.
37. Polack, F.M.: Management of anterior segment complications of intraocular lenses, Ophthalmology **87:**881, 1980.
38. Rich, W.J., and others: Early ocular hypertension after cataract extraction, Br. J. Ophthalmol. **58:**725, 1974.
39. Rowsey, J.J., and Gaylor, J.R.: Intraocular lens disasters: peripheral anterior synechiae, Ophthalmology **87:**646, 1980.
40. Savage, J.A., and Simmons, R.J.: Coaxial radiofrequency diathermy in anterior segment surgery. Submitted for publication.
41. Shaffer, R.N., and Rosenthal, G.: Comparison of cataract incidence in normal and glaucomatous population, Am. J. Ophthalmol. **69:**368, 1970.
42. Shields, M.B.: Combined cataract extraction and glaucoma surgery, Ophthalmology **89:**231, 1982.
43. Simmons, R.J.: Primary open angle glaucoma and cataract. In Chandler, P.A., and Grant, W.M., editors: Glaucoma, Philadelphia, 1979, Lea & Febiger.
44. Simmons, R.J., Thomas, J.V., and Singh, O.S.: Glaucoma surgical options with coexisting cataract and glaucoma. In New Orleans Academy of Ophthalmology: Symposium or glaucoma, St. Louis, 1981, The C.V. Mosby Co.
45. Simmons, R.J., and others: Surgical indications and options in the management of coexisting glaucoma and cataract, Glaucoma **4:**92, 1982.
46. Smith, J.A.: Editorial: glaucoma and the intraocular lens, Ann. Ophthalmol. **11:**1853, 1979.
47. Smith, J.A., and Anderson, D.R.: Effect of the intraocular lens on intraocular pressure, Arch. Ophthalmol. **94:**1291, 1976.
48. Spaeth, G.E.: The management of patients with conjoint cataract and glaucoma, Ophthalmic Surg. **11:**780, 1980.
49. Sugar, H.S.: Postoperative cataract in successfully filtering glaucomatous eyes, Am. J. Ophthalmol. **69:**740, 1970.
50. Taylor, D.M., and others: Intraocular lenses: 500 consecutive intracapsular cataract extractions with lens implantation compared with 500 intracapsular extractions—observations and comments, Ophthalmic Surg. **9:**29, 1978.
51. Van Buskirk, E.M.: Hazards of medical glaucoma therapy in the cataract patient, Ophthalmology **89:**238, 1982.

5

Current applications of the dye laser*

Francis A. L'Esperance, Jr.

To produce wavelengths of sufficient power for both photocoagulation and photodynamic (photoradiation) therapy, using wavelengths throughout the visible spectrum, a high-powered argon laser is required to "pump" the dye laser into full continuous-wave (CW) operation. Quasi-CW frequency-doubled neodymium:YAG lasers, excimer lasers, frequency-doubled ion lasers, and other lasers producing emissions in the short wavelength portion of the visible and ultraviolet spectrum can also be effectively used to produce operation throughout the visible spectrum with a dye laser, usually in a pulsed mode. The dye laser can function as an instrument for the treatment of all ocular lesions directly or as a catalyst for photodynamic therapy with certain photosensitizing substances (Fig. 5-1).

Basically the organic liquid dye is squirted across the path of a high-powered argon laser or similar pumping laser beam at a pressure of 40 to 50 psi (Fig. 5-2). This jet of organic liquid dye absorbs predominantly the green portion of the argon laser beam, which produces population inversion with most molecules in the excited state. As is typical with other laser systems, spontaneous and stimulated photons are produced, some of which strike a nearby mirror, which are then reflected by a perpendicular mirror at the end of the laser cavity. This cascading of photons eventually produces laser action and emission through the partially reflectant mirror (Fig. 5-3). The output beam of the laser is equal to approximately 25% to 30% of the power of the pumping argon laser beam, and the wavelength can be selected or "tuned" very accurately with a birefringent mirror (Fig. 5-4), which rotates slightly with a micrometer setting in a way that allows only photons of a certain wavelength to resonate within the laser cavity. Therefore, a typical liquid dye laser can produce laser emissions from the yellow portion of the spectrum throughout the deep-red portion of the spectrum with one dye, such as MD-631, or from the pea-green portion of the spectrum throughout the medium-red part of the visible spectrum with a dye such as Rhodamine 6G according to the output curves noted (Fig. 5-5). Each dye produces a strong power at a certain wavelength; the use of a particular dye must be considered with regard to the wavelength required for the particular ocular procedure.

Using a dual beam splitter system constructed in conjunction with Coherent Medical Group, Inc., the plane-polarized dye laser beam passes through a polarizing filter, a

---

*This chapter contains slightly modified sections from L'Esperance, F.A., Jr.: Ophthalmic lasers: Photocoagulation, Photoradiation, and Surgery, ed. 2, St. Louis, 1983, The C.V. Mosby Co.

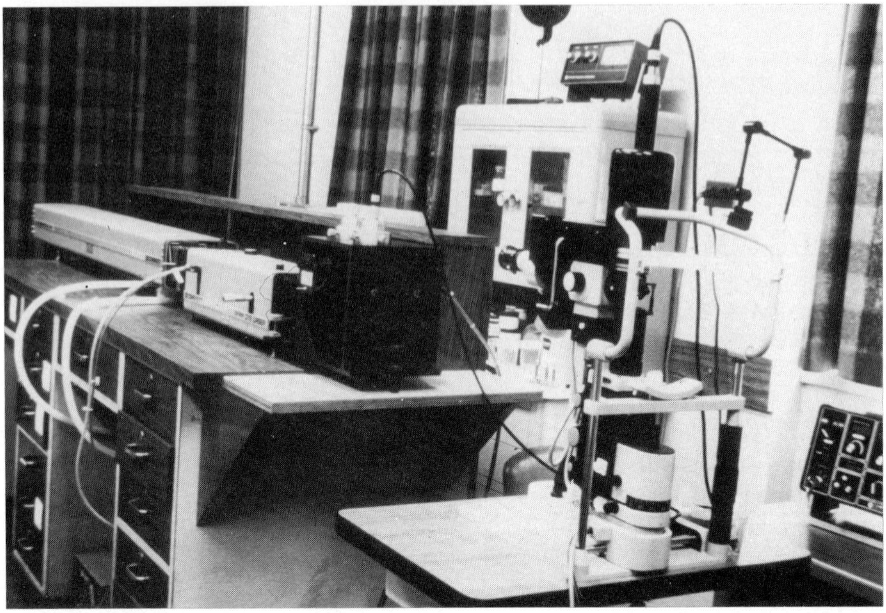

Fig. 5-1. Overall view of organic dye laser system showing pumping argon laser *(left)*, dye laser component *(center)*, and dual beam splitter apparatus *(right)*.

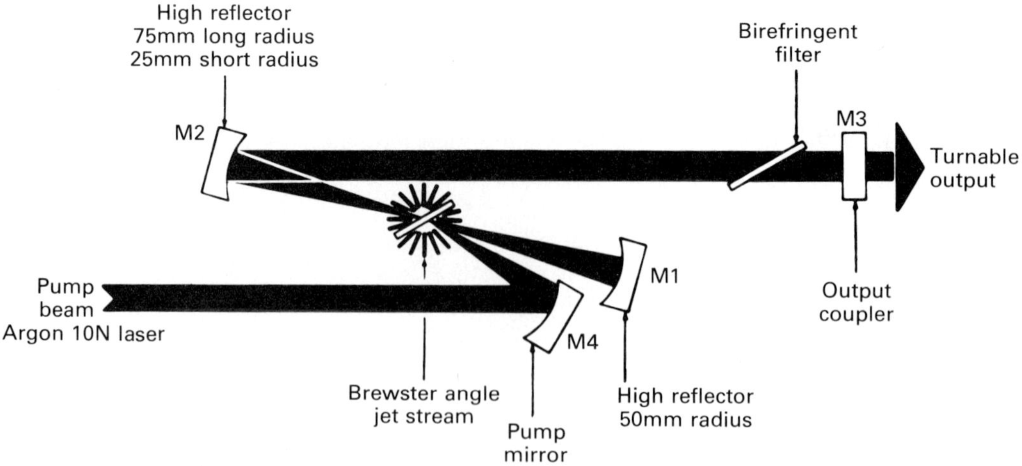

Fig. 5-2. Structural diagram of CW organic dye laser showing pumping argon ion laser beam *(lower left)* striking mirror 4, which impacts liquid dye jet stream, causing population inversion of organic dye molecules and laser action between mirrors 1 and 3.

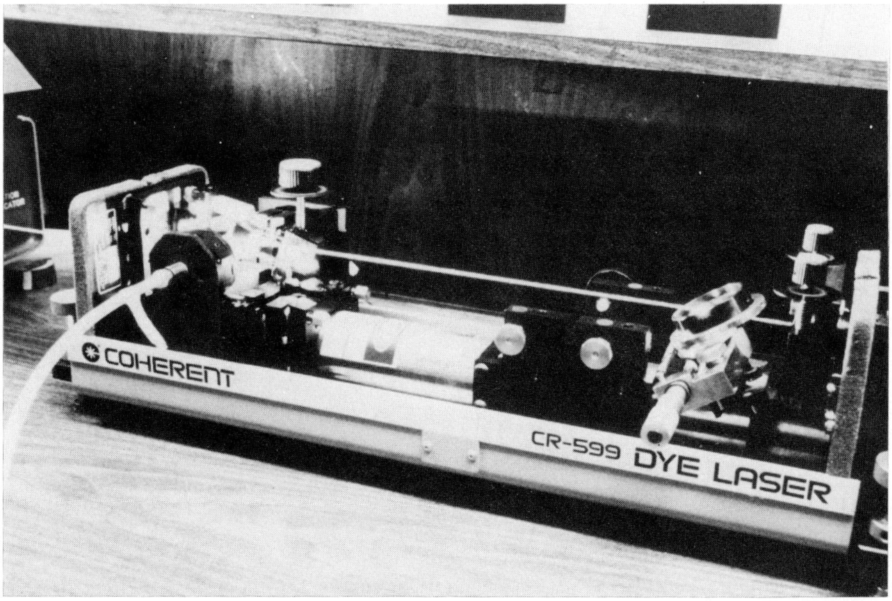

Fig. 5-3. Dye laser component showing pumping beam from argon laser *(far left)*, hose connecting organic dye pump with jet nozzle, mirror assemblies *(left)*, and birefringent filter *(right)*, which produces tunable laser action throughout the visible spectrum.

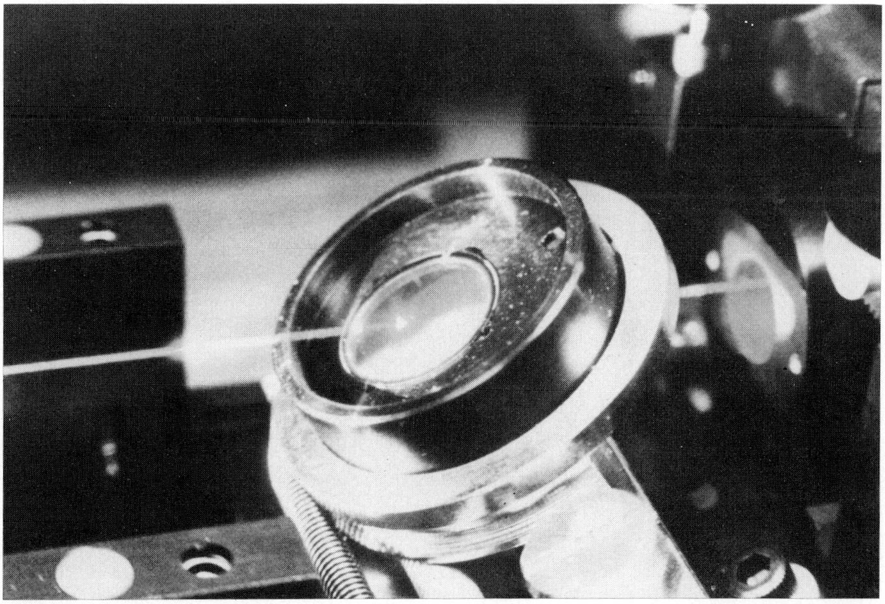

Fig. 5-4. Birefringent mirror. When tilted slightly by micrometer set screw, it selects wavelength for laser action and output.

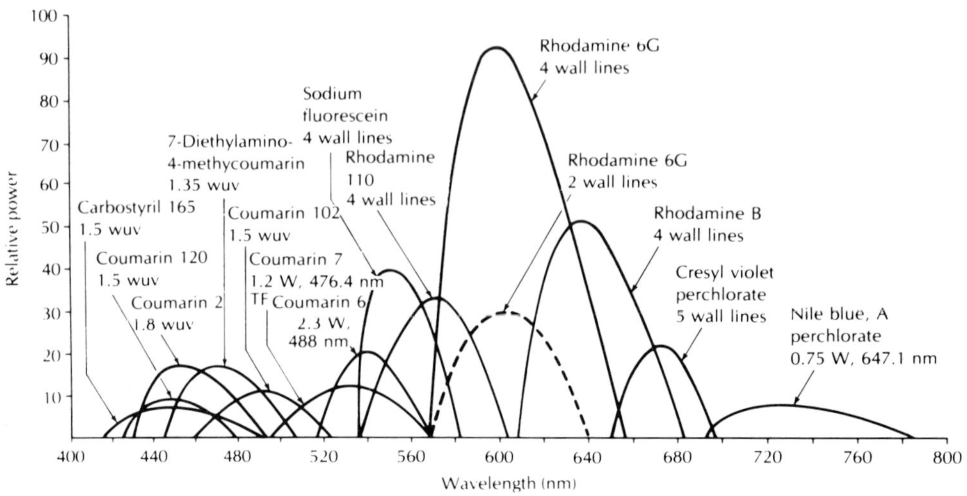

Fig. 5-5. Multiplicity of wavelenths, colors, and their relative powers that can be obtained from dye laser by using different dyes and concentrations in dye laser system.

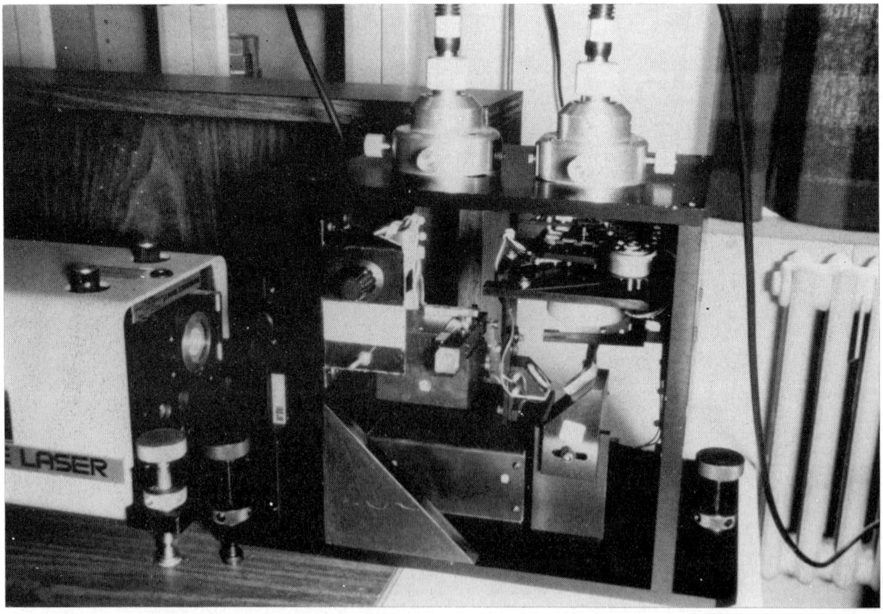

Fig. 5-6. Dual beam splitter mount. By varying the polarization of output laser beam, it can vary the percentage of laser beam directed to each fiberoptic cable between 0% and 100%.

beam splitter that is also polarized, and a power-sensing device and then strikes a totally reflecting mirror that angles the beam at 90 degrees to one of the fiberoptic ports (Fig. 5-6). A similar fiberoptic port is positioned directly above the beam splitter. With this combination of optical elements, the polarization of the dye laser beam can be rotated in such a manner that 0% to 100% of the beam will be reflected from the beam splitter to the first fiberoptic cable, and the rest transmitted to the second mirror and fiberoptic cable. In this manner any ratio of power can be obtained between the first and second fiberoptic delivery system. The dual fiberoptic cable system is used for photodynamic therapy, with 75% to 80% of the beam transmitted to the transscleral probe and 20% to 25% of the power transmitted to the transpupillary probe (Fig. 5-7). When photocoagulation is used with the dye laser, 100% of the beam is conducted to the photocoagulation slitlamp through either one of the fiberoptic cables. With this system, devised for us by Coherent Medical Group, Inc., any wavelength from the blue end to the deep-red portion of the spectrum can be selected within 1 minute, and the appropriate power distribution between the fiberoptic cables (for photodynamic therapy) or full power through a single fiberoptic cable (for photocoagulation therapy) can be adjusted within several seconds. Thus, even with this prototype dye system, the selection of wavelengths and power distribution to the fiberoptic cables can be quickly and accurately determined with photocoagulation powers approaching 1.5 W at most wavelengths in the visible spectrum.

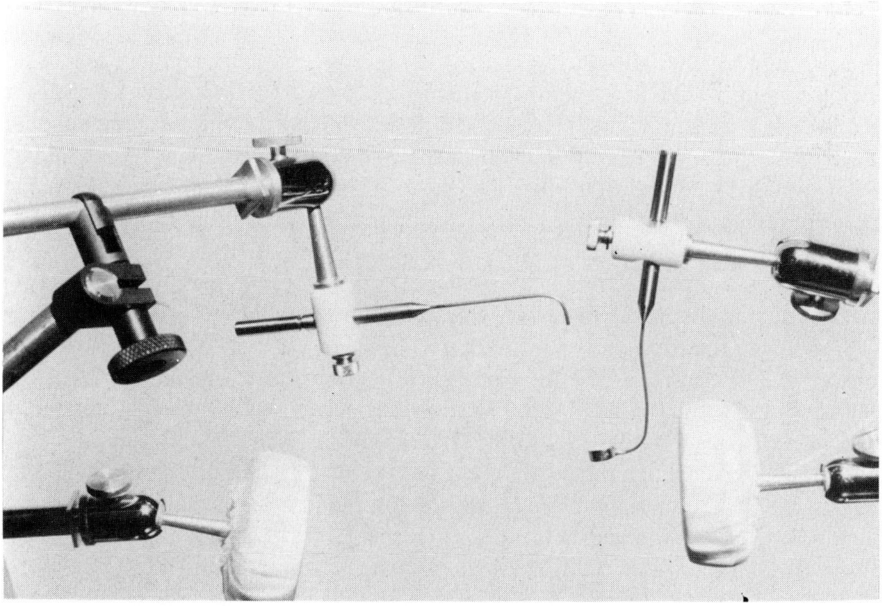

Fig. 5-7. Stereotactic mechanism and head stabilization mounts. These ensure accurate positioning of the transpupillary *(left)* and the transscleral *(right)* fiberoptic probes, which deliver laser energy to eye during photodynamic therapy.

PHOTODYNAMIC THERAPY

The term *photodynamic* (or *photoradiation*) *therapy,* in the context of this review by Dougherty and others,[10] describes the use of photosensitizing drugs to treat malignant tumors. A photosensitizer may be considered as a material capable of causing light-induced reactions in molecules that do not absorb the light. Phototherapy, photochemotherapy, and photodynamic therapy have all been used to describe the same procedure, but some of these terms have been used in a broader context to describe any therapy using light, sometimes with a drug and sometimes without; for example, phototherapy in the treatment of hyperbilirubinemia. Without attempting to judge the merits of any of these terms to refer to photosensitization as a treatment of malignant disease, the term *photodynamic therapy (PDT)* will be used exclusively for this purpose, since its meaning is unequivocal.

An ideal photosensitizer for treatment of malignant disease would (1) have no systemic toxicity, (2) be taken up and retained only by malignant tissue, and (3) absorb and be efficient in destroying malignant tissue at wavelengths not absorbed by normal tissue. Currently no such ideal photosensitizer is known. Until one is found, work progresses with certain photosensitizing drugs that approach the ideal closely enough to have therapeutic benefit in certain situations. Although no photosensitizer presently known can be taken up or retained only by malignant tissue, researchers claim several potentially useful photosensitizers possess such a tumor-specific characteristic: berberine sulfate,[23] fluorescein,[25] eosin,[28] tetracycline,[27] acridine orange,[31] and several porphyrins.[1,13,18,26,29] Among this group the porphyrins have been most extensively investigated.

Policard[26] first noted in 1924 that some human and animal tumors fluoresced on illumination with a Wood's lamp. The red fluorescence was attributed to endogenous porphyrins arising from secondary infection by hemolytic bacteria. In 1942 Auler and Banzer[1] noted characteristic red porphyrin fluorescence in rat tumors but not in normal tissues following systemic injections of hematoporphyrin, a nonmetallic porphyrin derived from hemoglobin. Figge, Weiland, and Manganiello[13] demonstrated the generality of this apparent tumor-localization characteristic of hematoporphyrin by examining various types of induced and transplanted tumors in mice. They found porphyrin fluorescence in several types of sarcomas and carcinomas, as well as in lymph nodes, traumatized tissues, and embryonic tissues. In 1960 Lipson[18] introduced hematoporphyrin derivative (Hpd), a material prepared by an acetic acid–sulfuric acid treatment of hematoporphyrin, according to Schwartz.[29] Hpd was shown to have a tumor-localizing property superior to that of hematoporphyrin.[18,20]

Fluorescence in human tumors as a result of systemically injected Hpd was demonstrated first in 1961 by Lipson in nine cases of bronchial and esophageal tumors[19] (Fig. 5-8). In a subsequent study by Lipson, Baldes, and Olsen[21] of 50 patients with suspected bronchogenic tumors, an 80% correlation of tumor fluorescence with biopsy-confirmed malignancy was found (Fig. 5-9). Lipson and others[22] also demonstrated Hpd fluorescence in cervical lesions. In a large study of Hpd localization reported in 1968, Gregorie and others[16] evaluated 226 patients with suspected squamous cell carcinoma or adenocarcinoma and found a 77% correlation of fluorescence with biopsy-confirmed malignancy for squamous lesions and an 84% correlation for adenocarcinomas. There were 23% false negatives for squamous cell and 16% for adenocarcinoma tumors. Except for fluorescence in traumatized tissues, embryonic tissues, and lymph nodes, all investigators indicated that normal tissues did not demonstrate fluorescence as a result of hematoporphyrin or Hpd. However, in 1979 Gomer and Dougherty[14] showed that following intraperitoneal injection of C-Hpd[15] or H-Hpd[3] in mice, distribution at 3 hours was as follows: liver-kidney > spleen > lung > transplanted mammary tumor > skin > muscle. At 24 hours a similar distribution was found, except that Hpd in the lung was lower than that in the tumor.

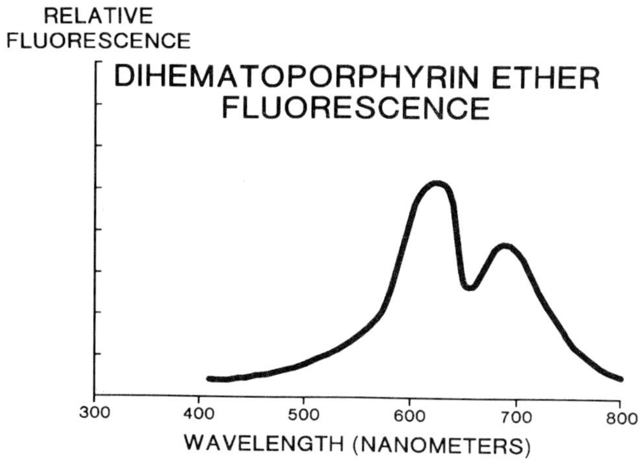

Fig. 5-8. Fluorescence curve of dihematoporphyrin ether (DHE) in solution, showing the peak fluorescences at 630 and 690 nm. (Courtesy T.J. Dougherty, Ph.D.)

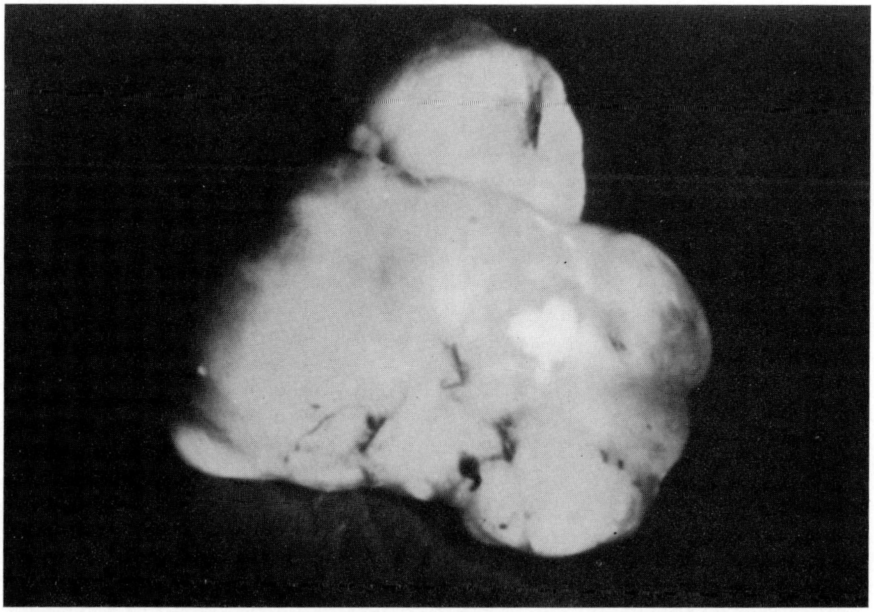

Fig. 5-9. Neurogenic sarcoma irradiated with deep-blue light, which creates bright-red fluorescence of Hpd-impregnated tumor mass. (Courtesy T.J. Dougherty, Ph.D.)

Having obtained a therapeutically useful level of a photosensitizer in a tumor, it is desirable to activate it using wavelengths not absorbed by tissue, but only by the photosensitizing drug itself (Fig. 5-10). However, since some tissue components—for example, melanin, hemoglobin, and oxyhemoglobin[11]—absorb throughout the entire visible spectrum, this requirement is not completely attainable, although it is approachable in some tissues. Visible wavelengths greater than 600 nm are least absorbed by skin and other tissue components and would be least attenuated if light were applied through the skin or other tissues to treat lesions. In this regard the porphyrins discussed earlier are again most useful, since nonmetallic porphyrins demonstrate weak absorption in red wavelengths (600 to 700 nm). Dougherty and others[8] measured the percent transmission of light from a helium-neon laser (632.8 nm) through an excised rat tumor. They found that approximately 10% of directly transmitted light reached 1 cm and approximately 30% of transmitted plus reflected light reached this distance. It should be noted that no skin or circulating blood was involved in these measurements. Measurements of this type are complicated by the large scattering component of the tissues and, aside from this rather crude measurement, no data relating to light dosimetry in tissue other than skin[12] are available.

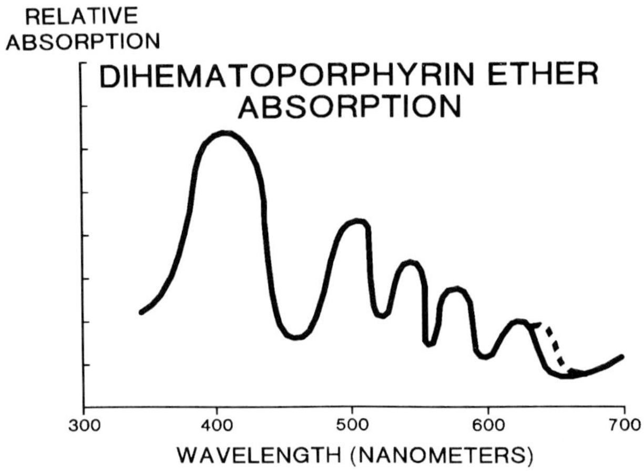

Fig. 5-10. Specific absorption spectrum of DHE, the active component of Hpd in solution. Note that in tissue peak absorption in red portion of spectrum shifts from 620 to 630 nm. (Courtesy T.J. Dougherty, Ph.D.)

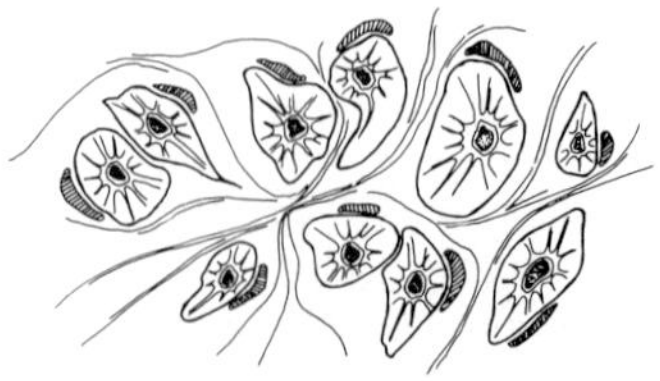

Fig. 5-11. Schematic drawing showing Hpd molecules close to the malignant melanoma cells in the neoplasm soon after intravenous injection.

TREATMENT OF TUMORS WITH PHOTOSENSITIZERS

The first attempt to use photosensitization to treat cancer was reported in 1903, when Tappenier and Jesionek[30] used topical eosin and sunlight to treat skin tumors. Although they noted some regression of the lesions, there were no further reports from this group. It was not until the early 1970s that interest in such therapy was revived. Diamond and others[3] in 1972 and Granelli and others[15] in 1975 reported that hematoporphyrin, injected systemically into rats bearing subcutaneously transplanted glioma tumors, caused extensive tumor necrosis when the lesion was exposed to white light. Neither the light nor the porphyrin had an effect alone. In 1973 and 1974 Dougherty[4,5] found that fluorescein and green light (488 nm) retarded the growth of subcutaneously implanted mammary tumors in mice. In 1974 Tomson, Emmett, and Fox[31] reported that acridine orange, given orally to mice with epithelial tumors, sensitized such tumors to light from an argon laser. Complete eradication of experimental tumors was first noted in 1975, when Dougherty and others[7] reported that Hpd in conjunction with locally applied red light, delivered 1 day after the drug, prevented recurrences for at least 90 days in about half of the mice with subcutaneous mammary tumors.[7]

Researchers at Roswell Park Memorial Institute have been studying the generally metastatic response of various malignant tumors in human beings to PDT, using Hpd as the photosensitizing drug (Fig. 5-11); first reports appeared in 1978 and 1979.[8,9] The initial study was designed primarily to assess toxicity and tumor response. Most patients had extensive, distant disease not treated by PDT and progressing disease following one or several conventional modalities such as surgery, radiotherapy, and chemotherapy.

Aside from skin toxicity caused by overtreatment with the therapeutic light, all patients in this study were ultrasensitive to bright light, especially sunlight, both outside and inside. They were cautioned to remain out of bright sunlight for at least 30 days and to then start exposure cautiously. Those who did not do so experienced mild to severe edema to exposed areas, and one patient also had slight sloughing of skin on the face. In this context a difference among patients in drug retention in skin is evident. Some patients experienced no difficulty in the sun 30 days after receiving the drug, whereas a few continued to experience difficulty for several months. Hepatic function appeared normal in all cases.

Besides this phototoxicity, patients treated by PDT with very extensive disease may experience mild to severe pain, usually controllable and of short duration, although in some cases discomfort may last several weeks. In addition, such patients may experience toxicity resulting from necrotizing tissue, such as spiking fever and infection.

MODE OF ACTION

Since Hpd is currently the only photosensitizer known to be effective against malignant tumors (besides methoxsalen), consideration of the mechanism is limited to this particular porphyrin. At this early stage in Hpd use that specific molecular mechanisms are largely unknown; however, information on certain aspects of its mode of action is available. The overall aspects are rather complicated and relate to the pharmacokinetics of the drug itself, the various chemical events elicited when the drug is photoactivated in tissue, and the biologic response of various tissues to these event (Figs. 5-12 and 5-13). Recently the active component of Hpd, dihematoporphyrin ether (DHE), was isolated and found to comprise about 45% of the Hpd substance.[6] Undoubtedly more potent action and less systemic toxicity and side effects will result from this purification process.

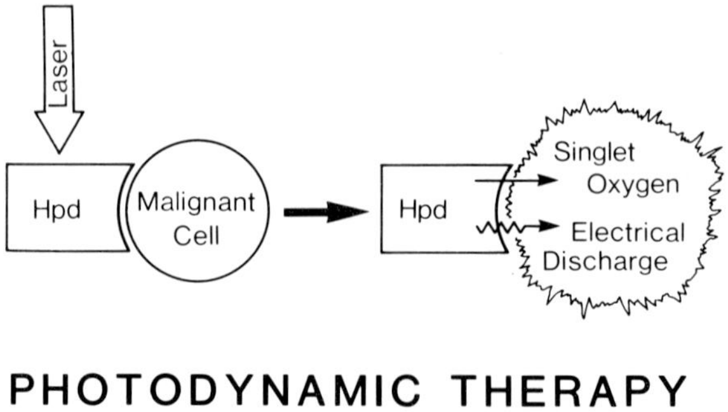

Fig. 5-12. Schematic drawing showing Hpd, containing active component DHE, closely attached to malignant cell following intravenous injection. Immediately on impact with photon at one of peak absorption wavelengths, Hpd releases singlet oxygen and probably an electric discharge that is cytotoxic to nearby malignant cells.

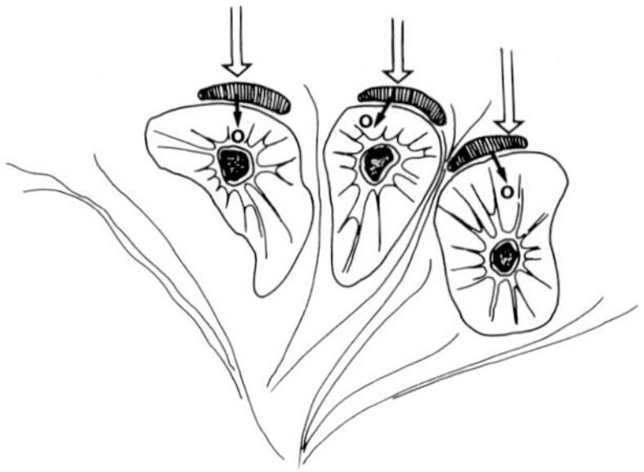

Fig. 5-13. Schematic drawing showing release of singlet oxygen by Hpd molecule to nearby malignant cells, causing their death.

When mouse tumors containing Hpd are exposed to light (600 to 700 nm), a series of changes can be seen starting immediately after exposure. The earliest changes detected histologically are around the tumor vessels, where the porphyrin level is highest, and consist of coagulation of red cells within the vessels and death of cells nearest the vessels. Tumor cells remote from the vessels, although not grossly damaged at this time, appear to be less well packed. Electron micrographs demonstrate that some tumor cells closest to the vessels have become devoid of cytoplasmic contents, which can be seen leaking into the interstitial fluid.[2] However, at this time the endothelial cells appear intact. By 3 hours after treatment the entire tumor shows gross hemorrhage and massive destruction of tumor cells.

The apparent cytotoxic agent responsible for cellular destruction is singlet oxygen by energy transfer from the excited porphyrin:

$$P + h\nu \rightarrow P^*(S)$$
$$P^*(S) \rightarrow P^*(T)$$
$$O_2 + P^*(T) \rightarrow P + {}^1O_2^*$$
$${}^1O_2^* \rightarrow O_2$$
$${}^1O_2^* + T \rightarrow T(O_2)$$

in which *P* is porphyrin; *P*(S)* and *P*(T)* are excited porphyrin singlet and triplet states, respectively; $^1O_2^*$ is singlet oxygen; *T* is cellular target; and $T(O_2)$ indicates oxidized target. Evidence for this mechanism is the protection from light of cells in culture containing both *Hpd* and isobenzofuran, an effective singlet oxygen trap.[32] However, this material may also be capable of trapping free radicals. In addition, Moan, Pettersen, and Christensen[24] have demonstrated an enhanced cytotoxic effect of photoactivated hematoporphyrin when D_2O is substituted for H_2O in the media of cultured cells, an effect frequently considered to be proof of singlet oxygen involvement. A similar experiment has not yet been reported for Hpd. Further, removal of oxygen from the atmosphere over cell cultures prevents destruction caused by Hpd and light combined, and clamping off blood flow in the legs of mice with leg tumors before and during illumination prevents tumor response resulting from the Hpd-light combination. It seems likely that formation of singlet oxygen is just the start of a long chain of events, probably including many oxygen radicals, leading to cell destruction.

OPHTHALMIC TUMOR APPLICATION

Instrumentation

A light source offering certain unique ophthalmic advantages is a dye laser operating at a wavelength of 630 ± 5 nm. Using a 12 W argon laser to pump the dye laser, approximately 2 W of red laser light can be obtained from the dye laser. The 12 W argon laser was used to pump the dye laser (Coherent Medical Group, Inc.; Model 59901), using MD-631 dye. The output beam from the dye laser was coupled to a single 200 μ quartz fiberoptic cable by means of a specially designed beam splitter mount mentioned previously. Coupling efficiencies of nearly 80% could be achieved over any desirable length of fiber (usually 10 to 40 feet). In most cases two fibers were coupled to the laser beam by passing the laser beam through a 75:25 beam splitter, producing two beams that were distributed to the transscleral and transpupillary probes, respectively (Fig. 5-14). Overall losses in the system were 20% to 30% from the laser to the fiberoptic delivery probes.

Patient selection

At present we have had the opportunity to treat four patients with choroidal malignant melanomas of the posterior pole.

Patient 1

The first patient was found to have a 6 × 8 disc diameter (DD) malignant melanoma of the posterior pole elevated approximately 4 mm into the vitreous body, as determined by ultrasonographic measurement (Fig. 5-15, *A* and *B*). The choroidal melanoma occupied the macular region and the zone temporal to the macula, but was in a position that could be irradiated clearly, with excellent visualization through a clear, refractive medium.

Since this patient was the first to undergo the combined Hpd-dye laser therapy for an intraocular or extraocular malignancy, we proceeded with great caution with the team at Roswell Park Memorial Institute.[17] After an initial intravenous Hpd injection of 1.5 mg/kg of body weight, we waited 3 days for Hpd washout from the normal tissue. We then proceeded with Rhodamine B dye laser (red) PDT for 10 minutes at a power density of 50 mW/cm^2, both directly through the pupillary space onto the anterior surface of the paramacular tumor and through fiberoptic irradiation transsclerally through a

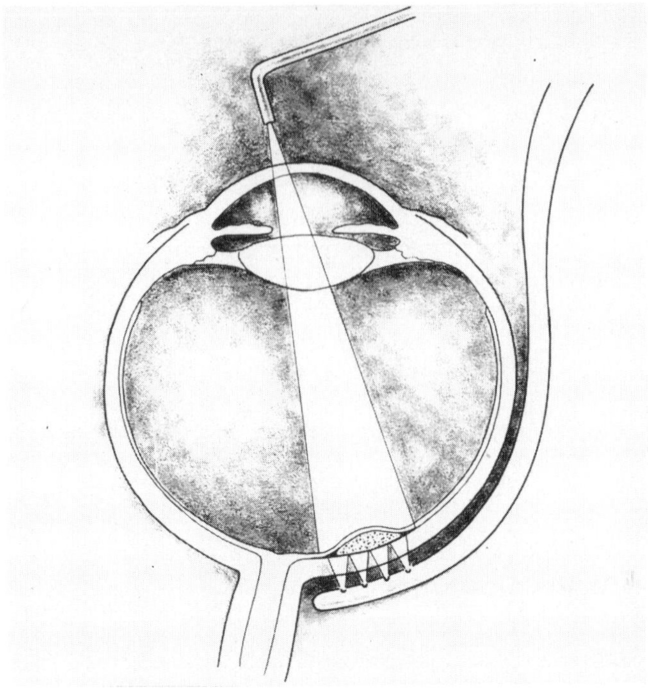

Fig. 5-14. Combination of transpupillary and transscleral photodynamic therapy of choroidal or retinal tumor sensitized by intravenous injection of Hpd. Transpupillary red dye laser radiation is channeled through pupil by fiberoptic cable while transscleral red dye laser radiation is conducted to that region by fiberoptic cable imbedded in curved probe to gain access to retrobulbar area.

A

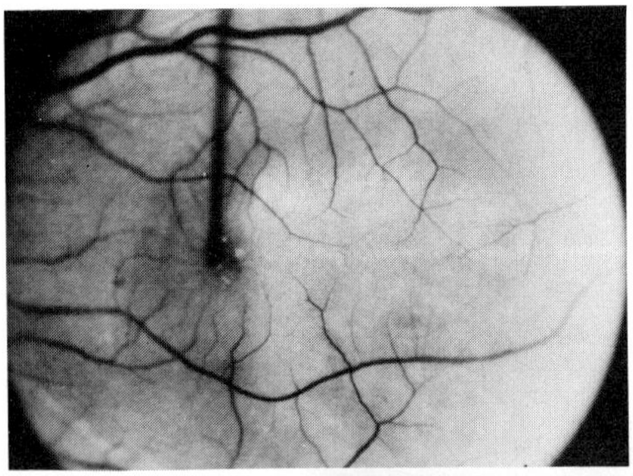

B

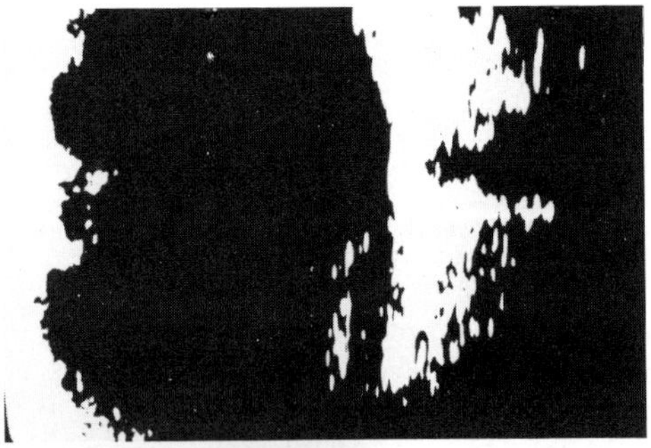

C

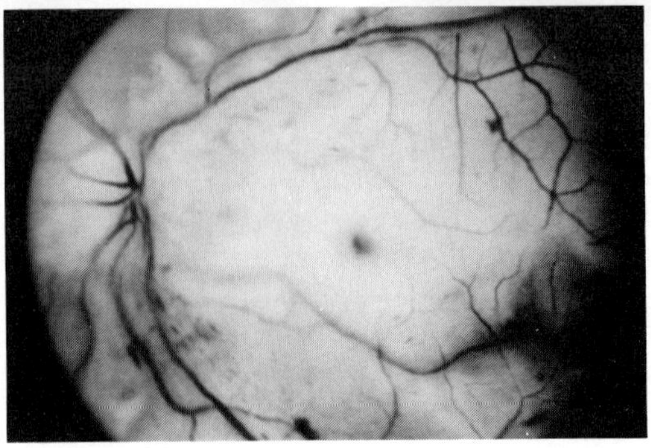

Fig. 5-15. A, Six DD choroidal malignant melanoma occupying macular and temporal paramacular region of left eye of 42-year-old blacksmith before Hpd and red-dye laser therapy. **B,** Ultrasonography demonstrating 4 mm elevation of tumor mass in choroidal plane. **C,** Posterior pole of treated eye showing destruction of melanoma and disappearance of most pigment tumor tissue approximately 5 weeks following red-dye laser irradiation of Hpd-sensitized tumor.

transconjunctival incision with the beam posterior and directed toward the tumor. In this manner the choroidal melanoma was irradiated by the red laser beam, which was transmitted simultaneously through fiberoptic cables through the pupil onto the anterior surface of the tumor and transsclerally from behind the tumor to the malignancy's posterior aspect. This combined anterior and posterior approach using fiberoptic delivery systems proved ideal, and the tumor and all vasculature in the tumor region were obliterated; acute necrosis occurred within the first day, and slow absorption and phagocytosis of the dead tumor cells took place over several months following treatment (Fig. 5-15,*C*).

During the 6 months after PDT the tumor appeared to be totally destroyed, although we still suspected a small portion of pigment in the inferotemporal area of the paramacular region. The patient was lost to follow-up for another 6 to 8 months, then returned with a moderately large, stalklike tumor extending directly into the vitreous from the area of suspicious pigmentation. Ultrasonography indicated the tumor regrowth's elevation to be approximately 3 mm. The physicians from the referring hospital then concluded that the eye should be enucleated, which was done. Histopathologic sections showed a completely destroyed tumor in all areas except for the one small area along the distal inferotemporal vascular arcade that had given rise to the tumor regrowth following PDT. Close observation during the months following PDT is essential in order to institute retreatment with one of the various antitumor modalities, including repeat PDT.

Patient 2

This 78-year-old woman had an 8 × 10 DD malignant melanoma of the choroid that extended approximately 6 to 8 mm into the vitreous body (Fig. 5-16, *A*). This enormous malignant tumor was subjected to PDT using 1.5 mg/kg of body weight of intravenously injected Hpd, followed 3 days later by radiation for 40 minutes by transscleral and transpupillary irradiation amounting to 100 to 150 mW/cm^2. We noted a tumor reaction almost immediately, although it was difficult to discern whether the internal portions of the tumor had been eradicated. We watched the tumor for several months and thought at that time that tumor growth might possibly be occurring. Because of the extent of the tumor, we employed a new procedure to debulk the central ocular tumor, with the ultimate purpose of eventually treating the remainder of the tumor again with PDT.

A

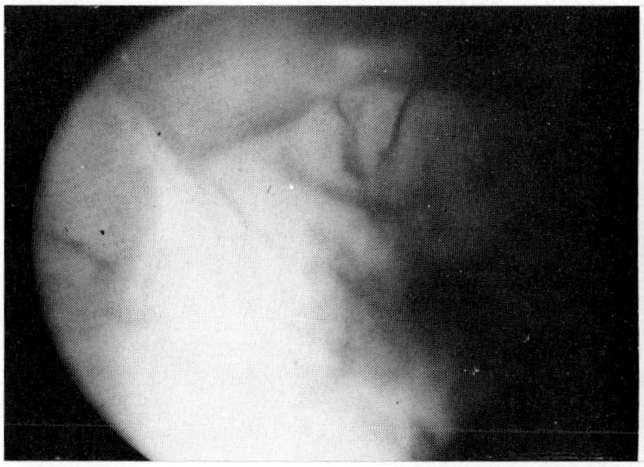

B

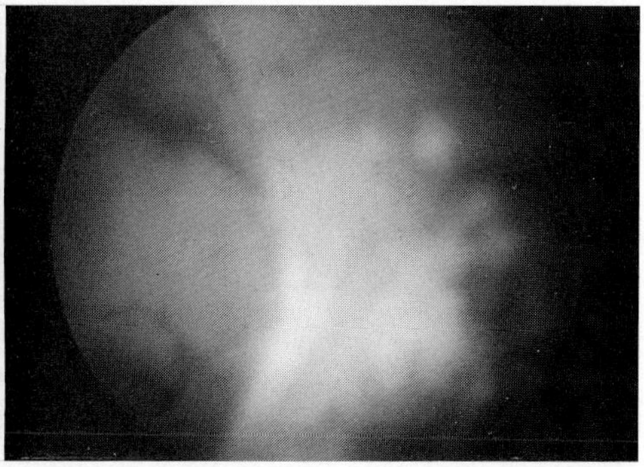

Fig. 5-16. A, Clinical appearance of extremely large choroidal malignant melanoma extending 8 mm into vitreous. **B,** Tumor's appearance following photovaporization therapy and PDT, with regression and stabilization of tumor mass.

An intracapsular cataract extraction was performed because of moderately dense cortical opacification of the patient's lens. The cataract wound was tightly sutured after a full iridectomy and inferior sphincterotomy. We then performed a pars plana vitrectomy using the standard Ocutome technique until we thought most of the vitreous had been removed from the tumor surface and the vitreous cavity. The vitreous body was then filled with medical-grade nitrogen that had been doubly filtered, and the entire eye was inflated to about 25 mm Hg pressure. A total inflow-outflow system had been designed to maintain the eye at normal pressure throughout the gas-fluid interchange procedure and for the forthcoming CO_2 laser photovaporization procedure.

When the eye had been totally filled with nitrogen, we introduced Co_2 laser probe, specially designed in collaboration with Coherent Medical Group, Inc., through the incision in the pars plana region; additional medical-grade nitrogen was gently wafted through the probe and into the vitreous cavity, exiting through a separate outflow portal. In this way, we could visualize the tumor clearly. The CO_2 laser was used in 0.2- to 0.3-second exposures, and the tumor was slowly vaporized and debulked (see Chapter 20). After each CO_2 laser photovaporization exposure, the vitreous cavity would fill with smoke and vapor, which was discharged through the exit port as nitrogen flowed through the probe into the vitreous cavity. When the tumor could again be visualized, it was resubjected to photovaporization and eventually was debulked to approximately 25% of its original size. At this time we placed a balanced salt solution in the eye and removed the nitrogen gas. The pars plana incision was closed, and prophylactic cryopexy was performed over the region of the pars plana incision. The patient proceeded extremely well, and her vitreous remained clear after the first postphotovaporization week.

We again treated the patient with PDT, using approximately 1.5 to 2.0 mg/kg of body weight of intraveneous Hpd, followed by transscleral and transpupillary PDT with the dye laser operating at a wavelength of 631 nm. The power density remained approximately 100 to 125 mW/cm^2, and the duration of the exposure for both probes was between 30 to 35 minutes. This patient continued to show progress without recurrence during the next 18 months (Fig. 5-16, *B*).

Patient 3

A 42-year-old female was sent to us from Europe with an enormous malignant melanoma infiltrating the conjunctiva and external surfaces of the left eye. This melanoma had been partially removed during seven previous surgical operations, all of which involved difficulties with hemorrhaging and maintaining hemostasis. Because of the tumor size, it was difficult for the patient to close her eyelid, and a small portion of the upper lid showed a typical "kissing melanoma."

We initially treated the patient with photovaporization, using the CO_2 laser to debulk most of the tumor from the conjunctiva, which resulted in complete destruction of the visually apparent melanoma completely down to bare scleral tissue. The corneal portions the tumor had grown onto were cauterized in a way so as to form a superficial keratectomy. The portion of the malignant melanoma that involved the central portion of the upper lid was destroyed so that none of the tissue remained visible; photovaporization had been carried inward from the conjunctival surface of the upper lid toward and involving the tarsal plate (Fig. 5-17, *A* and *B*).

At this point we intravenously injected Hpd, 3 mg/kg of body weight. Three days later, the entire region that had been previously cauterized by photovaporization was irradiated with the red liquid dye laser beam at a power density approximately 125 mW/sec for 35 minutes (Fig. 5-18). The purpose of the combined photovaporization and photodynamic therapy was (1) to physically destroy as many malignant cells as possible utilizing the former technique and (2) to photochemically destroy the remaining cells by Hpd-dye laser interaction. The patient appeared to do well, and the conjunctival wound and area healed without return of the malignancy during a 6-month follow-up.

A

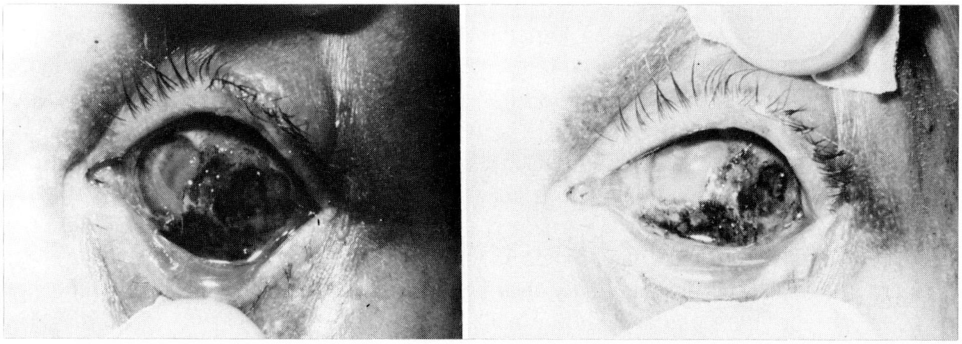

B

Fig. 5-17. A, Appearance of conjunctival malignant melanoma after photovaporization debulkment, with destruction of all visible pigment cells on conjunctiva and episcleral areas as well as on inner portions of upper lid. **B,** Appearance of eye 3 hours following PDT and 72 hours after intravenous Hpd injection. Note sloughing and destruction of many portions of extrabulbar tissues thought to contain residual malignant melanoma cells following photovaporization therapy.

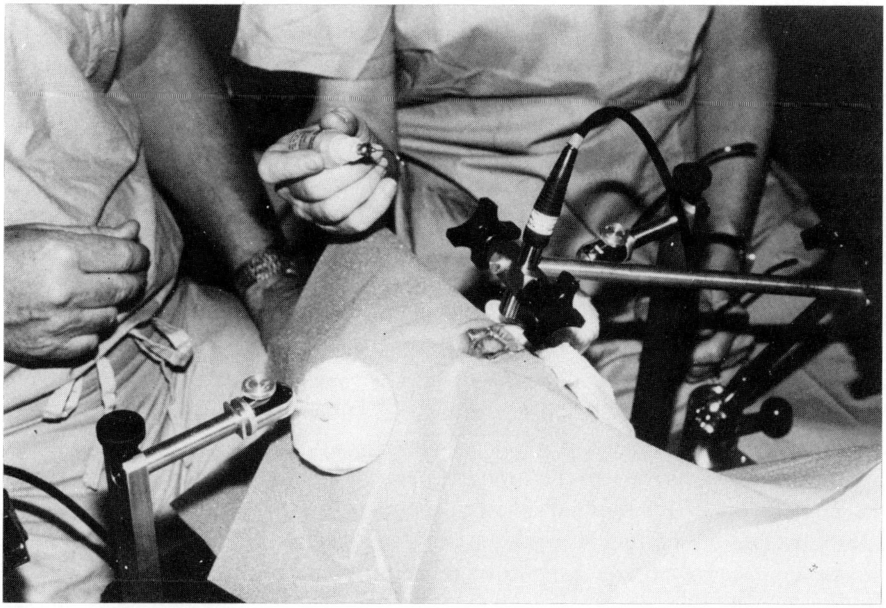

Fig. 5-18. Patient in Fig. 5-17 at the time of showing stabilization of head and irradiation of conjunctival area with red dye laser beam channeled through fiberoptic cable.

The patient was followed closely by ophthalmologists in France, who discovered regrowth of the conjunctival tumor approximately 9 to 10 months following PDT. Because of the long series of operative interventions and the extent of the tumor around the entire scleral surface, the eye was enucleated. Small areas of viable pigment melanoma cells were found in the conjunctival region close to the sclera, although most areas of previous tumor implantation had been destroyed by the combination of photovaporization and photodynamic therapy.

Patient 4

A 22-year-old white male was found to have a 5 × 6 DD malignant melanoma of the choroid that occupied the entire posterior pole between the temporal vascular arcades in the macular and the paramacular zones. Ultrasonography showed the malignant melanoma elevated approximately 3 mm into the vitreous, and a typical pattern consistent with a malignant melanoma was demonstrated by fluorescein angiogram (Fig. 5-19).

The patient was intravenously injected with *Hpd,* 3 mg/kg of body weight; we waited 72 hours for the *Hpd* to wash from the normal cells of the choroid and retina. The patient's head was placed rigidly in a head-stabilizing device, and the stereotactic arms used for the transpupillary and transscleral probes were brought into position (Fig. 5-20). We administered a retrobulbar injection of 0.75% Marcaine to the affected eye as well as individual injections to each recti muscle. We also gave a lid block of 2% xylocaine, using the Van Lint technique.

At this point we made a small incision just inferior and parallel to the insertion of the lateral rectus through the conjunctiva and Tenon's fascia and slipped the transscleral probe along the surface of the sclera until it was positioned directly over the posterior aspect of the tumor and firmly against the scleral wall. A Lo-Vac plano contact lens was then placed on the surface of the cornea and held in position with a slight vacuum using balanced salt solution. The transpupillary probe was then brought into position in such a way that the cone of light emitted from the fiberoptic cable was directed through the corneal contact lens, through the pupil, and impacted on the entire anterior surface of the tumor. Then we locked both stereotactic units into place. The cone of red dye laser light emerging from the fiberoptic cable at an angle of approximately 26 degrees was manipulated so that the entire light distribution covered the tumor in a homogeneous fashion without overlapping onto normal retinal tissue. Both the transpupillary and transscleral probes were in position to irradiate the tumor simultaneously—transclerally onto the tumor's posterior surface and transpupillarily onto the anterior surface. With 75% of the light channelled to the transscleral probe and 25% of the available red dye laser light channeled through the transpupillary probe, the laser was tuned to an emission that would create a power density of approximately 75 mW/cm^2 on the anterior surface and 100 mW/cm^2 on the posterior surface. These figures were estimates because of the difficulty in ascertaining the scleral scattering potential at this particular wavelength as well as the diffusion and scattering that occurred through the lens and other refractive elements of the eye with the transpupillary beam. The duration of treatment was 35 minutes, and the tumor appeared to be adequately bathed in extensive amounts of the red dye laser beam at a 631 nm wavelength.

Within 24 hours the choroidal malignant melanoma appeared to be necrotic on the anterior surface, although some patches of pigment could be seen interspersed with the

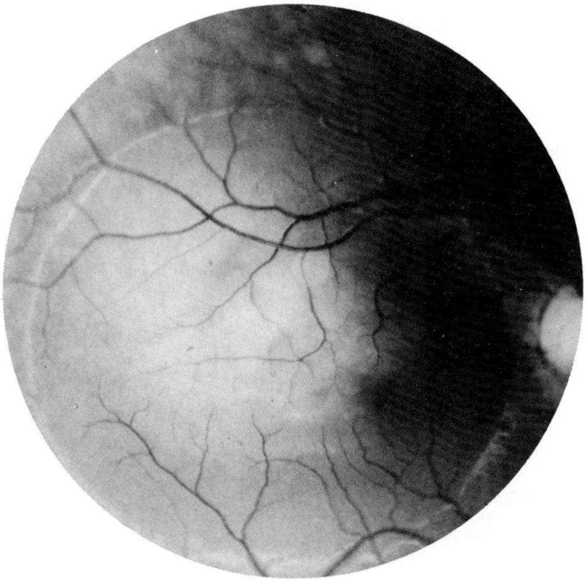

Fig. 5-19. A 5 × 6 DD choroidal malignant melanoma in macular region before PDT.

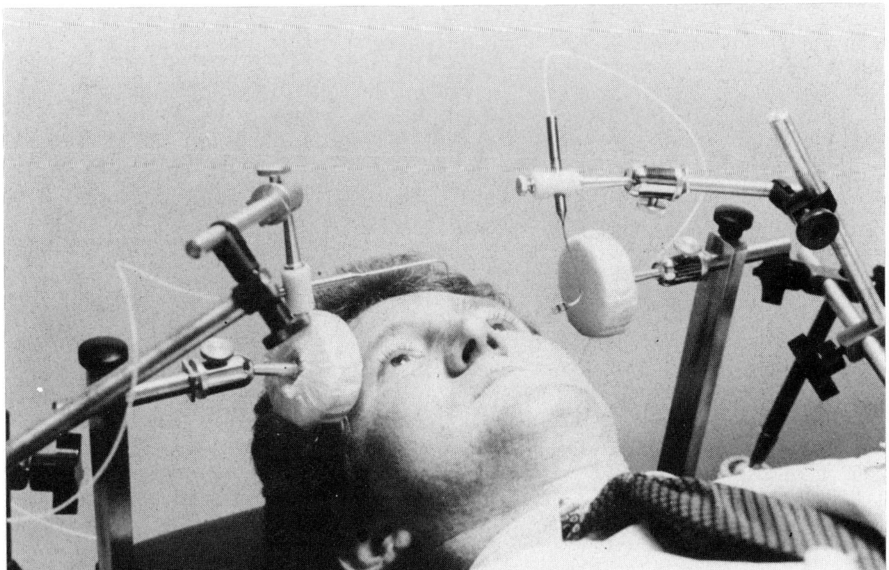

Fig. 5-20. Head stabilization device and stereotactic fiberoptic probes before adjustment for transpupillary and transscleral channeling of red laser beam.

white necrotic tissue (Fig. 5-21). It was difficult to determine the viability of the pigmented tissue, but the technique appeared to have been highly effective, even with relatively low-power density settings for each of the fiberoptic probes. On follow-up visit 2 months after PDT, the dual anterior and posterior bimural approaches appeared to have destroyed a large part of the tumor, but certain areas, although not growing, could well have been viable. Because the patient was from Canada, he was referred to a local ophthalmologist for further follow-up and possible treatment.

Conclusion

It is apparent that the power densities, the exact method of treatment, and the amount of intravenous Hpd (or the more active component DHE) are variables that must be adjusted for the particular tumor and for the area of the eye involved. Using the stereotactic system, we have been encouraged with the results from this initial series of patients. Although it would appear that the hematoporphyrin levels, power densities, and other factors affecting the delivery of the laser energy were calculated to be low, the stereotactic apparatus with the dual anterior-posterior bimural approach to the tumor with transpupillary and transscleral probes should prove to be a highly effective therapeutic approach. Higher levels of laser power and intravenous DHE will be used in future patients and carefully titrated with regard to tumor thickness, extent of tumor mass, and amount of malignant pigmentation. These factors should provide a more precise assessment of the amount of laser energy and other materials necessary to completely eradicate various types of malignancies within the eye.

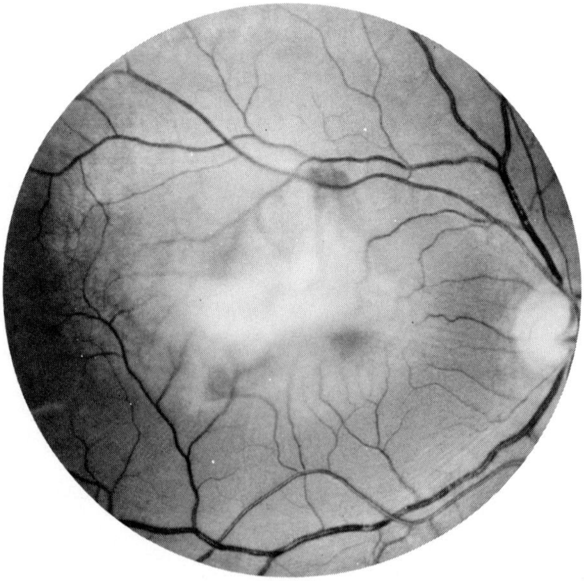

Fig. 5-21. Appearance of choroidal melanoma in Fig. 5-19 following transpupillary and transscleral PDT. Note only patchy necrosis of tumor rather than total cellular death, presumably caused by inadequate laser power density or low intravenous Hpd dosage.

PHOTOCOAGULATION THERAPY

Perhaps the most promising light source for photocoagulation therapy in ophthalmology is the tunable dye laser (Figs. 5-22 and 5-23). The great advantage of a dye laser is that its output wavelengths can be appreciably varied: about 100 nm with a single dye and through a spectral range of 360 to 960 nm with several dyes. By applying this wide assortment of wavelengths with strict monochromaticity and high-output powers, individual tissues in the retina or other portions of the eye can be selectively targeted for maximal absorption by using the particular laser or wavelength most highly absorbed by that tissue. Specific enzymes, elements of cells such as the mitochrondria, tissue planes such as the deep and superficial plexi and angiomatous lesions, pigmented layers or defects, cystic structures, and other tissue strata can be selectively destroyed by using several microsurgical laser techniques; this is possible only because of the monochromaticity and tunability of the dye laser. For instance, the following possibilities for selective photocoagulation are apparent:

1. A laser wavelength could be selected to impact a target tissue that most highly absorbs that wavelength, thereby converting the light energy to heat energy and coagulating at a high efficiency rate.
2. With a cyst or other more transparent structure the surrounding tissues could be selectively coagulated with the optimal wavelength to collapse the cystic or transparent tissue.
3. A wavelength could be shifted away from the maximal absorption point (lambda maxima) of the target tissue to avoid absorption by nearby tissue but still allow sufficient energy to be absorbed by the target tissue for effective coagulation. For instance, xanthophyll could be avoided with the coagulation of hemoglobin, or hemoglobin could be avoided with the coagulation of melanin or pigmented structures in the retina.
4. A combination effect could be produced whereby portions of two or more differently absorbent tissues could be cauterized in a ratio dependent on their particular absorption potential. Because of the well-known absorption potential of the main pigments of the eye, these ratios could be easily determined to produce optimal therapeutic results.

Applications of the dye laser to ophthalmology have become extremely practical and advantageous (see Figs. 5-24 to 5-29). Theoretically, for example, a dye laser that is tunable from 560 to 630 nm would offer the optimal wavelengths for photocoagulation of the fundus. The 560 nm wavelength is excellent for photocoagulation of hemoglobin and melanin granules, and lenticular scattering and absorption effects caused by early cataract formation are less than with the argon laser or with the frequency-doubled neodymium:YAG laser. By shifting these photocoagulation wavelengths between 620 and 630 nm, the absorption by hemoglobin is negligible, and the laser beam is primarily absorbed by choroidal pigment and the retinal pigment epithelial layer, much as is now recognized to occur with krypton red photocoagulation. With this wavelength in the 620 nm range) a deeper choroidal coagulation is apparent, with (1) obliteration of the feeder vessel to the subretinal subpigment epithelial neovascularization, (2) preservation of Bruch's membrane, and (3) moderate laser beam uptake by the pigment epithelium, with coagulum production that disrupts and destroys the outer third of the retinal tissue.

When an intermediate wavelength in the orange portion of the spectrum between 590 and 600 nm is used, the abnormal subpigment epithelial neovascularization (he-

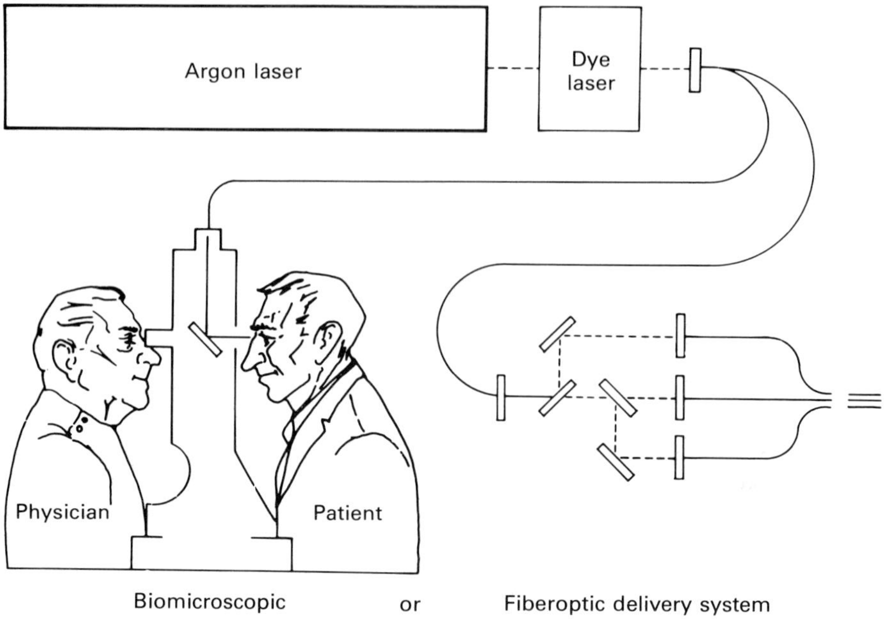

Fig. 5-22. Schematic drawing of fiberoptic delivery system to (1) biomicroscope and (2) fiberoptic triage terminal, from which beam channeled through original fiberoptic cable is broken into multiple fiberoptic cable delivery systems to transport to various portions of eye for PDT. Photocoagulation therapy can easily be accomplished by channeling entire output of dye laser through a fiberoptic cable, which conducts laser energy to biomicroscope. Photocoagulation parameters of spot size, exposure interval, and output power, and so on, can be varied as usual with this system.

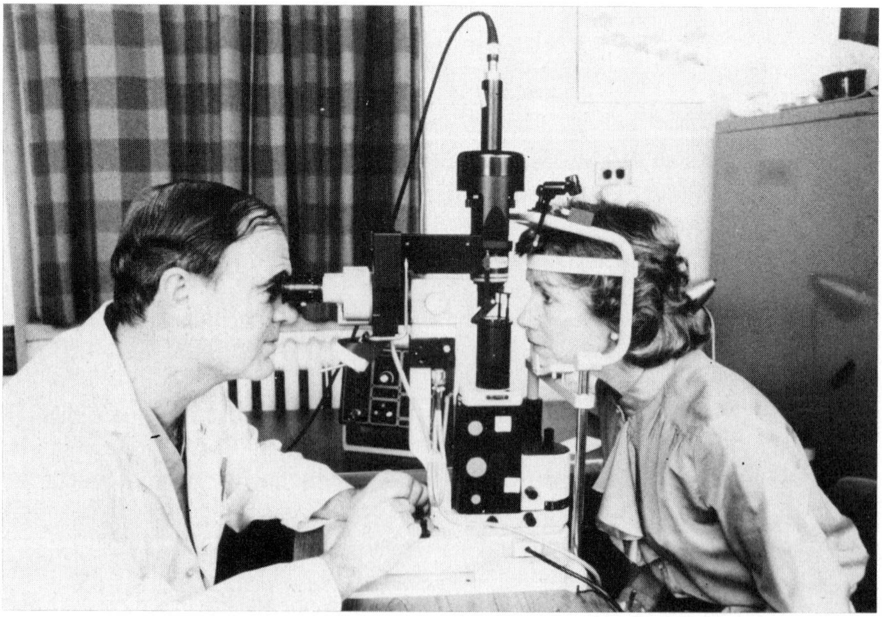

Fig. 5-23. Biomicroscopic dye laser photocoagulation system using fiberoptic cable to relay laser beam from dye laser to biomicroscope.

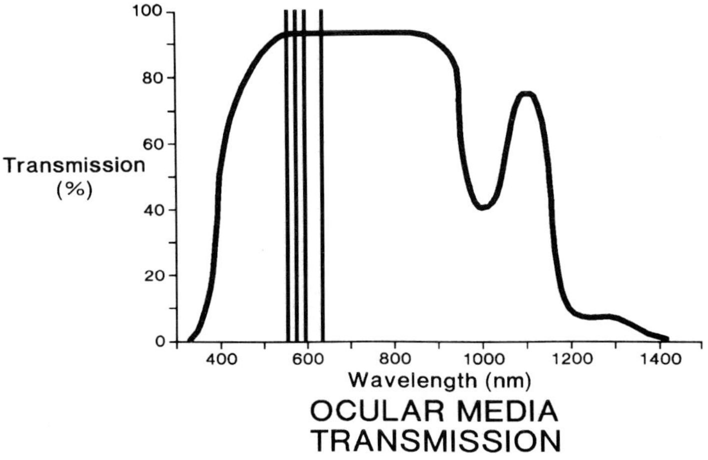

Fig. 5-24. Transmission of various wavelengths from organic dye laser (550, 570, 590, and 630 nm) through refractive ocular media.

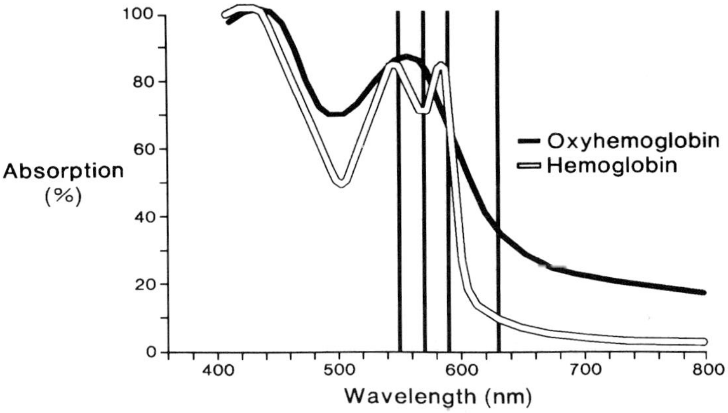

Fig. 5-25. Percentage of oxyhemoglobin and reduced hemoglobin absorption for representative wavelenths of organic dye laser in Fig. 5-24.

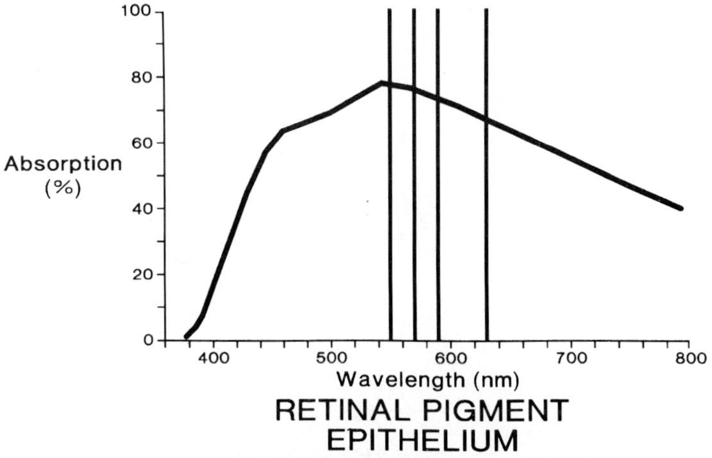

Fig. 5-26. Percentage of retinal pigment epithelium absorption for representative wavelengths of organic dye laser.

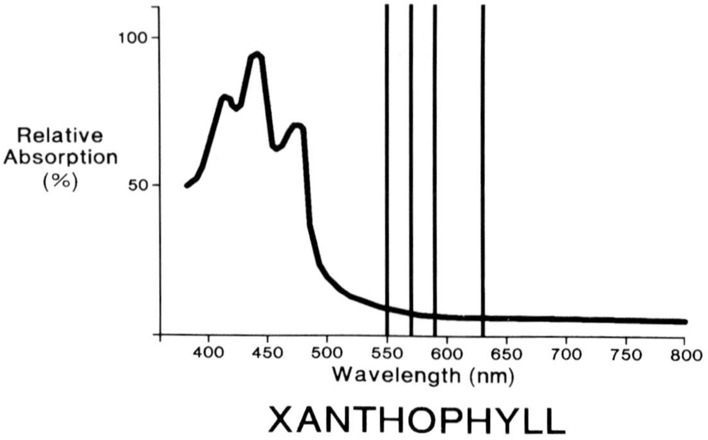

Fig. 5-27. Percentage of relative absorption of macular xanthophyll pigment for representative wavelengths. All wavelengths presently used for photocoagulation with organic dye laser are highly transmitted by xanthophyll pigment.

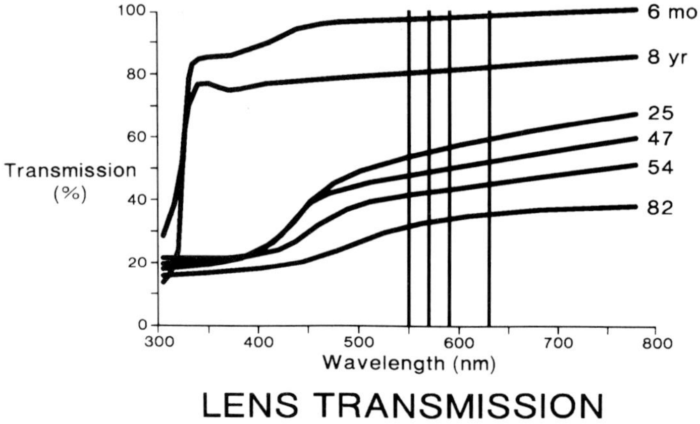

Fig. 5-28. Percentage of transmission of representative organic dye laser wavelengths through intact human lens at various ages. Percentage decreases substantially with increasing age because of filtration effect of yellow nuclear sclerotic lens.

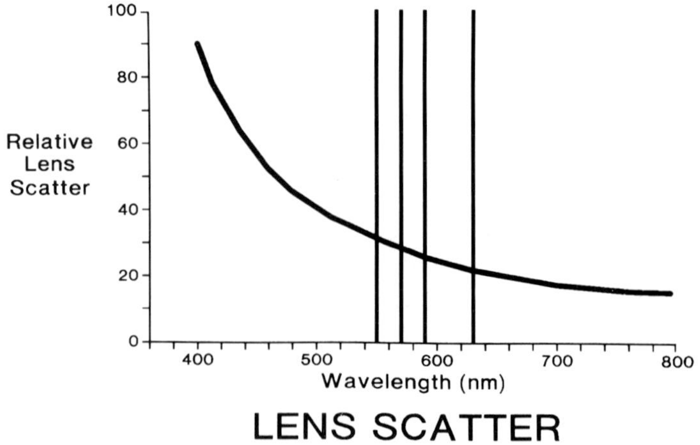

Fig. 5-29. Relative lens scatter of representative organic dye laser wavelengths. Scatter increases with shortness of wavelength.

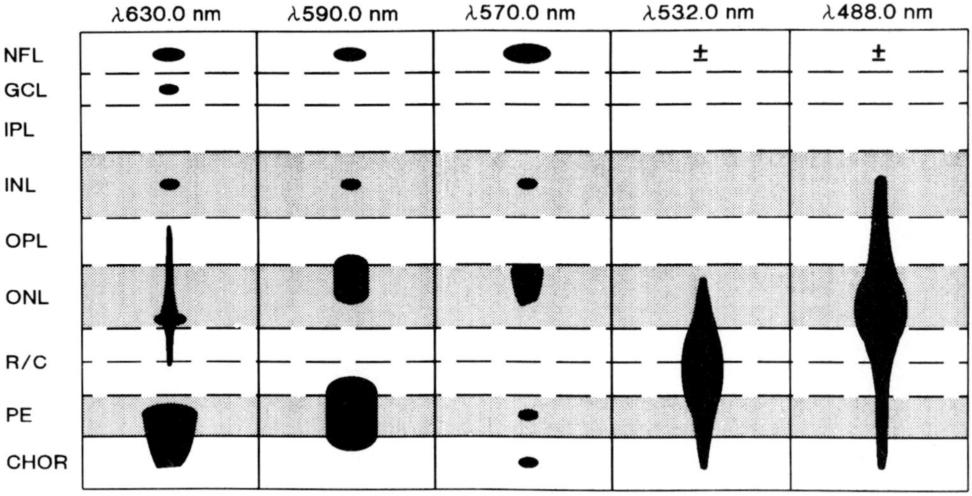

Fig. 5-30. Chorioretinal zones of maximal absorption and damage from laser photocoagulation according to various wavelengths: dye (630, 590, and 570 nm), frequency-doubled neodymium:YAG (532 nm), and argon (488 nm) laser radiations.

moglobin) and the overlying pigment epithelium absorb a moderately high portion of the incident radiation but allow part of the beam to enter the internal choroidal layers and create choroidal coagulation sufficient to obliterate the feeder vessel to the area of subretinal neovascularization (Fig. 5-30). Thus the orange wavelength from the dye laser—from a theoretic and more recently a practical basis—could prove to be the ideal wavelength when coagulating subpigment epithelial neovascularization that occurs in senile macular degeneration, histoplasmosis, and other forms of macular lesions.

Patient selection

Recently the dye laser has been used to coagulate a retinal lesion with a specific wavelength that would be most highly absorbed and most effective. For example, areas of surface or retinovitreal neovascularization were coagulated directly with the yellow dye laser beam at approximately 570 nm to illustrate the tremendous specificity as well as absorption by hemoglobin of the impinging yellow laser beam (Fig. 5-31). Coagulation, blockage, and destruction of the blood vessels were accomplished at relatively low-power levels and appeared to be more effective than the argon laser or the frequency-doubled neodymium:YAG laser.

In patients with subretinal neovascularization caused by senile macular degeneration or any other etiology, the orange dye laser (590 nm) beam (Fig. 5-32) was used to demonstrate that hemoglobin absorption in the subretinal neovascularization, as well as choroidal circulation, could be accomplished in a manner that would be difficult for the red krypton (647.1 nm) or red dye laser (630 nm) to simulate (Fig. 5-33). Coagulations in these structures and in the retinal pigment epithelium created a destructive nidus that appeared to effectively destroy the neovascularization. In this situation the coagulation directly surrounded the subretinal neovascularization rather than creating a coagulation (common with the krypton red laser) that was more localized and intense in the choroid than the pigment epithelial layer. In some cases red, orange, and yellow laser photoco-

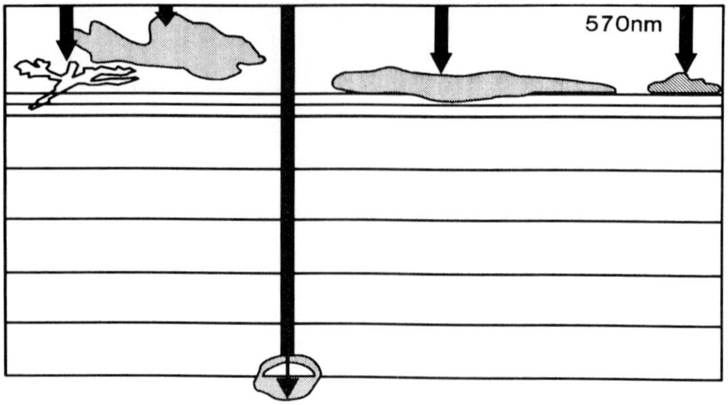

Fig. 5-31. Laser energy transmission at 570 nm wavelength through various periretinal and intraretinal defects. *Left* to *right,* retinovitreal neovascularization, vitreal blood, pigment epithelial and subretinal neovascularization, preretinal blood, and preretinal pigment accumulations.

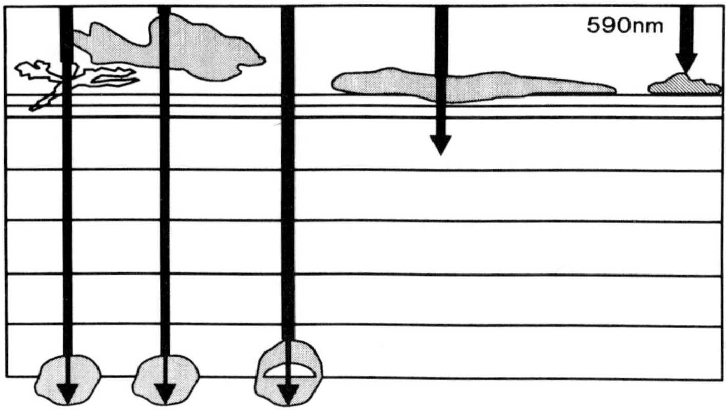

Fig. 5-32. Laser energy transmission at 590 nm wavelength through various periretinal and intraretinal defects. *Left* to *right,* retinovitreal neovascularization, vitreal blood, pigment epithelial and subretinal neovascularization, preretinal blood, and preretinal pigment accumulations.

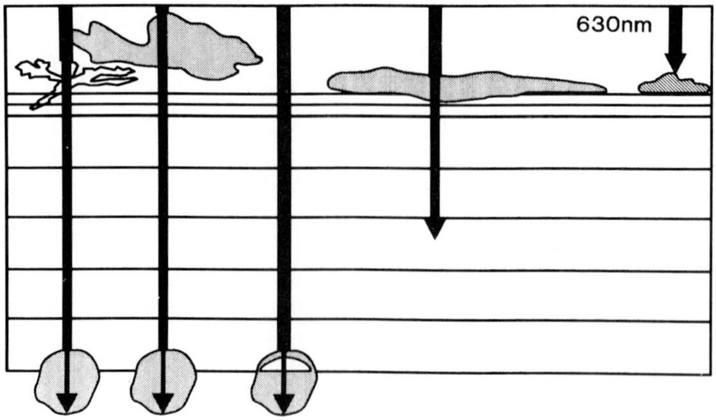

Fig. 5-33. Laser energy transmission at 630 nm wavelength through various periretinal and intraretinal defects. *Left* to *right,* retinovitreal neovascularization, vitreal blood, pigment epithelial and subretinal neovascularization, preretinal blood, and preretinal pigment accumulations.

Table 5-1. Photocoagulation with the dye laser (λ indicates wavelength)

Disease	*Yellow (λ 570 nm)*	*Orange (λ 590 nm)*	*Red (λ 630 nm)*
Senile macular degeneration	2	5	3
Diabetic retinopathy	2	2	2
Central retinal vein occlusion	0	1	2
Branch retinal vein occlusion	1	1	3
TOTAL	5	9	10

agulations were produced side by side to demonstrate the appearance and effectiveness of each wavelength.

The patients treated to date with the yellow, orange, and red dye laser photocoagulation are summarized in Table 5-1. All these attempts with various vascular diseases represent the first use of the continuous-wave organic liquid dye laser for photocoagulation. Although the series is short, the results definitely indicated the versatility and effectiveness of these laser wavelengths.

This new clinical research utilizing the yellow, orange, and red wavelengths of the dye laser (Rhodamine 6G and MD-631) appears to have enormous promise and may demonstrate that the liquid dye laser is the laser of choice for photocoagulation of many ocular defects. The effectiveness of the dye laser as a photocoagulation source results from the monochromaticity, tunability, relatively high output power, and wavelength versatility. Therefore, a target tissue can be selectively coagulated with minimal laser energy transmitted through the refractive media and with minimal damage to nearby normal tissues. The dye laser, as a photocoagulation system, should prove extremely valuable in treating most ocular diseases.

ACKNOWLEDGMENT

I would like to acknowledge the invaluable assistance of Beth Ann Hughes, Ruth J. Helmich, Paul Saivetz, and Virginia H. Cantarella.

REFERENCES

1. Auler, H., and Banzer, G.: Untersuchungen uber die Rolle der Porphine bei geschwiulstkranken Menschen and Tieren, Z. Krebsforsch **53:**65, 1942.
2. Bugelski, P.J.: Morphologic aspects of the photosensitizing effects and distribution of hematoporphyrin derivative in experimental tumors and cultured cells, doctoral dissertation, Buffalo, 1980, State University of New York.
3. Diamond, I., and others: Photodynamic therapy of malignant tumors, Lancet **2:**1175, 1972.
4. Dougherty, T.J.: Photoradiation therapy, abstracts of the American Chemical Society meeting, no. 014, Chicago, 1973, American Chemical Society.
5. Dougherty, T.J.: Activated dyes as anti-tumor agents, J. Natl. Cancer Inst. **51:**1333, 1974.
6. Dougherty, T.J., Potter, W.R., and Weishaupt, K.R.: The structure of the active component of hematoporphyrin derivative. In Doiron, D.R., editor: Porphyrin localization and treatment of tumors, New York, Alan L. Liss, Inc. (In press.)
7. Dougherty, T.J., and others: Photoradiation therapy. II. Cure of animal tumors with hematoporphyrin and light, J. Natl. Cancer Inst. **55:**115, 1975.
8. Doughtery, T.J., and others: Photoradiation therapy for the treatment of malignant tumors, Cancer Res. **38:**2628 (1978).
9. Dougherty, T.J., and others: Photoradiation in the treatment of recurrent breast carcinoma, J. Natl. Cancer Inst. **62:**231, 1979.
10. Dougherty, T.J., and others: Photoradiation therapy of malignant tumors, In Devita, V., Hellman, S., and Rosenberg S., editors: Principles and practices of oncology, Philadelphia, 1982, J.B. Lippincott Co.

11. Edwards, E., and Duntley, S.Q.: Spectrophotometry of living human skin, J. Invest. Dermatol. **16:**311, 1951.
12. Everett, M.A., Yeargers, E., Sayre, R.M., and Olson, R.L.: Penetration of epidermis by ultraviolet rays, Photochem. Photobiol. **1:**533, 1962.
13. Figge, F.H.J., Weiland, G.S., and Manganiello, L.O.J.: Cancer detection and therapy: affinity of neoplastic embryonic and traumatized regenerating tissues for porphyrins and metalloporphyrins, Proc. Soc. Exp. Biol. Med. **68:**640, 1948.
14. Gomer, C.J., and Dougherty, T.J.: Determination of $^{3}H^{-}$ and ^{14}C hematoporphyrin derivataive distribution in malignant and normal tissue, Cancer Res. **39:**146, 1979.
15. Granelli, S.G., and others: Photochemotherapy of glioma cells by visible light and hematoporphyrin, Cancer Res. **35:**2567, 1975.
16. Gregorie, H.B., Jr., and others: Hematoporphyrin derivative fluorescence in malignant neoplasms, Ann. Surg. **167:**820, 1968.
17. L'Esperance, F.A., Jr.: Ophthalmic lasers: photocoagulation, photoradiation, and surgery, ed. 2, St. Louis, 1983, The C.V. Mosby Co.
18. Lipson, R.L.: The photodynamic and fluorescent properties of a particular hematoporphyrin derivative and its use in tumor detection, master's thesis, Minneapolis, 1960, University of Minnesota.
19. Lipson, R.L., Baldes, E.J., and Olsen, A.M.: Hematoporphyrin derivative: a new aid of endoscopic detection of malignant disease, J. Thorac. Cardiovasc. Surg. **42:**623, 1961.
20. Lipson, R.L., Baldes, E.J., and Olsen, A.M.: The use of a derivative of hematoporphyrin in tumor detection, J. Natl. Cancer Inst. **26:**1, 1961.
21. Lipson, R.L., Baldes, E.J., and Olsen, A.M.: A further evaluation of the use of hematoporphyrin derivative as a new aid for the endoscopic detection of malignant disease, Dis. Chest **46:**676, 1964.
22. Lipson, R.L., and others: Hematoporphyrin derivative for the detection of cervical cancer, Obstet. Gynecol. **24:**78, 1964.
23. Mellors, R.C., Glassman, A., and Papanicolaou, G.N.: A microfluorimetric scanning method for the detection of cancer cells in smears of exfoliated cells, Cancer **5:**458, 1952.
24. Moan, J., Pettersen, E.O., and Christensen, T.: The mechanism of photodynamic inactivation of human cells invitro in the presence of hematoporphyrin, Br. J. Cancer **39:**398, 1979.
25. Moore, G.E.: Diagnosis and localization of brain tumors: a clinical and experimental study employing fluorescent and radioactive tracer methods, Springfield, Ill., 1953, Charles C Thomas, Publisher.
26. Policard, A.: Etudes sur les aspects offerts par des tumeurs experimentales examinee al lumiere de woods, Compt Rendu Soc. Bio. **91:**1423, 1924.
27. Rall, D.D., and others: Appearance and persistence of fluorescent material in tumor tissue after tetracycline administration, J. Natl. Cancer Inst. **19:**79, 1957.
28. Santamaria, L., and Prino, G.: The photodynamic substances and their mechanism of action. In Gallo, U., and Santamaria, L., editors: Research progress in organic biological and medicinal chemistry, Milan, 1964, Society Editoriale Farmacentia, vol. 1, p. 260.
29. Schwartz, S.: Personal communication, 1982.
30. Tappenier, H., and Jesionek, A.: Therapeutische Versuche mit fluoreszierenden Stoffe, Muench. Med. Wochenschr. **1:**2042, 1903.
31. Tomson, S.H., Emmett, E.A., and Fox, S.H.: Photodestruction of mouse epithelial tumors after acridine orange and argon laser, Cancer Res. **34:**3124, 1974.
32. Weishaupt, K.R., Gomer, C.J., and Dougherty, T.J.: Identification of singlet oxygen as the cytotoxic agent in photo-inactivation of a murine tumor, Cancer Res. **36:**2326, 1976.

6

Ophthalmic laser surgery: principles, technology, and technique

Martin A. Mainster

Selection and proper use of ophthalmic laser systems require familiarity with clinical instruments and background knowledge of lasers and their effects on ocular structures. This chapter presents an introduction to light, lasers, and laser-tissue interactions, with particular emphasis on photocoagulation and photodisruption in ophthalmic practice.

BASIC PRINCIPLES

Light

The electromagnetic spectrum is composed of a broad range of radiation, including ultraviolet radiation, visible light, and infrared radiation. Electromagnetic radiation has both wavelike properties, responsible for large-scale phenomena such as refraction and interference, and particle-like properties, which account for atomic-level phenomena such as light absorption and emission by atoms or molecules.[27]

Electromagnetic waves are characterized by their wavelength, λ, the distance between successive peaks of the waves. In free space all electromagnetic radiation travels at the same speed ($c = 3 \times 10^{10}$ cm/sec; c = speed of light) but radiation of different wavelengths interacts with materials in different ways. For example, the cornea is essentially opaque to ultraviolet radiation below 300 nm but transmits radiation between 300 and 1300 nm quite effectively.[10] Thus, if a corneal incision is to be performed with an ultraviolet laser, the wavelength must be well below 300 nm to avoid damage to the crystalline lens. Similarly, since the crystalline lens protects the retina from potentially hazardous near-ultraviolet light between 300 and 400 nm, cataract surgery increases the potential risk of the phakic or pseudophakic patient to photochemical retinal damage such as solar retinitis or welder's maculopathy.[24,25]

Wavelike properties of light are useful for analyzing how light will be affected by optical systems, but its particle-like properties are needed to explain how atoms or molecules acquire or release energy. If light is considered to be a stream of discrete particles, called *photons,* it is possible to explain atomic level phenomena such as light absorption or fluorescence by atoms. The energy of each photon is related to its wavelength by Planck's relationship:

$$E = hc/\lambda$$

where h is Planck's constant and c is the speed of light. The electrons of an atom can exist at only a limited number of energy levels, as first proposed by Niels Bohr in 1913. If an atom absorbs energy (is "excited"), an outer electron is generally moved from its normal ("ground") energy level, E_1, to a higher ("excited") energy level, E_2. If the atom absorbs enough energy, the electron may actually escape from the attraction of the nucleus, producing a free electron and an ion in a process called *ionization* (as in photodisruption with a neodymium:YAG laser, discussed in later sections). Ionization may be regarded as the state of an electron in which there is a continuum of allowed energy levels rather than the discrete number permitted when the electron is bound to the nucleus. This continuum is the basis for the "tunability" of a free-electron laser from the far-ultraviolet to the far-infrared regions of the spectrum.

An atom that is excited but not ionized returns quickly to its normal (ground) state when its excited electron falls from an excited energy level to the ground energy level. The excessive energy possessed by the excited atom can be given off in the form of a photon, whose energy is equal to the energy difference between the electron's excited and ground energy levels. This process is termed *spontaneous emission* or *fluorescence*. The energy of the emitted photon is simply equal to the energy difference between the excited and ground energy levels ($E_2 - E_1$), and the wavelength of the emitted photon, from Planck's relationship, is

$$\lambda = hc/(E_2 - E_1)$$

It should be noted that there is no preferred direction for the photons given off in fluorescence, so fluorescence itself does not produce coherent light.

In general the return of an electron from an excited, higher energy level to its ground energy level takes place not in a single jump ("transition"), but through alternative, competing pathways, each of which may consist of a sequence of photon-producing transitions and faster nonradiative transitions. Thus photons with several different wavelengths may be produced when a collection of excited atoms of a single type returns to ground state.

The time an atom spends in any one of its many possible excited states is termed the *fluorescent lifetime* of that state. Most lifetimes are very short, typically 10^{-9} second or less. Some atoms, however, have an excited energy level with a comparatively longer fluorescent lifetime, referred to as a *metastable* state. Atoms must have a metastable state to be a useful active medium for laser operation. Laser photons are generated when an electron makes the transition from the metastable energy state to the next lower energy. In most lasers, electrons (1) are excited to very high energy levels; (2) quickly fall through nonradiative transitions to a metastable state, E_2; (3) stay briefly in the metastable state before making the transition to the next lower level, E_1; and (4) fall from E_1 to their ground state by very rapid nonradiative transitions. This is the sequence of events in a "four-level" laser system, such as in an argon ion or neodymium (Nd):YAG laser. In a four-level system a collection of excited atoms tends to have more atoms with an electron in its longer-lived metastable state (E_2) than in the next lower state (E_1); this condition is called a *population inversion*.

If an atom absorbs a photon that has an energy (wavelength) equal to the difference in energy between two of its adjacent electron energy levels, an electron in the lower level may be excited from the lower to the higher energy level in a process called *stimulated absorption*. Photons causing stimulated absorption can arise from fluorescence or from a flashlamp that produces photons with a continuous range of wavelengths. A flashlamp is used to excite neodymium ions in a Nd:YAG laser. Atomic electrons can also be excited to higher energy levels by processes other than photon absorption. For example, collision with electrons from an electric current is used to excite active atoms in an ion (such as argon or krypton) or excimer (such as argon fluoride) laser.

In 1917 Albert Einstein postulated that if an atom with an excited electron were struck by a photon, and the photon has an energy equal to the difference between the electron's higher and lower energy levels, then the incoming photon could trigger the atom to return to its ground state by releasing a photon. This process is termed *stimulated emission,* and the photon released by the excited atom when the atom returns to its ground state would have the same wavelength, direction, and phase as the incoming photon that triggered its release. Thus a single photon can produce two identical photons, and stimulated emission has the potential for producing a chain reaction ("cascade") of photons with identical properties. T.H. Maiman first demonstrated light generated by stimulated emission in 1960 using a ruby crystal in a device that is now known as a laser. The term *laser* is an acronym for *l*ight *a*mplification by *s*timulated *e*mission of *r*adiation.[40]

Lasers

Most atoms or molecules of a crystal or gas are in their unexcited, ground state. For laser action to occur with a particular type of atom, the atom must have a comparatively long-lived metastable state, and enough energy must be supplied to a collection of those atoms so that more atoms have electrons in this excited metastable state than in the next lower energy level; that is, to produce a population inversion. This population inversion can be induced by transferring energy to the atoms ("pumping" them) in various ways, such as by using a flashlamp or electric current, as discussed.

A metastable state and population inversion are necessary but not sufficient conditions for laser action to occur. In addition, a *resonant cavity* is needed to preferentially produce light by stimulated emission along a single axis. Resonant cavities are usually constructed by placing atoms or molecules of a particular type in a cavity with a mirror at each end, as shown in Fig. 6-1. The material containing atoms or molecules with an appropriate metastable state is referred to as the laser's *active medium*. A variety of active media are used in gas, liquid, and solid state lasers (Table 6-1).

A pumping source, such as a flashlamp or electric current, may then be used to produce a population inversion in the resonant cavity. A certain number of the excited atoms, however, will return to their ground state by spontaneous emission (fluorescence). If a photon from fluorescence travels down the axis of the cavity and strikes an excited atom, this will produce two photons traveling down the axis of the cavity, and these photons will have essentially the same direction, wavelength, and phase. These photons in turn strike other excited atoms, eventually leading to a "cascade" of photons traveling along the axis of the cavity. Mirrors at the ends of the cavity redirect these photons back into the cavity along its axis to form the resonance that preferentially produces photons traveling along the cavity axis. Photons from fluorescence or stimulated emission that do not travel parallel to the axis of the cavity merely escape from the cavity. If one of the mirrors is only partially reflecting—known as the *output coupler*—then a fraction of the photons traveling along the axis will escape to provide the laser beam. If more than one wavelength is produced in this manner, as in an argon ion laser, all wavelengths other than the desired one, such as 514.5 nm green, can be suppressed by placing a prism in the cavity to deviate photons having any wavelength other than the desired one out of the cavity axis.

The design of the resonant cavity affects the energy distribution across the laser beam. This distribution is determined by the boundary conditions of the cavity, and it can have rectangular or cylindric symmetry. For example, the circular beam of a typical argon ion laser tube is produced by a longitudinal discharge between electrodes at both ends of the resonant cavity; that is, the electric discharge is used to pump electrons through the gas parallel to the cavity's axis. The square beam of an excimer laser, however, is produced by a transverse discharge perpendicular to the cavity axis; a much shorter path length is needed to obtain an electric discharge and effective laser action for excimers, even with extremely high voltages.

The energy distribution across the beam is characterized by its transverse electromagnetic mode (TEM) structure, which arises from cavity resonances.[40] If an aperture is placed in the beam to limit light output only to the fundamental TEM_{00} mode (a Gaussian or "bell-shaped" distribution of energy across the beam), the cavity produces less total energy, but the laser beam can be focused into a minimum spot size (maximum focal irradiance) for its wavelength. Thus using the fundamental TEM_{00} mode structure in a Nd:YAG laser permits a maximum focal irradiance for a particular cone angle. Thus for a particular focal irradiance, using the fundamental mode minimizes the exposure of structures anterior and posterior to the focal point.[35]

In addition to its transverse mode structure, a laser beam is characterized by its longitudinal mode structure. Each photon in a laser pulse may be thought of as having traveled back and forth between the ends of the laser cavity for a certain number of

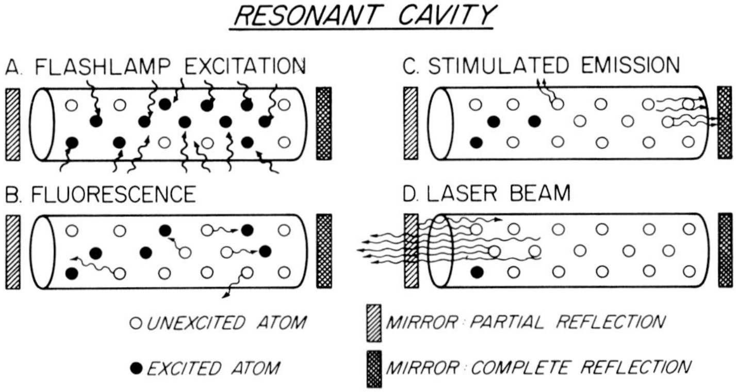

Fig. 6-1. Laser beam is produced in resonant cavity in following steps: **A,** Population inversion in active medium is created by photons from flashlamp or electrons from electric discharge. That is, enough energy is supplied to atoms or molecules in cavity so that more of them are in an excited metastable state than in their ground state. **B,** Atom stays briefly in excited state (its fluorescent lifetime) before returning to its ground state by spontaneous emission (fluorescence). **C,** If photon from fluorescence travels along the axis of cavity and strikes excited atom, stimulated emission will produce two photons traveling along axis of cavity with identical wavelength, direction, and phase. These photons strike other excited atoms, causing further stimulated emission and producing cascade of photons with identical properties. Mirrors at end of cavity redirect photons back into cavity along its axis, thereby producing cavity resonance. Photons not traveling along cavity axis (whether from spontaneous or stimulated emission) merely escape from cavity as excess fluorescence. **D,** One of two mirrors at ends of cavity is partly transmitting. This is the output coupler and is designed for specific cavity and active laser medium. Laser beam is formed when photons traveling along axis of cavity escape through this partly transmitting mirror.

Table 6-1. Ophthalmic laser sources

Name	*Primary wavelengths (nm)*	*Active species*	*Pumping type*	*Use**	*Status†*
Argon	488.0 blue	Ar ion	Electric discharge	PC	C
	514.5 green			PC	C
Carbon dioxide	10,600 infrared (IR)	CO_2 molecule	Electric discharge	PV, PC	I, C
Copper vapor	510 green	Cu atom	Electric discharge	PC	P
	578 yellow			PC	P
Organic dye	320-970 tunable	Various dyes	Ar, Nd:YAG or other lasers	PR, PC	I
Excimer	126-351 ultraviolet	Various excimers	Electric discharge	PA	E
Erbium:YLF	1228 IR	Er ion	Flashlamp	PD	I
Gold vapor	628 red	Au atom	Electric discharge	PR, PC	P
Helium-neon	632.8 red	Ne atom	Electric discharge	PD aiming, diagnosis‡	C
Krypton	531.0 green	Kr ion	Electric discharge	PC	I
	568.2 yellow			PC	I
	647.0 red			PC	C
Nd:YAG	532 green	Nd ion	Flashlamp	PC	E
	650 red			PC	P
	1064 IR			PD, PC	C
	1300 IR			PD	E
Ruby	694.3 red	Cr ion	Flashlamp	PD	I
				PC	H

*PA, photoablation; PC, photocoagulation; PD, photodisruption; PR, photoradiation; PV, photovaporization.
†C, clinical; E, experimental; H, historical; I, investigational; P, possible clinical use.
‡Laser retinal interferometry, laser Doppler velocimetry, and automated lensometers.

transits before leaving the cavity. Separation of the longitudinal modes by *mode-locking* provides a beam with a series (''train'') of brief spikes.[35] Each spike in the train consists of a group of photons that have made a particular number of intracavity transits. The peak power of the spikes is considerably higher than the average power output that the cavity would have produced without mode locking.

In general, laser action in a resonant cavity commences almost as soon as pumping begins. If the atoms of the active laser medium have a sufficiently long fluorescent lifetime in their metastable state, an opaque shutter placed in the resonant cavity can prevent laser action until an extremely high population inversion is produced. This shutter is known as a *Q-switch*. In Q-switched laser operation, pumping begins (that is, the flashlamp is turned on), but since the Q-switch is closed, a very high population inversion quickly occurs. Then, when the switch is opened very briefly (that is, made transparent) shortly after pumping begins, an extremely brief light pulse of very high power escapes from the cavity. Without the Q-switch, (1) only a smaller population inversion is achieved; (2) light production commences almost as soon as pumping begins; and (3) a lengthier light pulse with lower peak power is produced. The comparatively lengthy 0.25 msec fluorescent lifetime [44] of the neodymium ion in a Nd:YAG laser is quite useful for Q-switched operation, whereas the much shorter 5 nanosecond (1 nsec = 10^{-9} second) lifetime of the argon ion's metastable state is not suitable. Other techniques, such as ''cavity dumping,'' can be used to increase the power output of an ion laser.

Two types of Q-switches are commonly used: a Pockels cell, which is a solid-state device that is switched electronically (''active'' Q-switching); and a dye cell that bleaches, or becomes transparent, when exposed to very high irradiances (''passive'' Q-switching).[35] In addition to Q-switching, the dye cell can also serve to mode-lock the laser output, thereby splitting the Q-switched pulse into a train of even briefer spikes (usually 7 to 9), each of which has a higher peak power than that of the Q-switched pulse without mode-locking.

Laser light

Since a laser's resonant cavity amplifies only photons traveling along its axis, a laser beam is highly directional and has little divergence. Low divergence permits effective focusing of the beam into a small spot of high *irradiance*. (Irradiance is power per unit area and is also termed, less properly, ''power density.'') Most surgical applications of lasers require very high focal irradiances, as discussed in the next section. The spot size into which a laser beam can be focused is directly proportional to (1) the wavelength of the laser light and (2) the focal length of the focusing lens. Thus, 193 nm ultraviolet radiation can be focused into a smaller spot than 1064 nm infrared radiation, and Nd:YAG laser radiation can be focused into a smaller spot size with a short than with a long focal length lens, as discussed in the section on photodisruptors.

Light scattering in the intraocular transit of a laser beam and aberrations in an optical delivery system or in the eye itself can both increase spot size, thereby reducing focal irradiance. For example, the increased Nd:YAG laser focal spot size arising from light scattering caused by an irregular cornea can be reduced by using a contact lens. Light scattering also diminishes contrast in a surgeon's microscopic image. In general an image is more readily improved by altering the orientation of the slitlamp beam or by reducing the height and width of the slit beam, rather than by increasing slitlamp illumination, since increasing illumination only increases veiling back-scattered light. Scattering in ophthalmic laser systems is presented in greater detail elsewhere.[27]

In addition to its directionality, laser light is also monochromatic and spatially and temporally coherent. Monochromaticity means that laser light is composed of one or several individual wavelengths (lines), since there are only a limited number of efficient electronic transitions from metastable to lower-lying electron energy levels. Although no line is completely monochromatic (that is, the spectral line width is not zero), laser light is effectively monochromatic for all current surgical applications in ophthalmology. Monochromaticity permits the selection of particular wavelengths for specific applications or tissue targets, as discussed in the section on photocoagulators. The irradiance at a particular wavelength that is obtainable with a laser is millions of times greater than that attainable by filtering the broad spectral output of a conventional incandescent or arc lamp.

Spatial coherence means that there is good phase correlation across the laser beam. That is, if there is a peak in the electromagnetic wave in the center of the laser beam as it crosses an imaginary plane perpendicular to the path of the laser beam, there will also be a peak in the peripheral part of the laser beam as it crosses the plane. Spatial coherence is primarily caused by the geometry of the resonant cavity.[40] Temporal coherence means that the wavelength of the laser beam does not change in time, since differences between electronic energy levels do not change with time. Neither spatial nor temporal coherence is perfect, but they are characterized by a coherence length that is quite long for a highly coherent beam. For example, the coherence length of a He-Ne laser is 1000 m (for single-mode operation), whereas that of a typical Nd:YAG laser is only 1 cm. Spatial and temporal coherence are essential for diagnostic applications in which laser beams are divided and subsequently recombined, as in retinal interferometry, or compared, as in Doppler velocimetry. Whereas laser beams of high spatial coherence do have low divergence, current surgical applications of the laser do not specifically require spatial and temporal coherence.

LASER EFFECTS

Laser interactions

Laser light entering biologic tissue is either absorbed or scattered. Scattering affects the distribution of photons in the tissue target,[27] but absorption determines the effect of the light. As noted earlier, the absorption of a photon may alter the electronic structure of a molecule, that is, the energy state of electrons circulating around its nuclei. In particular, if irradiances are lower than those produced by Q-switched lasers, photons from ultraviolet or visible radiation generally excite outer shell electrons to higher energy levels; these are the electrons involved in chemical reactions. An excited molecule usually loses this excess electron energy when (1) it participates in a chemical reaction, that is, a photochemical reaction; (2) it collides with another molecule or atom; (3) it releases a photon in spontaneous emission, or (4) the excess electron energy is converted into increased relative motion of the molecule's constituent atoms—a thermal effect. In this latter thermal process, photon absorption has resulted in an increased rate of vibration of atoms relative to their molecule's center of mass, thereby increasing the molecule's vibrational energy level.

Photons from infrared radiation differ from ultraviolet and visible light photons because, in addition to depositing their energy by exciting molecular electrons to higher energy levels, they can also directly transfer energy to the vibrational energy levels of irradiated molecules. Regardless of whether photons induce molecular vibration indirectly by first exciting molecular electrons, or directly as with infrared radiation, the net effect of this transfer of photon energy is an increase in the average vibrational motion of the irradiated molecules. Since the large-scale phenomenon of "heat energy" is equivalent at an atomic level to the kinetic energy of atoms and molecules, light absorption converts photon energy into heat energy, and target tissue "temperature" increases. Furthermore, since vibrating molecules collide with and transfer energy to neighboring molecules, heat energy quickly diffuses over an area much larger than that initially irradiated, in a process known as *heat conduction*. In this effect entropy (crudely, "disorderliness" or "randomness" in the universe) increases, as it must in any natural, irreversible process in an isolated system.

In general molecules in biologic tissues are opaque to ultraviolet radiation at wavelengths shorter than 300 nm and have strong vibrational absorption bands for infrared radiation at wavelengths greater than about 1000 nm.[18] Between 300 and 400 nm only a limited number of biomolecules have moderate absorption. Most biomolecules, however, are effectively transparent between 400 and 1000 nm. Differences in the spectral absorption properties of different molecules permit selective damage to specific components of a target tissue.[27,31] For example, macular xanthophyll in the inner and outer plexiform layers of the neural retina has good absorption below but not above 500 nm. By using argon green (514.5 nm) or krypton red (647.1 nm) rather than argon blue (488.0 nm) laser light, inner retinal damage can be avoided, as discussed in the section on photocoagulators.[42]

Laser effects in biologic tissues may be divided into three general categories: (1) photochemical, (2) thermal, and (3) ionizing. Clinical applications of these effects are summarized in Fig. 6-2.

1. For exposures longer than roughly 1 microsecond (one millionth of a second) and low to moderate irradiances, laser radiation below 320 nm produces primarily photochemical reactions.[18] In these reactions photon absorption by outer electrons is needed to provide the excited molecular electronic state from which the chemical reaction can occur.

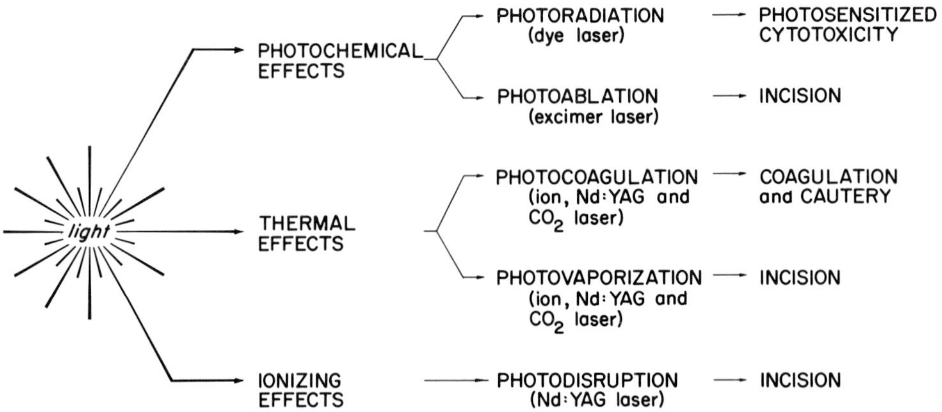

Fig. 6-2. Laser-tissue interactions may be divided into photochemical, thermal, or ionizing effects. (See section on laser effects.)

2. For similar irradiances and exposure durations, laser radiation at longer wavelengths generally produces thermal effects. Thermal effects occur when photon absorption by outer electrons or molecular vibrations produces enough temperature rise to denature biomolecules by breaking the weak van der Waals forces that help to stabilize their complex structures.
3. At very high irradiances, generally produced by exposure durations shorter than 20 nanoseconds, enough energy is provided to tear electrons from atoms and molecules, thereby ionizing them and inducing secondary mechanical effects.[35]

Although it is useful conceptually to differentiate between photochemical, thermal, and ionizing processes, it is also important to recognize that more than one of these processes may be responsible for clinical effects observed at intermediate values of irradiance and exposure time.

Photochemical effects

Photoradiation

Hematoporphyrin derivative (HpD) is selectively taken up and retained by metabolically active tumor tissue, predisposing this tissue to photochemical damage if the tumor is subsequently irradiated with light between 625 and 635 nm. The exposure of photosensitized tumor tissue is termed *photoradiation therapy* (PRT). Current clinical ophthalmic PRT studies are directed toward the treatment of large choroidal melanomas, which are exposed to 630 nm red light from a rhodamine B dye laser 72 hours after intravenous HpD administration.[22] This irradiation produces an excited state of porphyrin, which interacts with oxygen to produce cytoxic singlet oxygen. The gold vapor laser producing 628 nm red light is a potentially useful alternative light source for PRT.

Photoablation

Ultraviolet light at wavelengths shorter than 300 nm generally causes photochemical reactions in biologic tissues, and tissues are effectively opaque in this wavelength region. This is true for the cornea, and excimer lasers producing ultraviolet light below 300 nm can provide precise experimental corneal incisions to predetermined depths.[43] This process may be termed photoablation, and photochemical reactions at the target site not only fragment exposed molecules but also volatilize them.

Carbon dioxide lasers produce infrared radiation to which the cornea or any other water-containing tissue is also opaque, but CO_2 lasers incise the cornea by thermal effects, primarily vaporization but with associated coagulation and cautery.[22,26,32] Thus, whereas CO_2 lasers are useful in tractionless incision of vascular tissue, excimer lasers producing ablation but not cautery would have limited value in that application. On the other hand, an excimer laser has the potential to produce much more precise incisions of avascular tissue because photoablation apparently leaves adjacent tissue unaffected, and its short wavelength radiation can be focused into a much smaller spot size.

Significant questions yet to be resolved regarding excimer laser photoablation include: (1) Which of the available excimer laser wavelengths (listed in Table 6-2) is most appropriate for corneal incision? (2) Does ultraviolet excimer laser radiation have any mutagenic potential? (Questions 1 and 2 are related, and experimental studies probably should address the relative vulnerability of DNA and collagen to specific ultraviolet excimer laser wavelengths.) (3) What is the optimal repetition rate for excimer laser pulses? (Tissue fragments being volatilized could absorb and interfere with incident radiation if the repetition rate were too high.) (4) If there are specific advantages for

Table 6-2. Excimer laser sources*

Laser medium	*Wavelength (nm)*	*Comments*
Fluorine	157	Very limited range in air restricts use
Argon fluoride	193	Experimental corneal photoablation[43]
Krypton chloride	222	Potential corneal photoablation
Krypton fluoride	248	Potential corneal photoablation
Xenon chloride	308	Transmitted by cornea
Nitrogen	337	Transmitted by cornea
Xenon fluoride	351	Transmitted by cornea
Carbon dioxide	10,600	Potential corneal photovaporization[26]

*An excimer is a molecule that forms only when one of its constituent atoms has an electron in an excited state; the molecule does not form under normal conditions when both atoms are in their ground state. In an excimer laser a transverse electric discharge—perpendicular to the axis of the resonant cavity—creates excimer molecules from a mixture of a rare gas and a halogen. The excimer molecules are in a resonant cavity and emit ultraviolet radiation as they return to their ground state. A population inversion occurs because the lower energy level (E_1) of the excimer molecule is depleted immediately when atoms of an excimer molecule dissociate as the molecule returns to its ground state. Pulse lengths for excimer lasers range from 6 to 25 nanoseconds, with repetition rates of 50 to 200 Hz. Energy output depends on the laser size and type of medium, with available pulse energy ranging from 500 mJ for ArF to 5000 mJ for CO_2. Precise ablation of intraocular structures may be feasible with an appropriate intraocular probe.

photoablation over conventional surgical techniques, are they sufficient to warrant the expense, complexity, and potential hazards (toxic gases) of excimer laser instrumentation?

Thermal effects

Photocoagulation

Denaturation of biomolecules occurs at an appreciable rate when ambient temperatures are sufficiently high to overcome weak van der Waals forces stabilizing their structure. Whereas some denaturation may occur even at normal body temperature, renewal processes maintain a physiologic equilibrium unless destabilization is favored by a temperature increase or change in chemical milieu.[18,23,47] In general, (1) nucleic acids are more resistant to thermal injury than collagen; (2) thermal tissue damage requires a 10° to 20° C increase in corneal or retinal temperature [39,45]; and (3) the extent of thermal injury is proportional to the magnitude and duration of a temperature increase, that is, increasing the temperature rise in a target tissue reduces the exposure interval required to produce a given burn severity, and thus "reciprocity" exists between temperature rise and exposure time.[2,7] It should also be noted that a higher temperature rise is required for an immediate photocoagulation lesion than for one that becomes apparent several hours later. Thus a photocoagulation lesion may appear to "spread" because the immediate burn is surrounded by a zone of tissue that has had a temperature rise high enough to produce a delayed but not an immediate lesion.[35]

For a particular spot size and exposure duration, tissue temperature rise from a laser beam is proportional to irradiance, which is the ratio of light power delivered to the area exposed. That is,

$$T \propto E$$

where T is temperature rise of the exposed tissue, and

$$E = P/A$$

where E is irradiance, P is the light power delivered to the surface of the tissue, and A is the tissue area exposed.

Temperature rise in an irradiated tissue is also proportional to light absorption in that tissue,[27,31,33] which in turn is determined by how effectively its constituent molecules absorb incident photons of a particular wavelength. For example, the excellent absorption of visible light by melanin in the trabecular meshwork or retinal pigment epithelium make these tissues excellent targets for argon ion laser photocoagulation. However, the poor absorption of visible light by corneal collagen helps make the cornea an effective window for vision and for photocoagulation or photodisruption. The transparency of the cornea to visible light is primarily a result of the fact that variations in the density of scattering particles are so small relative to the wavelength of light that light scattered in any direction other than forward undergoes destructive interference.[6,27]

Closure of blood vessels by photocoagulation is most likely caused by light absorption in the blood column, which heats the hemoglobin to a temperature high enough to produce thrombus formation[9] and collagen shrinkage in the wall of a blood vessel and its surrounding connective tissue.[16] Since the blood column is moving, vessel effects are often located downstream from the actual exposure site or the site of damage to underlying tissues.[46] It is important to note that light absorption by hemoglobin varies with wavelength and oxygen saturation, as well as other parameters, as shown in Fig. 6-3.[12] For example, the photon penetration depth in hemoglobin is 60 μm for argon green light (514.5 nm) but more than 400 μm for Nd:YAG infrared radiation (1064 nm). Thus argon green light is well absorbed in small intraocular blood vessels and is therefore a good selection for closing them,[3] whereas Nd:YAG infrared radiation deposits only a small fraction of incident radiation in the small vessels.[35] On the other hand, continuous-wave or long-pulse (0.2 to 0.5 second) Nd:YAG lasers are useful for treating very large blood vessels, such as in esophageal varices,[14] because infrared light provides uniform bulk heating. Ideally photon penetration depth of the laser wavelength selected for vessel closure should be the same order of magnitude as the vessel's diameter so that an irradiance can be used that provides effective bulk heating of the blood column without causing superficial damage to the vessel wall at the radiation site.

Photovaporization

If very high laser irradiances are used, tissue temperature can quickly reach the boiling point of water, and rapidly expanding water vapor will cause tissue disruption (photovaporization) before denaturation can cauterize the tissue. In most situations, however, photovaporization (cutting) is accompanied by photocoagulation (cautery). For example, in CO_2 laser surgery, cautery during incision can provide a virtually bloodless operating field.[4,37] Water vaporization tends to stabilize tissue temperature until all the water is boiled off, at which point the temperature increases rapidly again, and carbonization occurs. Pulsed operation of a CO_2 laser at high repetition rates permits higher peak tissue irradiances than continuous-wave operation and should therefore offer a higher ratio of incision to cautery, with a corresponding decrease in thermal damage to surrounding tissues.

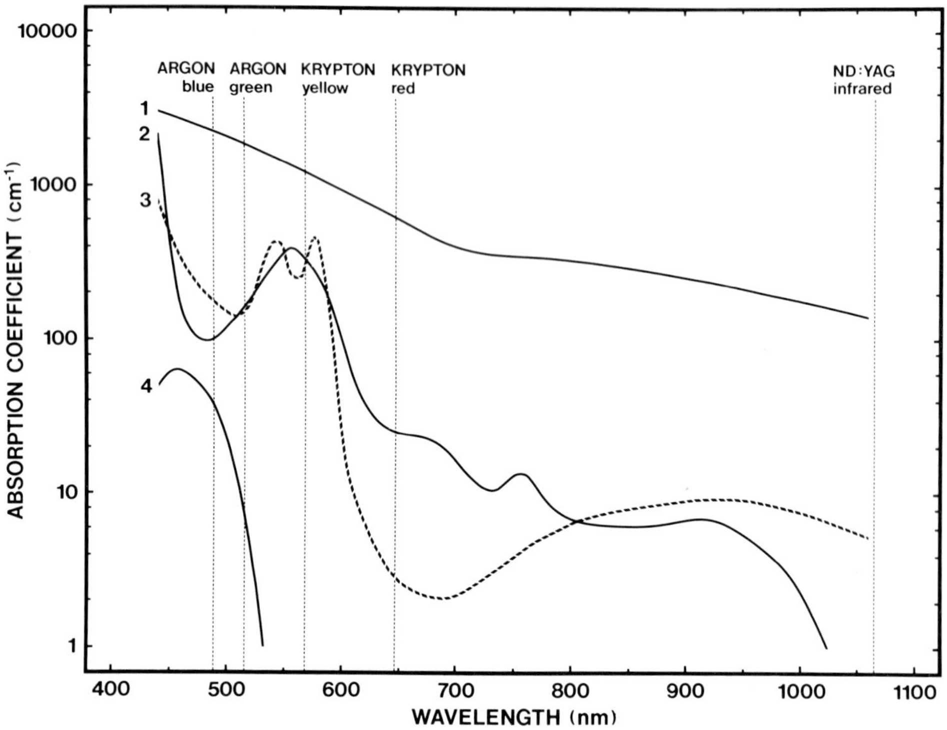

Fig. 6-3. Three primary light absorbers in ocular tissues are melanin *(curve 1),* hemoglobin (reduced, *curve 2;* oxygenated, *curve 3*), and macular xanthophyll *(curve 4)*. Absorption coefficients are presented as function of wavelength, based on data from reference 12.

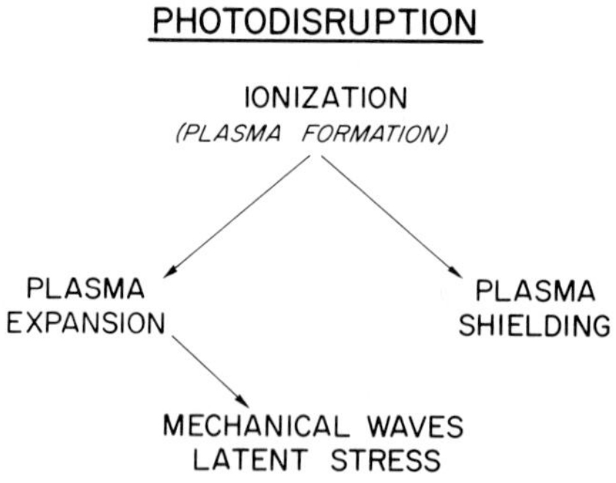

Fig. 6-4. Photodisruption of transparent ocular tissue involves three nonlinear mechanisms.[35] Very high irradiances disintegrate target tissues in focal volume by stripping electrons from atoms and molecules, thereby creating transient plasma of free electrons and ions. (See text.)

The CO_2 laser produces 10,600 nm (10.6 μm) infrared radiation, which is absorbed in water-bearing tissue at a rate comparable to the absorption of argon green light in the retinal pigment epithelium.[26] More than 99% of CO_2 laser radiation is absorbed in the first 50 μm of water-containing tissue that is encountered. Thus the cornea is opaque to CO_2 laser radiation, and intraocular applications require an intraocular probe. The limited range (photon penetration depth) of the CO_2 laser can be an advantage in intraocular applications, however, allowing vitreous syneresis and vaporization, or tractionless cautery and incision of fibrovascular bands without damage to adjacent retina.[11,26,37]

Ionizing effects

Short-pulse Nd:YAG lasers disrupt even transparent tissues by delivering enormous near-infrared (1064 nm) irradiances to tissue targets.[1,15] These irradiances are obtained by using small spot sizes, and extremely brief pulses ranging from 30 nanoseconds down to 20 picoseconds (1 psec = 10^{-12} second). The high irradiance ionizes material in a small volume of space at the laser beam focus, disintegrating it into a collection of ions and electrons called a *plasma*. Plasma may be considered a fourth state of matter that has the mechanical properties of a gas and the electric properties of a metal. Once formed, the plasma (1) absorbs or scatters radiation arriving later in the pulse, thereby shielding underlying tissues; and (2) expands rapidly, producing shock and acoustic (pressure) waves that mechanically disrupt tissue adjacent to the region of disintegration. Additional tissue disruption occurs because of latent stress present in the tissue when the laser incision occurs. Photodisruption is summarized in Fig. 6-4, and details of plasma production and materials effects have been presented previously.[35]

Hazards

The eye is vulnerable to photochemical, thermal, or ionizing damage from inadvertent exposure to intense light sources, but safety standards have been developed for ocular exposures to ultraviolet, visible, and infrared radiation.[41] It is clear that standard clinical photocoagulators and photodisruptors are potentially hazardous and that the characteristics of each clinical instrument and procedure must be fully understood to maximize the benefit-to-risk ratio of any laser operation. It is not as widely understood, however, that reflected laser light could pose a hazard to operating room personnel. The surgeon's eyes are effectively protected against "flashback" by a fixed filter in the operating slitlamp or by a filter with "fail-safe" switching into the field of view during exposures, but unprotected personnel adjacent to the surgeon are vulnerable to potentially hazardous specular reflections from the surface of a contact lens used in the procedure, even if the lens has an antireflection coating. For example, in conventional laser photocoagulation, this hazard extends to a distance of 1.6 m from the coated contact lens,[20] and nearby personnel should wear eye protection appropriate for the laser wavelength being used.

For the past two decades accumulating evidence suggests that photochemical damage from lifelong exposure to ordinary environmental radiation may play a role in the development of certain age-related ocular problems in susceptible individuals. For example, single oxygen formation from photochemical reactions—induced by the ultraviolet light between 300 and 400 nm that passes through the cornea but is absorbed in the crystalline lens—has been implicated in cataractogenesis in experimental animals and in human beings.[21] Similar photochemically generated cytotoxic agents in the retinal pigment epithelium are probably responsible for solar retinitis and welder's maculopathy and may play a significant role in the development of macular degeneration.[17,28,47] Cataract extraction places the aphakic or pseudophakic patient at greater risk to photochemical retinal damage, since potentially hazardous ultraviolet light between 300 and 400 nm previously absorbed by the crystalline lens can now reach the retina.[24,25] This emphasizes the need for properly designing intraocular lenses with an absorption spectrum similar to that of the original adult crystalline lens,[24] and for cautioning aphakic or pseudophakic patients (1) to avoid observing the midday sun or welding arcs and (2) to wear appropriate spectacle filters in unusually bright environmental conditions, such as when boating or snow skiing.[25,28]

PHOTOCOAGULATORS

Light absorption in a target tissue determines the efficiency with which laser light energy is converted to heat energy for photocoagulation. The three primary absorbers in ocular tissues are (1) melanin, (2) macular xanthophyll, and (3) hemogloblin. (See Fig. 6-3.[12])

Melanin is the best absorber, but since its absorption does not vary substantially between 400 and 700 nm, its absorption spectrum is not a principal factor in selecting a surgical laser system producing visible light. Thus there should be little difference between argon blue plus green, argon green, and even krypton red in laser trabeculoplasty, in which melanin in the trabecular mesh is presumably the primary absorber. On the other hand, melanin's absorption definitely decreases with increasing wavelength, which is one of the reasons that a chorioretinal burn becomes deeper as wavelength increases. In general the deeper the burn, the more painful and less ophthalmoscopically prominent it is. Argon green is absorbed at the level of the pigment epithelium and choriocapillaris, krypton red produces a deeper lesion, and Nd:YAG causes primary choroidal and even scleral effects.

When using longer wavelengths, it is important to remember that the ophthalmoscopic appearance of a burn is different from that of an argon lesion. If a similar burn appearance is obtained—a markedly suprathreshold burn—choroidal damage will be much more extensive than that produced by the argon laser. Thus it is often safer with longer wavelengths to use longer and lower power exposures, which produce safer lesions that have a lower ratio of temperature rise in the burn center to that at the burn periphery as a result of heat conduction.[27,31] By using longer exposures that minimize this ratio, peak temperature rise in the center will be lowest for a lesion of a particular size, and thus the probability of iatrogenic hemorrhage will be minimized in posterior segment photocoagulation.

Macular xanthophyll absorbs well in blue, poorly in green, and minimally in yellow and red light. Thus, if blue light is used for macular photocoagulation, direct inner retinal damage will be produced in addition to the desired pigment epithelial and subretinal lesion.[36] This inner retinal damage not only is a source of needless nerve tissue loss, but also obscures posttreatment fluorescein angiographic detection of persistent or recurrent choroidal neovascularization and obstructs retreatment of neovascularization when present.[42] In addition, blue light is scattered more in intraocular transit (Rayleigh scattering increases with decreasing wavelength[27]) and is absorbed more in an aging lens than other wavelengths in the visible spectrum, thereby necessitating higher corneal irradiances when ocular media are hazy. Thus blue light has fundamental disadvantages for macular photocoagulation, and argon green and krypton red lasers are preferred now for macular applications. The relative merits of alternative laser wavelengths for macular photocoagulation are detailed elsewhere,[19,27] but both argon green and krypton red lasers appear to be useful, and only further clinical and experimental studies can determine the most appropriate applications for each.

Hemoglobin absorbs well in blue, green, and yellow but poorly in red. As shown in Fig. 6-3, red light has better absorption in reduced than in oxygenated hemoglobin, which is one reason why retinal veins are more prominent than retinal arteries in monochromatic red ophthalmoscopy. The disadvantages of Nd:YAG infrared radiation for treating small intraocular blood vessels have been discussed earlier. The poor absorption of Nd:YAG radiation in both melanin and reduced hemoglobin may be useful, however, in photocoagulating through heavily pigmented structures or long-standing hemorrhages, provided that very-long-pulse (0.2 to 0.5 second) or continuous-wave Nd:YAG sources are used so that the potentially hazardous high irradiances of shorter exposures are avoided. In this latter application it is interesting to note that Nd:YAG infrared radiation actually has better absorption in oxygenated hemoglobin than krypton red light (see Fig. 6-3) and may therefore be more effective in treating pigmented, vascularized structures. It is important, however, to reemphasize that the safety margin between lesion and iatrogenic hemorrhage becomes progressively smaller as pulse length is shortened.[8,35] This is a main reason why pulsed ruby laser photocoagulators were superseded by continuous-wave argon laser systems, and why current commercial Nd:YAG photodisruptor systems offering 0.0002 to 0.02 second exposures in a non-Q-switched thermal mode are potentially hazardous for retinal applications.[35]

Clinical laser photocoagulators generally consist of (1) an argon or krypton laser source, (2) a fiberoptic or mirror arm apparatus to deliver the laser source output to the slitlamp delivery system, and (3) a slitlamp to view the target tissue and to direct the aiming and treatment beam to a desired location on the target tissue.[30] Fiberoptic delivery systems provide flexible slitlamp movement and reasonably uniform distribution of power across the focal spot. Mirror arm systems are less flexible but preserve the transverse mode structure of the laser beam and thus can provide smaller spot sizes than fiberoptic systems.

Photocoagulator use is simplified by contact lenses designed for specific clinical applications, and lenses currently available for anterior and posterior segment photocoagulation are analyzed in a previous report.[13] These lenses generally have a broad-spectrum antireflection coating that reduces light reflection in the visible spectrum from approximately 4% to less than 1% for normal incidence. The purpose of this coating is to reduce reflected (1) slitlamp (white) light and (2) laser light.

1. Slitlamp light scattered back from the surface of a contact lens reduces the contrast in a surgeon's microscopic image. Since tissue targets or localizing structures are often small and subtle features, it is useful to minimize this scattered white light by using antireflecting coatings. As already noted, regardless of the contact lens, reducing slit height and width is usually more effective than increasing slitlamp illumination for improving microscopic image quality when ocular media are hazy (to minimize veiling back-scattered light). Computerized image enhancement of a video image[34] of target structures could also expedite target structure visualization through hazy media in future photocoagulator systems.

2. Although clinical photocoagulators have enough power for most applications, a coated contact lens surface does reduce back-scattering of laser light, thereby increasing target tissue irradiance for a particular power setting. More significantly, however, coating a contact lens surface reduces the potential hazard to an observer standing behind

the surgeon, as discussed previously. It is also important to recognize that light scattering from media opacities can cause the laser aiming beam to flicker. If higher power settings are used to treat through rather than around opacities, there are two dangers. First, when the laser beam is displaced off the opacity, scattering will decrease, spot size at the target will also decrease (that is, irradiance will increase), and a hemorrhage could result if power is not reduced appropriately. Second, light absorption by an opacity in the path of the laser beam, such as pigment on the crystalline lens, can produce enough heat to damage a contiguous structure. Thus a flickering aiming beam is a warning to use the beam manipulator, when feasible, to treat around rather than through opacities.

Wavelengths of current commercial laser photocoagulator systems are shown in Fig. 6-5. Argon laser systems provide bichromatic blue plus green (488 nm blue plus 514.5 nm green) or green-only (514.5 nm) light, whereas commercial krypton lasers provide red-only (647 nm) light. Laser systems are now available in argon-only, krypton-only, or argon plus krypton configurations. Other potentially useful laser sources not currently available commercially include (see Table 6-1): high-power krypton (531 nm green, 568 nm yellow or 647 nm red); copper vapor (510 nm green or 578 nm yellow); frequency-doubled Nd:YAG (high-frequency, pulsed operation producing 532 nm green); organic dye (tunable, including 631 nm for post–HpD irradiation); gold vapor (628 nm red); and continuous-wave or very-long-pulse Nd:YAG (1064 nm infrared).

Clinical argon and krypton photocoagulators have power, pulse duration, and spot-size settings. Spot-size selector systems are either of the defocus or parfocal type. The cone angle of the beam in a fiberoptic system is generally larger than that in a mirror arm system, and therefore a small axial (anterior or posterior) slitlamp movement can

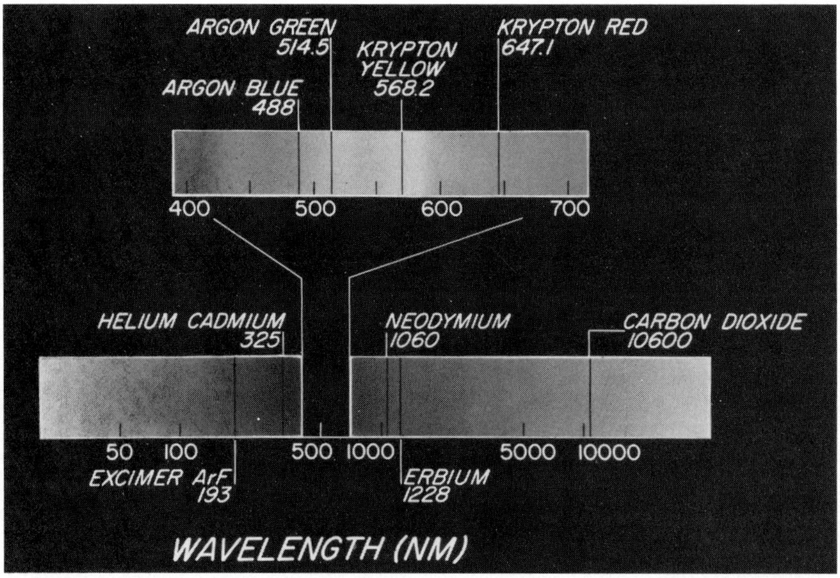

Fig. 6-5. Current clinical photocoagulators use laser sources that produce visible light, but Nd:YAG lasers in photodisruptor systems generate invisible near-infrared radiation. CO_2 lasers produce much longer wavelength infrared radiation, whereas experimental excimer lasers generate ultraviolet radiation.

cause a marked change in the spot size diameter. For this reason most fiberoptic systems use a parfocal-type spot size selector, at least for smaller spot sizes, in which spot size is varied by changing magnification; the spot size selected is the smallest spot size that can be achieved. Mirror arm systems often use defocus spot size selectors, in which spot size is increased merely by posteriorly displacing the focal plane of the treatment beam; since the cone angle is smaller with a mirror arm system, spot size is less sensitive to small axial slitlamp movements.

As noted earlier, tissue temperature increase is proportional to irradiance (''power density''). Thus, for a given power setting and exposure time, spot size determines temperature increase, and therefore uniformity and reproducibility of clinical results require accurate spot size selection. Regardless of the type of spot size selector that a photocoagulator has, it is important to realize that spot size settings are not correct unless the target tissue is properly located at the working distance of the slitlamp microscope. Since the operator may accommodate and the slitlamp has a considerable depth of field, it is imperative that a surgeon determine the proper ocular settings for each instrument and that the instrument itself be properly aligned.

Perhaps the simplest way of being sure that the ocular settings are correct is to use the aiming bar or reticle supplied by the manufacturer, fog (add excess plus power in the ocular), and then slowly decrease ocular power until the aiming bar or reticle first appears sharp. With those ocular settings the surgeon's unaccommodated retina is conjugate with the working distance of the slitlamp. If the slitlamp is then moved forward, with the control stick directed back toward the surgeon, until the target tissue is sharply in focus, then the target tissue will be at the slitlamp working distance, and spot size settings will be valid. Furthermore, any forward movement of the control stick can only increase spot size, thereby reducing irradiance and producing a larger spot size of lower peak temperature rise. This maneuver is useful for decreasing irradiance quickly to surround a retinal hemorrhage if one occurs during treatment. Hemorrhages can be virtually eliminated, however, if the surgeon is familiar with the ophthalmoscopic end point for each wavelength used and if irradiance is minimized for each region treated. Areas of increased subretinal pigmentation that are not apparent ophthalmoscopically can still pose a rare problem, although they can be detected with monochromatic red ophthalmoscopy. Nonetheless, if improper ocular settings are used, difficulties may arise—regardless of the type of spot size selector in the photocoagulator—if slitlamp movement inadvertently reduces spot size and increases focal irradiance.

PHOTODISRUPTORS

Commercial laser photodisruptors generally consist of (1) a high-power, Q-switched, Nd:YAG laser (with or without mode-locking) that produces invisible, 1064 nm infrared radiation; (2) an articulated or directly coupled mirror system that delivers the infrared radiation to the slitlamp (irradiance is too high for fiberoptic transmission); (3) a low-power, continuous-wave (CW), aiming/focusing, helium-neon (He-Ne) laser that produces 632.8 nm red light; (4) a lens system for focusing the Nd:YAG beam into a small spot size at the working distance slitlamp; and (5) a slitlamp for aiming and focusing the visible He-Ne beam and hence the Nd:YAG treatment beam on selected tissue targets.[29,35]

Q-switched, non-mode-locked lasers produce single pulses or bursts of one to nine pulses, each of which is 2 to 14 nanoseconds, depending on the individual photodisruptor. Q-switched, mode-locked lasers produce a train of seven to nine 30-picosecond spikes over roughly a 30-nanosecond pulse interval and can also be used in multiple-pulse, burst operation. Mode-locked photodisruptors are generally more complex instruments, requiring a long resonant cavity and periodic replacement of the dye in the cell used for Q-switching and mode-locking, whereas non-mode-locked systems can be much smaller and use a simple, solid-state Pockels cell for switching. Mode-locked and non-mode-locked systems have been compared in a previous report.[35]

The treatment beam in an ion laser photocoagulator is merely an intensification of the aiming beam, so there is no possibility of disalignment of the two beams. In a photodisruptor, however, aiming/focusing and treatment beams are produced by two separate sources, the treatment beam is invisible, and the clinician must depend on the manufacturer to accurately and reliably align the aiming/focusing beam with the treatment beam. Most manufacturers minimize the number of mechanical linkages connecting the laser sources to the slitlamp to reduce the possibility of disalignment of the laser beams. Disalignment would be manifested as ''beam walk'' of the treatment beam around the aiming/focusing beam—differences in their relative positions for different slitlamp orientations—and the aiming beam would then no longer identify the exact location of the treatment beam. Ideally all components should be connected directly to or mounted on the slitlamp to eliminate disalignment. One simple method of checking alignment is to make test spots on photographic paper that has been exposed and developed, but the manufacturer should be consulted promptly any time trouble is suspected.

The photodisruptor aiming/focus beam must not only provide a visible spot for selecting tissue targets, as in a photocoagulator, but must also provide an accurate and reliable method for placing the beam waist (focal spot) at the axial location of the tissue target. Current photodisruptors use either single- or multiple-beam aiming/focusing systems. With a single-beam system, the slitlamp control stick is moved forward and backward to minimize the size of a red aiming spot on the target tissue. With a multiple-beam system (double or triple beam), the control stick is moved forward or backward until the multiple (two or three) spots fuse into one on the target tissue.

Although multiple-beam aiming/focusing systems have an easier and more reproducible end point for axial focusing than single-beam systems, even with a single-beam system it is usually possible to open an opacified posterior capsule directly apposed to the posterior surface of a posterior chamber intraocular lens without marking the lens. This can be accomplished by locating the first exposure just posterior to the capsule and using low-energy settings just above breakdown threshold, usually less than 1 mJ. The first exposure not only initiates discission but displaces the capsule posteriorly and provides optically inhomogeneous borders where breakdown threshold is reduced. Regardless of the aiming/focusing system used, accurate focusing requires spending enough time before actual exposures to determine an orientation of the slitlamp beam that provides effective direct or retroillumination of the capsule but minimizes the bright specular reflex from the polymethylmethacrylate lens. As with photocoagulators, proper slitlamp ocular settings should be used at all times, as already described.

High irradiances are achieved at the working distance of the slitlamp, where the aiming/focusing beam is also focused, by using a converging lens to focus the treatment beam into a small spot. Since spot size is proportional to lens focal length, a short focal length lens that provides a large cone angle will produce a small focal spot and high irradiance. Thus increasing the cone angle increases the focal irradiance and decreases the irradiance at structures anterior and posterior to the focal plane.[35] If the focal length is too short, however, there is little room for a contact lens between the photodisruptor and the patient's cornea, and part of the Nd:YAG beam may be lost at the border of the pupil when midvitreous structures are treated. On the other hand, a long focal length lens provides a small cone angle that facilitates contact lens use and vitreous applications but produces a larger spot size with a lower irradiance in the focal plane and higher irradiance at structures posterior to the focal plane. Clinical Nd:YAG photodisruptor systems represent a balance between the advantages of short and long focal length lenses, with most companies selecting cone angles ranging from 14 to 17 degrees to ensure high focal volume irradiances and low retinal irradiances.[29,35] Additional details of photodisruptor instrumentation and clinical applications have been presented in other publications.[5,35]

NEW DEVELOPMENTS

In ophthalmic laser applications, demonstration of clinical efficacy has often preceded firm comprehension of the reasons for that efficacy. Although fundamental improvements in clinical instrumentation must await better understanding both of the interaction of laser radiation with ocular tissues and of the pathophysiology of successful laser therapy for specific ocular problems, certain improvements in current laser instrumentation are promising.

Multiple laser tube photocoagulators that permit rapid switching between different wavelengths are now becoming available, such as argon green plus krypton red. These systems should permit (1) selection of appropriate wavelengths for specific tissues or media properties; (2) analysis of the efficacy of posttreatment with a different wavelength; (3) prompt response to intraoperative problems (for example, treating a hemorrhage from krypton red with argon green light that is well absorbed in hemoglobin); and (4) intraoperative monochromatic ophthalmoscopy to detect potential hazards (for example, using monochromatic red to inspect subretinal features not apparent in white light ophthalmoscopy).

As laser technology progresses, the cost of current instrumentation should decrease and its reliability should increase. New types of lasers, such as the copper vapor and frequency-doubled Nd:YAG lasers, may be useful for ophthalmic photocoagulation, and the continuous-wave Nd:YAG laser may be effective for treating densely pigmented structures, such as intraocular tumors.

Control of exposure duration by monitoring the light reflected from a tissue target (fundus reflectometry) could provide a more objective end point for photocoagulation than the subjective appearance of a retinal burn to the surgeon.[8,38] Furthermore, if difficult technical problems can be solved, characteristic changes in the reflectance of an evolving lesion could be used to shut off a laser exposure at an appropriate point on the curve of reflectance vs. time, as in ordinary exposure-controlled flash photography. Effective reflectometry control could improve both the safety and the uniformity of conventional photocoagulation with various wavelengths that produce retinal burns of different ophthalmoscopic appearance.

Scanning laser ophthalmoscopy is a new technique that provides a real-time television image of the retina with light levels less than $1/1000$ of that required for indirect ophthalmoscopy.[34] By varying the intensity of the scanning laser beam as it sweeps across the retina, test stimuli may be placed on specific retinal loci and observed directly on the television screen so that the exact anatomic locus of visual deficits can be determined. Scanning laser ophthalmoscopy could provide an integrated system for macular perimetry, fluorescein angiography, macular photocoagulation, and low vision rehabilitation.

REFERENCES

1. Aron-Rosa, D., and others: Use of the neodymium-yag laser to open the posterior lens capsule after lens implant surgery: a preliminary report, Am. Intraocul. Implant Soc. J. **6:**352, 1980.
2. Arrhenius, S.: Uber die reaktionsgeschwindigkeit bei der inversion von rohrzucker durch sauren, Z. Physik Chemie **4:**226, 1889.
3. Bebie, H., and others: Theoretical estimate of the temperature within irradiated retinal vessels, Acta Ophthalmol. **52:**13, 1974.
4. Beckman H., and Fuller, T.A.: Carbon dioxide laser scleral dissection and filtering procedure for glaucoma, Am. J. Ophthalmol. **88:**73, 1979.
5. Belcher, C.D., III, Mainster, M.A., and Buzney, S.M.: Current status of Neodymium:YAG lasers in ophthalmology, part 1, Ann. Ophthalmol. **15:**997, 1983; part 2, **15:**1097, 1983, part 3, **16:**13, 1984.
6. Benedek, G.B.: Theory of transparency of the eye, Appl. Opt. **10:**459, 1971.
7. Birngruber, R.: Thermal modeling in biological tissues. In Hillenkamp, F., Pratesi, R., and Sacchi, C.A., editors: Lasers in biology and medicine, New York, 1980, Plenum Publishing Corp.
8. Birngruber, R., Gabel, V.-P., and Hillenkamp, F.: Fundus reflectometry: a step towards optimization of retinal photocoagulation, Mod. Probl. Ophthalmol. **18:**383, 1977.
9. Boergen K.-P., Birngruber, R., and Hillenkamp, F.: Laser-induced endovascular thrombosis as a possibility of selective vessel closure, Ophthalmic Res. **13:**139, 1981.
10. Boettner, E.A., and Wolter, J.R.: Transmission of the ocular media, Ophthalmology **1:**776, 1962.
11. Bridges, T.J., and others: Syneresis of vitreous by carbon dioxide laser radiation, Science **219:**1217, 1983.
12. Bursell, S.E., Mainster, M.A., and Sliney, D.H.: Spectral properties of ocular pigments. (Unpublished data.)
13. Dieckert, J.P., Mainster, M.A., and Ho, P.C.: Contact lenses for laser applications, Ophthalmology **90S:**55, 1983.
14. Dwyer, R.M.: The technique of gastrointestinal laser endoscopy. In Goldman, L., editor: The biomedical laser: technology and clinical applications, New York, 1981, Springer-Verlag New York, Inc.
15. Fankhauser, F., and others: Clinical studies on the efficiency of high power laser radiation upon some structures of the anterior segment of the eye, Int. Ophthalmol. **3:**129, 1981.
16. Gorisch, W., and Boergen K.-P.: Heat-induced contraction of blood vessels, Lasers Surg. Med. **2:**1, 1982.
17. Ham, W.T., Jr., and others: The nature of retinal radiation damage: dependence on wavelength, power level and exposure time, Vision Res. **20:**1105, 1980.
18. Hillenkamp, F.: Interaction between laser radiation and biological systems. In Hillenkamp, F., Pratesi, R., and Sacchi, C.A., editors: Lasers in biology and medicine, New York, 1980, Plenum Publishing Corp.
19. Ho, P.C., and Mainster, M.A.: Macular photocoagulation: which laser, J. Ocul. Therapy Surg. **2:**78, 1983.
20. Jenkins, D.L.: Hazard evaluation of the Coherent model 900 photocoagulator laser system, non-ionizing radiation protection special study no. 25-42-0310-79, (NTIS no. ADA 068713). Aberdeen Proving Ground, 1979, U.S. Army Environment Hygiene Agency.
21. Lerman, S.: Radiant energy and the eye, New York, 1980, Macmillan Publishing Co.
22. L'Esperance, F.A., Jr.: Ophthalmic lasers: photocoagulation, photoradiation, and surgery, ed. 2, St. Louis, 1983, The C.V. Mosby Co.
23. Mainster, M.A.: Destructive light adaptation, Ann. Ophthalmol. **2:**44, 1970.
24. Mainster, M.A.: Spectral transmittance of intraocular lenses and retinal damage from intense light sources, Am. J. Ophthalmol. **85:**167, 1978.
25. Mainster, M.A.: Solar retinitis, photic maculopathy and the pseudophakic eye, Am. Intraocular Implant Soc. J. **4:**84, 1978.
26. Mainster, M.A.: Ophthalmic applications of infrared lasers—thermal considerations, Invest. Ophthalmol. Vis. Sci. **18:**414, 1979.
27. Mainster, M.A.: Macular photocoagulation: laser principles and applications. In Yannuzzi, R.A., Gitter, K.A., and Schatz, H., editors: The macula: a comprehensive text and atlas, ed. 2, Baltimore, 1984, Williams & Wilkins.
28. Mainster, M.A., Ham, W.T., Jr., and Delori, F.C.: Potential retinal hazards: instrument and environmental light sources, Ophthalmology **90:**927, 1983.
29. Mainster, M.A., Ho, P.C., and Mainster, K.J.: Nd:YAG laser photodisruptors, Ophthalmology **90S:**45, 1983.

30. Mainster, M.A., Ho, P.C., and Mainster, K.J.: Argon and krypton laser photocoagulators, Ophthalmology **90S:**48, 1983.
31. Mainster, M.A., White, T.J., and Allen, R.G.: Spectral dependence of retinal damage produced by intense light sources, J. Opt. Soc. Am. **60:**848, 1970.
32. Mainster, M.A., White, T.J., and Tips, J.H.: Corneal thermal response to the CO_2 laser, Appl. Opt. **9:**665, 1970.
33. Mainster, M.A., and others: Transient thermal behavior in biological systems, Bull. Math. Biophys. **32:**303, 1970.
34. Mainster, M.A., and others: Scanning laser ophthalmoscopy: clinical applications, Ophthalmology **89:**852, 1982.
35. Mainster, M.A., and others: Laser photodisruptors: damage mechanisms, instrument design and safety, Ophthalmology **90:**973, 1983.
36. Marshall, J., Hamilton, A.M., and Bird, A.C.: Intra-retinal absorption of argon laser irradiation in human monkey retinae, Experientia **30:**1355, 1974.
37. Miller, J.B., and others: Transvitreal carbon dioxide laser photocautery and vitrectomy, Ophthalmology **85:**1195, 1978.
38. Pomerantzeff, O., and others: Time and location analysis of lesion formation in photocoagulation, Arch. Ophthalmol. **101:**954, 1983.
39. Priebe, L.A., Cain, C.P., and Welch, A.J.: Temperature rise required for the production of minimal lesions in the Macaca mulatta retina, Am. J. Ophthalmol. **79:**405, 1975.
40. Ready, J.F.: Industrial applications of lasers, New York, 1978, Academic Press, Inc.
41. Sliney, D.H., and Wolbarsht, M.L.: Safety with lasers and other optical sources, New York, 1980, Plenum Publishing Corp.
42. Trempe, C.L., and others: Macular photocoagulation: optimal wavelength selection, Ophthalmology **89:**721, 1982.
43. Trokel, S.L., Srinivasan, R., and Braren, B.: Excimer laser surgery of the cornea, Am. J. Ophthalmol. **96:**710, 1983.
44. Weber, M.J.: CRC handbook of laser science and technology, vol. 1, lasers and masers, Boca Raton, Fla., 1972, CRC Press, Inc.
45. White, T.J., and others: Chorioretinal temperature increases from solar observation, Bull. Math. Biophys. **33:**1, 1971.
46. Wieder, M., Pomerantzeff O., and Schneider, J.: Retinal vessel photocoagulation: a quantitative comparison of argon and krypton laser effects, Invest. Ophthalmol. Vis. Sci. **20:**418, 1981.
47. Young, R.W.: A theory of central retinal disease. In Sears, M.L., editor: New directions in ophthalmic research, New Haven, 1981, Yale University Press.

7

Pigmentary glaucoma

David G. Campbell
John W. Boys-Smith*

Pigmentary glaucoma (PG)[6,14,20,21] is one of the more fascinating open-angle glaucomas. The disease generally strikes early in life and is seen most commonly in young myopic males. In some fortunate instances the disorder can resolve spontaneously. The characteristic signs involve dispersion of pigment in the anterior and posterior chambers. This dispersion can manifest as a Krukenberg's spindle (Fig. 7-1), as a pigment line on or above Schwalbe's line, or as new pigment on the anterior surface of the iris. It may also appear as a circular posterior lenticular line (Fig. 7-2), representing pigment caught in the angle of the hyaloideocapsular ligament, as pigment within the aqueous, or occasionally as pigment on the zonules (Fig. 7-3). The most serious aspect of the pigment dispersion is seen gonioscopically as pigment collecting heavily within the trabecular meshwork (Fig. 7-4), obstructing outflow, and causing pressure elevation.

The source of the pigment[3,19] is the neuroectodermally derived posterior surface of the iris. Characteristic peripheral radial, slitlike transillumination defects (Fig. 7-5) develop as the pigment leaves this posterior surface. The slits can occasionally enlarge at their midportions and connect, forming a continuous transillumination ring through which the shadow of the lens edge can often be seen.

The etiologic basis of pigmentary glaucoma has long been debated. Some investigators believe that the glaucoma is a form of congenital glaucoma[11,15,16,18,23]; others maintain that it is a variant of chronic open-angle glaucoma[1,2]; and still others think that pigment itself is the cause of the glaucoma.[10,20]

THE NEW THEORY

Recently I proposed a new theory reaffirming the belief that the pigment is the cause of the problem in pigmentary glaucoma.[7] The theory states that rubbing between the posterior surface of the iris and anterior packets of zonules in predisposed eyes is the cause of pigment loss from the posterior surface of the iris. I noted that almost all patients with early pigmentary glaucoma have a concavity in the peripheral iris, most easily seen gonioscopically, that contrasts to the more normal flat or slightly convex iris seen in most eyes. In this configuration the iris could then rub against anterior zonules. Anatomic studies showed that whereas normal eyes with flat irides do not exhibit contact between the posterior surface of the iris and zonules, only a small separation exists—a

*M.D., Department of Ophthalmology, Tulane University School of Medicine, New Orleans, La.

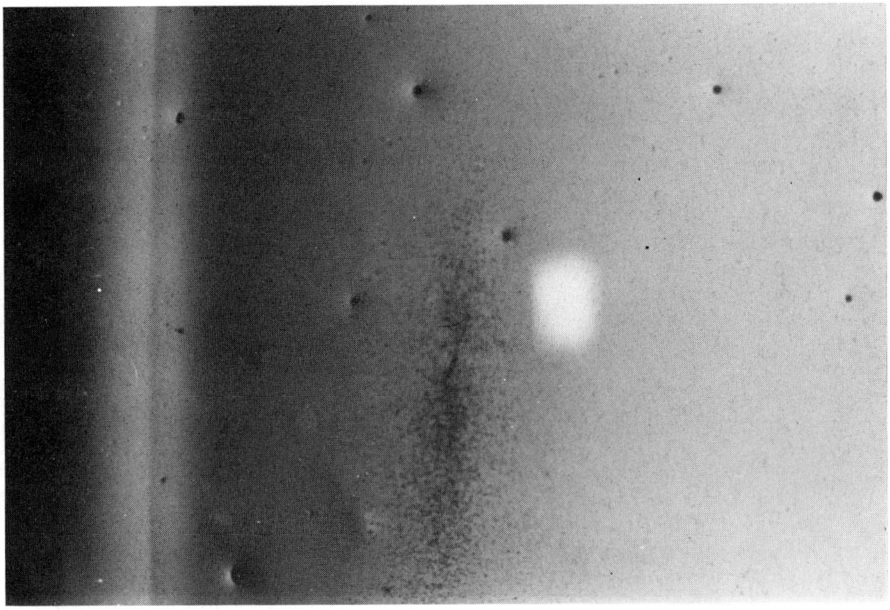

Fig. 7-1. Krukenberg's spindle in patient with pigmentary glaucoma.

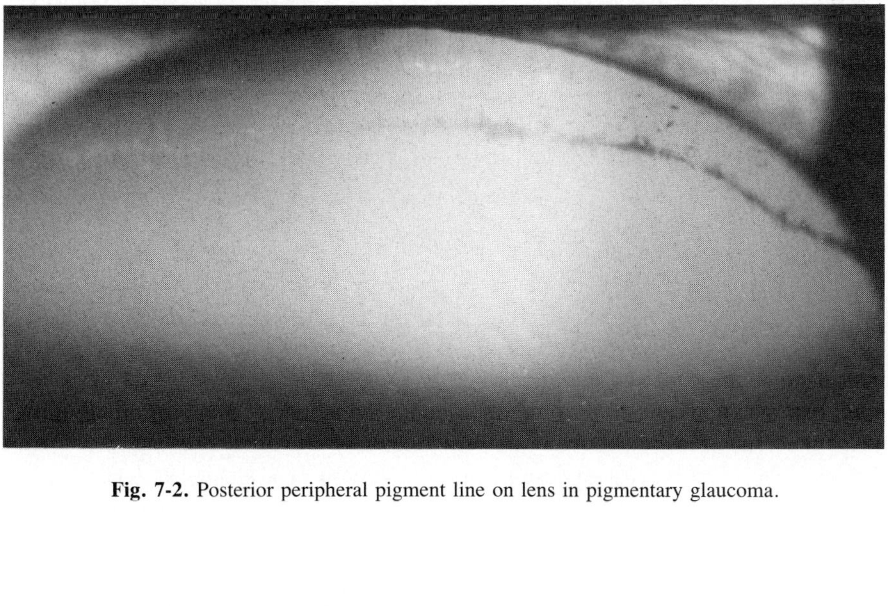

Fig. 7-2. Posterior peripheral pigment line on lens in pigmentary glaucoma.

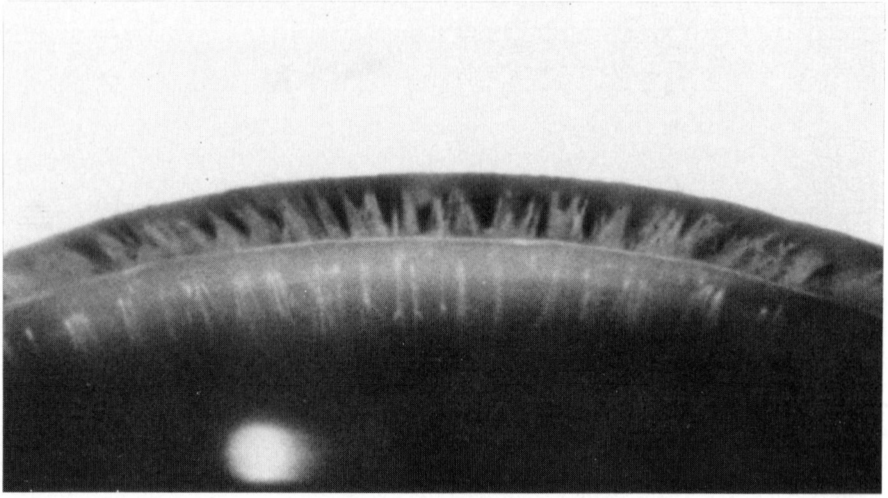

Fig. 7-3. Heavy and unusual deposits of zonules in pigmentary glaucoma. (Courtesy E.M. Van Buskirk, M.D.)

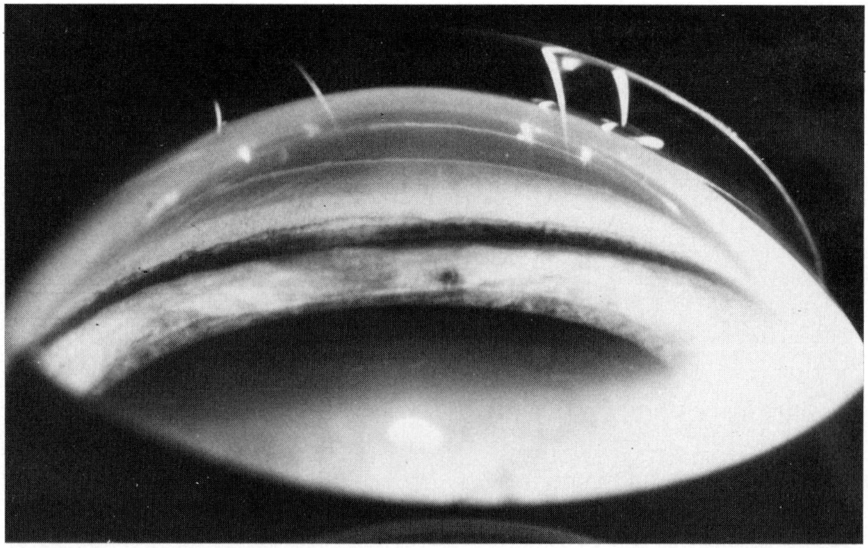

Fig. 7-4. Dark pigment band in trabecular meshwork in pigmentary glaucoma.

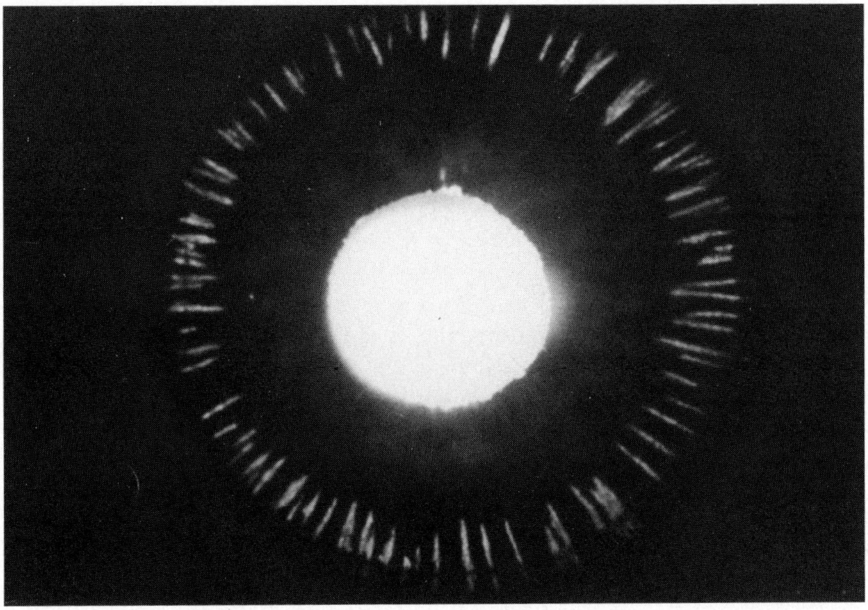

Fig. 7-5. Peripheral radial, slitlike transillumination defects of iris in pigmentary glaucoma (Courtesy Robert C. Allen, M.D.; photograph by Mark Maio.)

separation easily overcome by slight posterior iris displacement. These studies also demonstrated that the zonules do not insert on the anterior lens surface singly, but rather in groups or packets, approximately one packet or more per ciliary process. Such packets would be strong enough to rub pigment off the posterior surface of the iris.

Additional studies have shown a correlation between the total number of peripheral radial slits that develop in a fully transilluminating iris and the total anterior packets in the normal eye. Finally studies of enucleated eyes with characteristic peripheral, slitlike transillumination defects have shown extreme proximity between the iris and the zonules, along with an anatomic correlation between the defects and underlying packets. Histologic examination of these defects has lent further confirmation to the mechanical theory in that no iris pathology other than that which might be expected from mechanical rubbing have been observed; the iris was normal except in the defect areas. In these areas mechanically created grooves in the iris were occasionally noted. Pigment-filled macrophages were seen frequently and represented macrophages removing pigment that had been rubbed into the stroma of the iris. Occasional hypertrophy of the dilator muscle was presumed to be a cellular reaction secondary to the frictional rubbing. The initial studies reported from our laboratory have been confirmed.[9]

If correct, this theory explains some of the previously more puzzling aspects of the disease. The disease tends to occur in myopic eyes because these larger eyes provide space between the lens and the enlarged ciliary body ring, in which the peripheral iris may drape posteriorly, predisposing the iris to rubbing. In addition, the disease generally begins in early adult life (ages 20 to 30), since at this time or shortly before the myopic eye reaches its full size. Finally men may tend to develop the disease more frequently than women because they have larger eyes in general.

Spontaneous resolution of the disease would then occur with aging, when the peripheral irides of all eyes tend to move forward as a result of increased lens size, increased miosis, and resultant increased relative pupillary block. In pigmentary glaucoma, such peripheral, forward bowing of the iris separates the iris from the zonules and halts the rubbing of pigment from the posterior surface of the iris, in turn stopping the alluvial flow of pigment that can be so damaging to the trabecular meshwork. Forward bowing of the iris also explains why pigmentary glaucoma rarely develops in the elderly, a proposition borne out by fact.

MODE OF TRABECULAR OBSTRUCTION

The manner in which pigment obstructs the trabecular meshwork is both interesting and unexpected. Although the investigator might initially suppose that the pigment would cause primary obstruction of the intertrabecular spaces, leading to increased resistance to outflow and consequential elevation of intraocular pressure, electron microscopic studies have shown that the obstruction seems to result from obstruction by cellular debris[12,17] and trabecular beam collapse (Fig. 7-6).

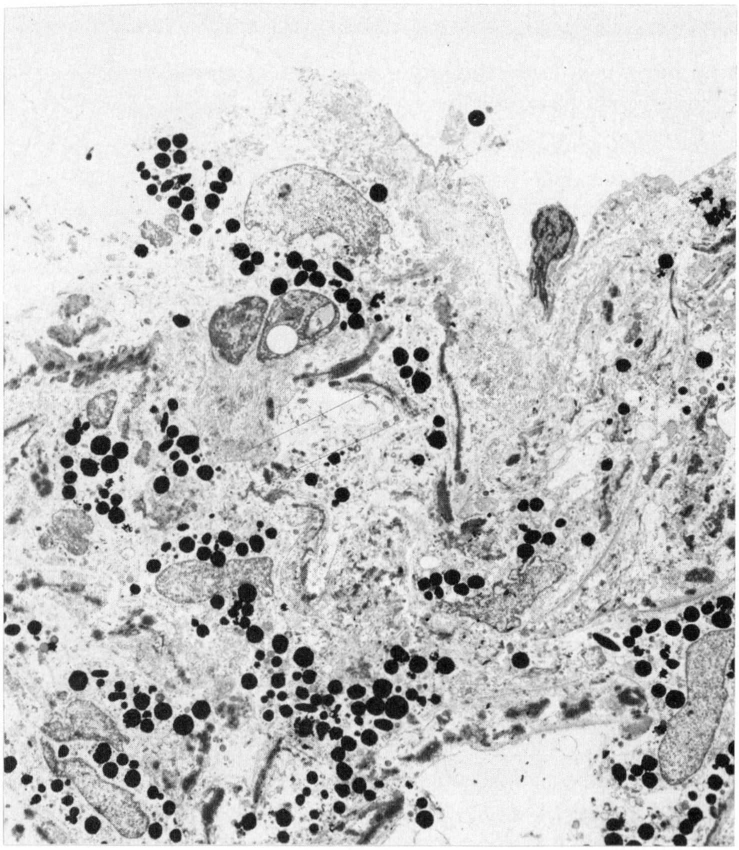

Fig. 7-6. Trabecular meshwork specimen of pigmentary glaucoma, with Schlemm's canal *above*. Cellular disorganization and trabecular beam collapse predominate.

Confirmatory studies[9] done in our laboratory have shown that when perfused pigment strikes the trabecular meshwork, it is quickly phagocytized by the endothelial cells that line the trabecular beams. It appears that if too much pigment is presented, the cells disintegrate and migrate off the beams, leaving them bare and prone to collapse. The disintegrated cells collect in the juxtacanicular region, further obstructing outflow. The process of phagocytosis and secondary obstruction can be reversed if too much permanent damage has not been done; this can be contrasted to the trabecular meshwork pathology in ghost cell glaucoma,[13] another glaucoma caused by particles. In this disease, ghost cells do cause primary obstruction of the trabecular channels, and phagocytosis with secondary disruption of the trabecular meshwork seems to play almost no role.

PATIENT CLASSIFICATION AND EVALUATION

The new theory has led to new ways to evaluate and follow patients with pigmentary glaucoma. My current recommendation is that specific parameters should be evaluated on initial examination, as they will be helpful in determining the stage of the disease. These parameters are based on the view that there are three stages of pigmentary glaucoma with regard to pigment dispersion: (1) an initial or advancing stage, characterized by an increase in the number of transillumination defects and pigment dispersion; (2) a stabilization stage, in which the number of transillumination defects stabilizes and the pigment dispersion either slows or stops; and (3) a resolution phase, in which the iris transillumination defects heal, causing a decrease in the number of the defects and in the levels of pigment dispersed throughout the anterior portion of the eye.

In evaluation of a patient with pigmentary glaucoma, the degree of corneal, iris, and lenticular pigmentation should be noted. More importantly the degree of pigmentation in the trabecular meshwork should be recorded. To do this, a new gonioscopy lens incorporating a pigment scale has been developed in our laboratory. It is very important that the exact number of peripheral iris transillumination defects be recorded, as this number can increase, stabilize, or decrease with time. The baseline intraocular pressure and tonographic facility of outflow (*C* value) should be determined as well. In addition, of course, the status of the optic nerve head and visual field should be recorded. By following these parameters over 1 or 2 years, the ophthalmologist can often determine whether the patient is in the advancing, stabilization, or resolution phase of the disease.

TREATMENT

In regard to treatment, either standard medical, laser, or surgical glaucoma therapy may be used. Early evidence[8] indicates that chronic miotic therapy, which flattens the peripheral iris and lifts it away from the zonules, may cause or hasten a reversal of the disease. With respect to chronic parasympathomimetic therapy, pilocarpine ocuserts seem to create the least disruption and are best tolerated by these often young patients. Some young patients can tolerate parasympathomimetic therapy in only one eye because of the severe accommodative blur. I recommend that if the patient cannot tolerate bilateral miotic therapy, and the disease is in the advancing phase and pressure is high, the worst eye should be treated with chronic miotic therapy. Miotic treatment needs to be maintained for many years before it can be effective in causing reversal of pigment dispersion, healing of the iris transillumination defects, lightening of the pigmentation within the trabecular meshwork, and an improvement in the baseline intraocular pressure and facility of outflow. In the future thymoxamine,[22] an alpha-adrenergic blocking agent that can cause miosis without accommodation, may prove to be beneficial.

Standard laser trabeculoplasty therapy has been helpful for some patients but should only be used when increasing disc or visual field damage occurs despite maximum-tolerated medical therapy. Care should be taken to avoid overtreatment in the heavily pigmented meshwork, and low-energy settings should be used, which cause only a blanching or very slight bubble formation. Laser therapy to the peripheral iris to cause flattening has been initially unpromising, both elsewhere[24] and in my experience, but new techniques may offer hope.

PIGMENTARY GLAUCOMA FOLLOWING INTRAOCULAR LENS IMPLANTATION

In view of the new theory just described, it might be expected that intraocular lenses (IOLs), particularly those that can rub against the posterior surface of the iris, might occasionally cause pigmentary glaucoma. We[4] have recently found this to be the case in four eyes. In one patient the offending lens was a mobile iris clip lens whose haptics had rubbed considerable pigment off the posterior surface of the iris. In three other patients the offending lenses were posterior chamber IOLs. In one of these the superior haptic and the superior portion of the optic were tilted anteriorly, causing rubbing and pigment loss in these areas. In the other two the posterior chamber IOLs were in good and normal position, but had been placed with the convex face posteriorly, exposing the flat edge of the lens to the posterior iris surface; this flat face and sharper edge had rubbed off considerable pigment.

In all patients the glaucoma was unilateral and occurred in eyes that had not had high pressures before cataract surgery. The glaucoma developed fairly rapidly, within 1 to 2 years after surgery, and was severe, with advanced glaucomatous disc damage and visual field loss. In addition, the fellow eyes were without glaucoma. One patient's glaucoma could not be controlled despite maximum-tolerated medical therapy, laser trabeculoplasty, and required filtration surgery. Electron microscopic evaluation of the filtration specimen confirmed the diagnosis of pigmentary glaucoma in that it showed pigmentation, endothelial cell disruption, and beam collapse, all characteristic findings.

Diagnosis

Pigmentary glaucoma secondary to an IOL should be suspected when elevation of intraocular pressure (IOP) is found postoperatively in an eye with an iris clip or posterior chamber IOL and no evidence of causes such as inflammation or angle closure. However, pigment can be chronically dispersed in the postoperative period, and the ophthalmologist should not mistake these particles of pigment for inflammatory cells and institute steroid treatment. Signs of pigment dispersion in the anterior chamber may be present in the form of a mild Krukenberg's spindle, pigment in the aqueous, or pigment on the anterior surface of the iris. There will also be a heavy unilateral trabecular meshwork pigment band. Transillumination examination may show defects at the edge of the optic or along the haptics, indicating rubbing (Fig. 7-7). These defects must be distinguished from those benign defects that occur at the time of surgery; thus it is important to note the location of surgically created, benign defects in the immediate postoperative period so that these can be distinguished from any new defects.

Posterior chamber IOLs, now the most popular lens in the United States, pose a real threat of pigmentary glaucoma. For this reason all patients with posterior chamber lenses should be examined at 6-month intervals for 3 years to be sure the IOP remains normal.

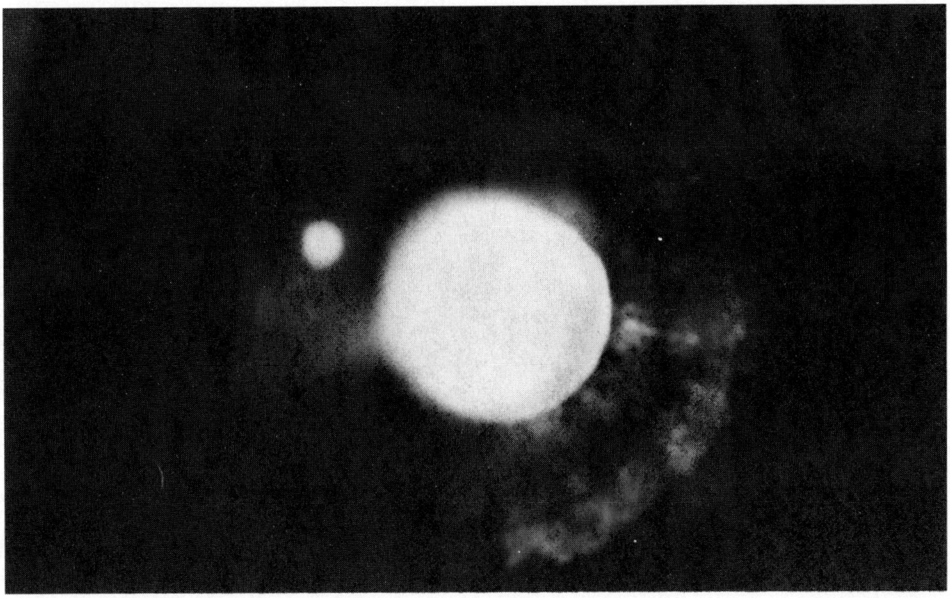

Fig. 7-7. Transillumination defects surrounding edge of posterior chamber intraocular lens in patient with pigmentary glaucoma caused by placing lens with flat edge anterior.

Prevention

In regard to avoiding this complication, posterior chamber lenses should only be placed when their stability can be assured. Thus, if it appears at the time of surgery that the posterior chamber lens will fit poorly, or if there is reason to think that there has been zonular or posterior capsular weakening or disruption, consideration should be given to the omission of the lens. The lens should be placed with the convex face anterior to prevent rubbing between the posterior surface of the iris and the flat surface of the lens. The clinician should strongly consider the routine use of 10-degree angulated lenses, which may sit more posteriorly and away from the iris surface and thus are less likely to cause pigment dispersion and glaucoma.

Treatment

Once pigmentary glaucoma secondary to an IOL is diagnosed, treatment should consist of surgical stabilization of the mobile IOL. If this cannot be accomplished, the lens should be removed if it is continuing to cause pigment dispersion and secondary elevation of IOP. If the lens is stable but causing dispersion of pigment, immobilization with a chronic miotic agent such as pilocarpine should be considered. If the glaucoma continues to worsen, however, then the ophthalmologist should again consider removing the lens. Elevation of IOP can be treated with standard glaucoma medications, and in some cases these patients will respond to laser trabeculoplasty. To date, one patient has undergone successful filtration surgery.

All ophthalmologists should be aware of this potential complication of the IOL and its severity, as delayed diagnosis in our cases resulted in advanced disc damage and visual loss.

REFERENCES

1. Becker, B., and Podos, S.M.: Krukenberg's spindles and primary open angle glaucome, Arch. Ophthalmol. **76:**635, 1966.
2. Becker, B.: Round table discussion. In New Orleans Academy of Ophthalmology: Symposium on glaucoma, St. Louis, 1967, The C.V. Mosby Co.
3. Blick, M.W.: Pigmentary glaucoma in females, Arch. Ophthalmol. **58:**483, 1957.
4. Boys-Smith, J.W., Aiken, D., and Campbell, D.G.: Pigmentary glaucoma secondary to intraocular lenses. (Submitted for publication.)
5. Boys-Smith, J.W., and others: A new gonioscopy lens for the gradation of trabecular meshwork pigmentation. (Accepted for presentation at the 1984 meeting of the Association for Research in Vision and Ophthalmology.)
6. Calhoun, F.P., Jr.: Pigmentary glaucoma and its relation to Krukenberg's spindles, Trans. Am. Ophthalmol. Soc. **50:**103, 1952.
7. Campbell, D.G.: Pigmentary dispersion and glaucoma: a new theory, Arch. Ophthalmol. **97:**1667, 1979.
8. Campbell, D.G.: Improvement of pigmentary glaucoma and healing of transillumination defects with miotic therapy, Invest. Ophthalmol. Vis. Sci. **23**(suppl.):173, 1983.
9. Campbell, D.G., Woods, W.D., and Aiken, D.G.: Studies concerning glaucoma caused by pigment particles in the trabecular meshwork, Invest. Ophthalmol. Vis. Sci. **22**(suppl.):192, 1982.
10. Chandler, P.A., and Grant, W.M.: Pigmentary glaucoma. In Chandler, P.A., and Grant, W.M., editors: Lectures on glaucoma, Philadelphia, 1965, Lea & Febiger.
11. Etienne, R.: L'atrophie essentielle des couches epitheliales de l'iris et du corps ciliaire, ses relations avec le glaucome. II, Ann. Ocul. **193:**224, 1960.
12. Hoffman, F., Dumitrescu, L., and Hager, H.: Pigment glaucom (Rosterelektronenmikiroskopische Befunde), Klin. Monatsbl. Augenheilkd. **166:**609, 1975.
13. Lambrou, F.H., and others: The production and mechanism of ghost cell glaucoma in the cat and primate, Invest. Ophthalmol. Vis. Sci. **23**(suppl.):136, 1983.
14. Lichter, P.R., and Shaffer, R.N.: Diagnostic and prognostic signs in pigmentary glaucoma, Trans. Am. Acad. Ophthalmol. Otolaryngol. **74:**984, 1970.
15. Malbran, J.: Le glaucome pigmentaire ses relations avec le glaucome congenital, Bib. Ophtalmol. **47:**132, 1957.
16. Nordmann, J., Gerhard, J.P., and Payeur, G.: A propos du glaucomae dit pigmentaire, Bull Mem. Soc. Fr.. Ophtalmol. **66:**651, 1966.
17. Richardson, T., Hutchinson, B.T., and Grant, W.M.: The outflow tract in pigmentary glaucoma: a light and electron microscopy study, Arch. Ophthalmol. **95:**1015, 1977.
18. Sampaolesi, R.: Le glaucome dit pigmentaire; son rapport avec le glaucome congenital (22 cas), Bull. Mem. Soc. Fr. Ophtalmol. **81:**434, 1968.
19. Scheie, H.F., and Fleischhauer, H.W.: Idiopathic atrophy of the epithelial layers of the iris and ciliary body, Arch. Ophthalmol. **59:**216, 1958.
20. Sugar, H.S.: Pigmentary glaucoma: a 25-year review, Am. J. Ophthalmol. **62:**499, 1966.
21. Sugar, H.S., and Barbour, F.A.: Pigmentary glaucoma: a rare clinical entity, Am. J. Ophthalmol. **32:**90, 1949.
22. Wand, W., and Grant, W.M.: Thymoxamine hydrochloride: effects on the facility of outflow and intraocular pressure, Invest. Ophthalmol. **15:**400, 1976.
23. Weekers, R., and Watilon, M.: Hypertensions oculaires attributables a l'action conjuguee d'une anomalie mesodermique et d'une migration pigmentaire, Bull Mem. Soc Fr. Ophtalmol. **66:**637, 1966.
24. Zimmerman, T.: Personal communication.

8

The pathogenesis of optic nerve damage in glaucoma

Harry A. Quigley

The cause of blindness in glaucoma has been a subject of great interest in ophthalmology for many years. It was discussed at the NOAO symposium the previous two times that glaucoma was the topic. Much new information has been accumulated in the last several years that was not previously summarized. This chapter attempts to place this new information in perspective.

DEFINITION OF GLAUCOMA

Glaucoma is characterized by a progressive optic neuropathy consisting of a typical optic disc appearance and a particular pattern of retinal sensitivity loss with visual field testing. The disc appearance associated with glaucoma includes enlargement of the disc cup toward the rim, undercutting of the rim tissue, and deepening of the cup floor. All of these features are included in the term *glaucomatous cupping,* although the extent to which each is present varies. Whereas some normal eyes and some eyes with other disorders can successfully simulate aspects of this typical glaucoma appearance, the pattern can be recognized in a large proportion of eyes known to be glaucomatous from other criteria. By present field-testing methods, visual sensitivity in glaucomatous optic neuropathy first becomes abnormal between 5 and 30 degrees from fixation. This scotomatous area then expands into an arcuate shape, ultimately isolating the central and temporal field into islands. Again, other disorders can simulate this pattern, but these simulating conditions are not typically progressive and are rarely associated with a disc resembling that of glaucoma.

Glaucomatous optic neuropathy most often appears in eyes with abnormal intraocular pressure (IOP) dynamics. These eyes have higher than normal mean IOP, wider than normal diurnal fluctuations in IOP, and poorer than normal outflow facility.[20,24,28] These simple generalizations have exceptions. For example, all eyes with elevated IOP do not have glaucomatous optic neuropathy, if we define the neuropathy chiefly by the presence of field loss.[6,19,35] Some of these eyes have not yet had elevated IOP long enough to be damaged. Others are already damaged, but the visual field test is too insensitive to detect it.[40] It is therefore inaccurate to define glaucomatous optic neuropathy solely by the results of field testing. The opposite contradiction is an eye with apparently normal IOP and glaucomatous nerve damage (low-tension glaucoma). This group is considered later in this discussion. It is quite incontrovertible, however, that under many circumstances chronic IOP elevation leads to glaucomatous optic neuropathy. For example, high IOP after steroid use, trauma,[34] or inflammation leads to typical glaucoma damage. Whereas the eyes of infants and children respond to elevated IOP in some unique ways, the optic nerve damage that they develop is similar to that of adult glaucoma eyes.[49] If one artificially increases IOP in a primate eye, the disc and optic nerve develop glaucomatous optic neuropathy indistinguishable from that of a human eye.[36,37] Thus there is a typical damage pattern that defines glaucoma. This pattern is most often associated with abnormal IOP and can be produced by chronic IOP elevation. This report examines the mechanism by which this optic neuropathy occurs.

SITE OF GLAUCOMA DAMAGE

If the clinician wishes to know how glaucomatous neuropathy occurs, it is helpful to start by locating the site of damage. Ten years ago there was room for vigorous debate on this subject; at that time few human glaucoma eyes had been examined by modern histologic techniques. With the aid of Drs. W. Richard Green, A. Edward Maumenee, and others who generously provided material, I have examined 75 human glaucoma eyes with known clinical data.[39,40,43] These ranged from early glaucoma suspects without definitive damage to eyes with advanced neural loss. This material demonstrates that the site of nerve fiber damage in glaucoma is within the optic nerve head at the level of the sclera, the scleral lamina cribrosa (Fig. 8-1).

The optic nerve head is the channel for 1 million axons of retinal ganglion cells.[3] Nerve fibers form into bundles that are separated from each other in the superficial nerve head by astrocytes (glial cells). The nerve head has a continuous plexus of capillaries that surrounds the neural bundles. A series of 10 perforated sheets crosses the canal at the level of the sclera.[44] The zone defined by these collagenous sheets is the scleral lamina cribrosa; the nerve bundles pass through pores in the scleral lamina's sheets. Just behind the scleral lamina is the myelinated optic nerve outside the eye.

When I examined human glaucomatous eyes, it was clear that the nerve fibers were abnormal in the scleral lamina cribrosa.[43] Individual axons were swollen with membranous vesicles and mitochondria (Fig. 8-2). One could look from superficial nerve head to myelinated nerve and see that this site was obviously where the fibers were injured. Vrabec has studied human glaucomatous eyes using silver staining, a method that shows the course of individual axons.[57] He also concluded that the scleral lamina was the location of damage.

A second source of information is the chronic glaucoma model in monkey eyes. Two methods have proved useful: (1) injection of fixed red blood cells into the anterior chamber[36] and (2) laser destruction of the trabecular meshwork[16,45] Both methods produce elevated IOP, glaucomatous cupping, and a pattern of neural loss similar to human glaucoma. The location at which the earliest cellular abnormalities occur is also the scleral lamina cribrosa.[37] After extended injury it is there that axon segments show permanent degeneration. In the monkey the clinician can study the movement of radioactive tracers within the nerve fiber from cell body to brain terminals, the process called *axonal transport*. The intracellular contents that accumulate in human and monkey axons at the scleral lamina are organelles that were moving in axonal transport. Such studies have shown axonal transport to be blocked at the scleral lamina with acute IOP elevations, both for material moving out of the eye (orthograde)[5] and back to the cell body (retrograde).[32] Axonal transport is the means by which the cell body communicates

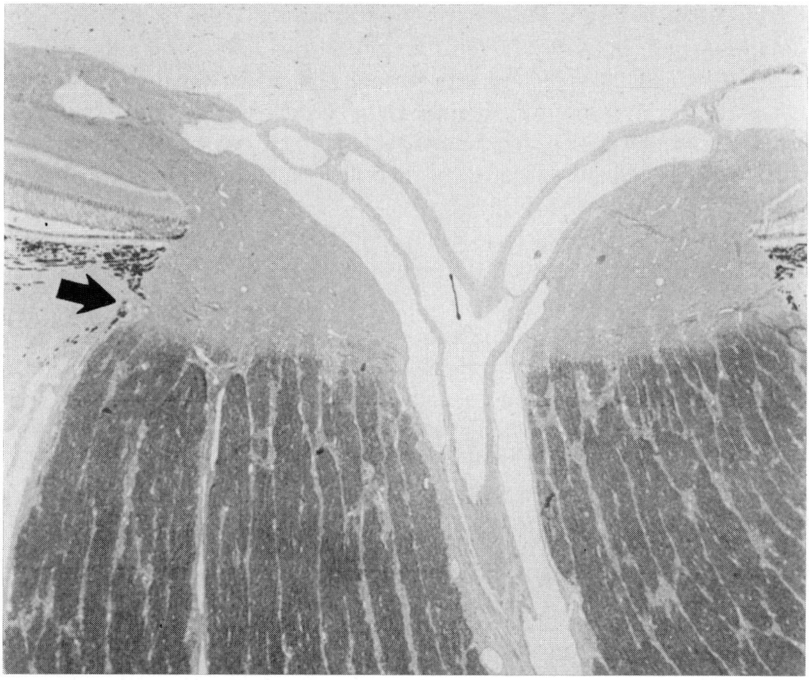

Fig. 8-1. Histologic section of optic nerve head, with vitreous cavity at *top* and dark, myelinated optic nerve at *bottom*. The site of earliest damage to nerve fibers in glaucoma is scleral lamina cribrosa—band crossing just in front of myelin line and indicated by *arrow*. (×40, paraphenylenediamine stain.)

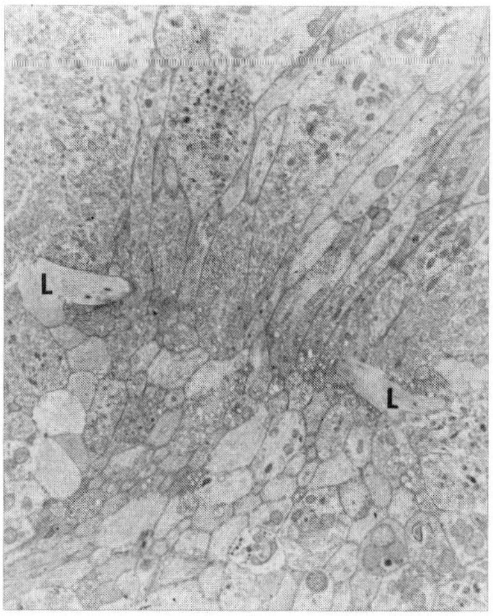

Fig. 8-2. Electron microscopic photograph of zone of damage in human glaucoma: scleral lamina cribrosa. Bundle of nerve fibers is passing between edges of pore through lamina's connective tissue, sides of which are indicated by *L*s. Nerve fibers are swollen by accumulation of intracellular contents, whose movements in axonal transport were interrupted by elevated IOP. (×11,000.)

with its extended process and by which supply of nutrients and clearance of spent products is accomplished. Interference with this process is a serious insult to cell integrity and, if severe enough, is sufficient to lead to cell death. Thus, in human and primate eyes with chronic glaucoma, nerve fiber injury occurs at the scleral lamina cribrosa. Furthermore, the appearance of the injured human axons is identical with monkey axons that have obstructed axonal transport; this may represent the feature of cellular function whose interruption leads to cell death.

It must be stressed that axonal transport might be interrupted at this site by anoxia, mechanical compression, or toxic substances.[33] Axonal transport blockade is thus present in glaucomatous optic neuropathy, but this does not of itself establish the intervening links between elevated IOP and cell death.

It is worth reemphasizing that the sole cell type lost from the retina in human or primate glaucoma eyes is the ganglion cell. Previously there was an ingenious hypothesis that glaucoma caused dysfunction of the radial peripapillary capillaries in the superficial retina.[2,29] We found no axonal abnormalities in the retinal nerve fiber layer to confirm this suggestion.[37,39,40,43] Others have failed to detect a correlation between position and extent of peripapillary capillary loss and field defects.[9]

RELATION OF SCLERAL LAMINA ANATOMY TO GLAUCOMA DAMAGE

The collagenous sheets of the lamina conduct 1 million nerve fibers out of the eye without kinking them. To do so, the axons divide into 200 to 400 bundles and pass through the successive laminar sheets that are loosely in register. Astrocytic glial cells surround the bundles,[3] maintaining the proper ionic concentration for neural impulse transmission. Serial section reconstruction of the collagenous sheets by Wilczek[59] first showed the lovely latticework of the lamina. Scanning electron microscopy allowed Emery and co-workers[11] to illustrate how laminar structure collapsed outward in human glaucoma eyes. Radius, Maumenee, and Green[48] were impressed that some glaucoma eyes developed pitlike excavations that were especially frequent at the superior and inferior disc poles. The nerve head appeared to rupture into an ectatic area with loss of the laminar cross-struts.

My study of optic nerve cross-sections from human glaucomatous eyes showed a particular pattern of nerve fiber loss.[39,40] We have noted that arcuate area scotomas are typical for glaucoma. The cells that subserve this field area send their axons into the upper and lower poles of the nerve head. Human glaucomatous nerves show loss of fibers throughout the nerve, but loss at the vertical poles is selectively greater. The shape of the most susceptible region is that of an hourglass (Fig. 8-3). This confirms clinical observation of Kirsch and Anderson[27] that some glaucoma eyes lose the vertical disc rim first, producing vertically oval cup shape or a local notch of rim loss at 12 or 6 o'clock. Since the site of damage is the scleral lamina and the pattern of vulnerability is hourglass-shaped, we examined the laminar anatomy for features that would explain the characteristic nerve loss pattern.[38] In advanced glaucoma cups the pores of the most anterior lamina cribrosa sheets appear as dark dots, which are often larger in the upper and lower poles of the lamina. With the scanning electron microscope, I confirmed that the upper and lower poles of the lamina have consistently larger pores for the passage of nerve bundles. The temporal and nasal quadrants have smaller pores and hence more structural connective tissues per unit area. This regional difference in the structure of the human lamina was confirmed by Radius and Gonzales.[47]

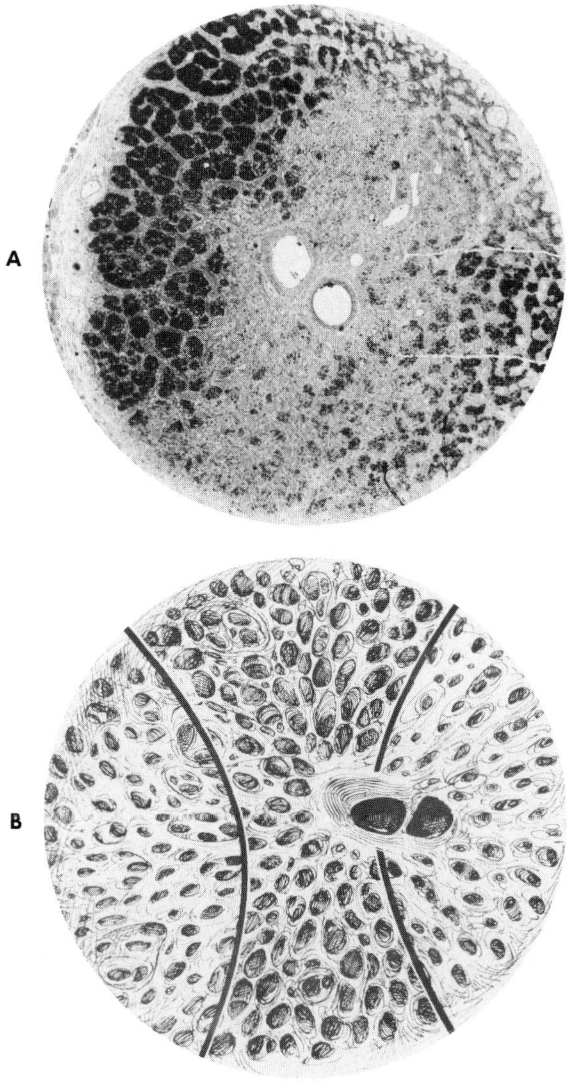

Fig. 8-3. A, Cross-section of glaucomatous human optic nerve taken 2 mm behind globe. Normal myelin bundles are *black,* and atrophic areas are *light* in color. Central artery and vein are seen in middle of nerve. Superior pole is at *top,* nasal at *right,* and temporal at *left*. In this nerve most of its inferior pole is atrophic, and much of superior nasal pole is likewise gone *(light)*. Pattern is similar to number of other human and primate specimens, in which most damage is in hourglass shape. **B,** Structure of connective tissue of scleral lamina cribrosa. Note that this schematic points out lower density (larger pores) of structural support that corresponds to hourglass shape of neural atrophy. (**A** ×45, paraphenylenediamine.)

A

B

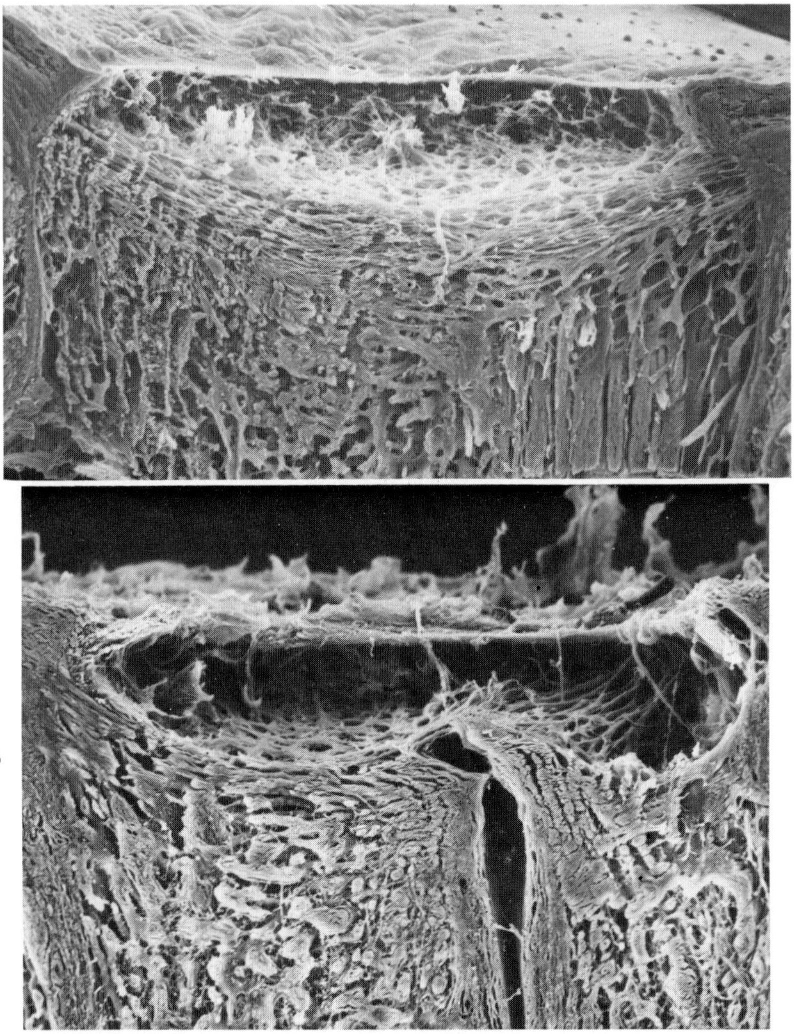

Fig. 8-4. Scanning electron microscope views of human optic nerve head. Tissue was digested to remove all elements except connective tissue, then divided in half. Vitreous cavity is at *top,* myelinated nerve at *bottom,* and inlet into nerve head (scleral canal) is semicircular rim. **A,** Normal adult nerve head; **B,** glaucomatous eye with advanced damage. Scleral lamina stretches across nerve head as about 10 plates, through which pores for nerve bundles pass. In comparing **B** to **A,** lamina is compressed and has taken on shape of a W, indicating that compression was greatest at superior and inferior poles (*left* and *right* sides), compared to the middle nerve head *(center).* (× 60.)

The conclusion drawn from these observations is logical. If IOP increases, two forces act on the lamina. First, there would be an inside-out push, tending to compress the nerve head's successive laminar sheets and bow them outward. Second, the increased IOP would increase the tension in the scleral wall, pulling on the rim of the scleral canal to which the laminar sheets are attached. Since it is unlikely that this force would be uniform in all directions, the shape of the lamina would distort. In either case new forces would be exerted on both the nerve bundles themselves and their nutrient capillaries, which are always located within the laminar sheets. Since there are differences within the lamina in the amount of structural connective tissue, resistance to being distorted would vary. The upper and lower poles of the nerve head, containing the lowest collagen density, would distort or compress first or most, leading to greater damage to the bundles passing through their zones. In this way the pattern of hourglass atrophy is explained by the regional laminar architecture.[38,47]

This hypothesis that the vertical poles of the lamina are more susceptible to distortion is directly supported by examinations of human glaucomatous eyes.[44] I found that even in glaucomatous eyes from patients who had no field loss, there is compression of the 10 successive laminar sheets, as in collapse of an accordion. Laminar compression worsens with each succeeding stage of optic nerve damage. The change was indeed greater at the superior and inferior poles than in the temporal nasal axis (Fig. 8-4). Interestingly, whereas we often refer to laminar bowing as typical of glaucoma, the cause of the clinical deepening of the cup appeared to result mostly from loss of anterior nerve fiber tissue and compression of laminar sheets. Backward movement of the posterior limit of the lamina—essentially the whole nerve head moving out of the eye—was a late and inconstant finding.

Another feature of laminar structure measured in this study was the diameter of the scleral canal. Even in eyes with advanced damage, the diameter at Bruch's membrane was unchanged from the mean normal diameter in adult glaucomatous eyes. Hence the cup enlargement in adult glaucoma eyes is definitely not caused by permanent increase in scleral canal diameter.

This is the first hypothesis that successfully relates the anatomy of the damage site to the pattern of damage in glaucoma. Although there were previous attempts to specify a regional blood flow pattern, the evidence was based on observations of fluorescein angiography of the choroid.[22] It is increasingly clear, as is detailed in the next section, that if one wishes to understand the site of damage in glaucoma, one must study the lamina cribosa and its features.

ROLE OF ASTROCYTIC GLIAL CELLS IN GLAUCOMATOUS CUPPING

Nearly 75 years ago Fuchs reported that glaucomatous eyes studied histologically had an early loss of glial cells.[15] Since there was at that time no accurate tonometry, gonioscopy, or field testing, we have no way of knowing how the eyes he examined would be classified today. This statement was, however, repeated as fact throughout the literature and formed the basis for an hypothesis about glaucomatous cupping.[52] Since cup size increase was often seen to precede detectable field loss, it was suggested that the early cup size increase was not caused by loss of neuronal tissue, but rather by loss of glial cells. Since the glia were believed to represent an important part of the physical support of the nerve head, a further extension of this concept hypothesized that early loss of glia would compromise either capillary function or axonal health and lead to neuronal death.[5]

The human glaucomatous eyes examined in my laboratory are well characterized as to diagnosis, stage of damage, and lack of associated disorders. They have been examined by light, scanning, and transmission electron microscopy. I have found that at no stage in the glaucoma damage process is there a disproportionate loss of astrocytic glial cells from the nerve head.[37,39,43] In eyes with an early stage of damage, neural fibers can be seen to have disappeared, leaving behind less organized groups of astrocytes. After atrophy of large numbers of axons, astrocytes fill in the spaces previously occupied by axons and can be seen to be phagocytosing dead cell debris. Astrocytes synthesize extracellular matrix during the later phases of glaucoma damage, filling in spaces with collagen. We have observed astrocytes synthesizing protein from injected radioactive amino acids at artificially elevated levels of IOP that are damaging to the nerve fibers.[37] Thus there is little support either in primate or human eyes for early loss of glia as a cause of glaucomatous neuropathy or as an explanation of early cup size increase.

Why, then, did it appear to Fuchs and others that glial cells were lost? Possibly this derived from several facts regarding normal nerve head anatomy and its change with glaucoma. Astrocytes make up only about 10% of the nerve head volume. Once all the nerve fibers are gone, the nerve head would look empty, even if all the glia were preserved. Second, it is possible that there is a proportionate loss of glia as there is of capillaries of the nerve head as nerve fibers die. Although no evidence exists to support this, it would certainly further contribute to the appearance of few remaining nuclei in a glaucomatous disc. Next, in advanced glaucoma eyes with large, bean-pot cups, the lamina is compressed and expanded outward into the choroid and sclera. The actual surface area of the nerve head on the vitreous side therefore must be three times normal. The remaining glia are spread out over a bigger area and would look few in number, even if the original number were present. Finally, it is likely that the glial loss in glaucoma was most obvious in comparing glaucomatous eyes with eyes that had suffered optic atrophy from other causes. In the latter eyes the lamina would not be compressed, and the surface area increase just mentioned would not have occurred. Even if there were the same number of glial cells in eyes with the two diagnoses, the number in glaucomatous eyes would appear fewer.

SUBSEQUENT STEPS IN THE DAMAGE PATHWAY

If the early abnormality induced in the nerve head by elevated IOP is distortion or compression of the laminar structure, there are a number of possible consequences that might be relevant to the pathogenesis of glaucoma damage. In my view we cannot yet say which of these next steps does occur—we must maintain an open mind until further data are available. One possibility is that the distortion of the lamina causes a direct compressive force on the axons themselves, leading to cell injury and death. Second, the laminar change in shape could conceivably hinder the vascular nutrition of the neural bundles, with consequent damage. Other possibilities exist, but these first two are considered in detail.

We have already seen that the pores of the lamina can and do change shape in response to elevated IOP. These changes are only those that remain in the fixed, enucleated eye. Since they are easily and quantitatively separated from normal, age-matched eyes, they do not represent an artefact. It is possible that the distortions are greater in vivo and reversibly return more toward normal before fixation of the eye.

Some experimental evidence suggests that such shifts in tissue position occur.[31] Forces generated by laminar shape changes could far exceed the simple increase in pressure gradient across the nerve head caused by the increase in IOP. The normal gradient is IOP minus optic nerve tissue pressure, or about 10 mm Hg. With the usual range of IOP in glaucoma, this would increase to 20 at an IOP of 30 mm Hg. However, the shearing force, caused by pinching of two adjacent laminar sheets or by changing shape of a laminar pore, could exceed this considerably. These forces have not been measured directly. It is well established that compressive force applied to neurons is injurious and potentially fatal because it interrupts vital cell functions.[53] This possible pathway is now being investigated in our laboratory by special studies on the type of derangement in intracellular function induced by experimental glaucoma. Since this is the simplest possible pathway, it is intuitively attractive.

The majority opinion for many years has been that glaucoma damages neurons by affecting their blood supply.[22] We now know that it is the vasculature of the scleral lamina that we wish to investigate to determine if this occurs. To look at the direct evidence that the blood supply in this area is affected by glaucoma, we must decide what feature of nutrition we wish to examine. Many publications on this subject speak of ischemia without defining what is meant by the term. Other reports show angiograms with no definable vessels and state that this shows ischemia. Still further discussions have implied that if blood flow decreases, there must be inadequate nutrition to nerve fibers. We actually know very little about which vascular functions are most important to axons along a white matter tract of the central nervous system. The information that is available, however, suggests that the axons supply themselves with much of what they need by axonal transport.[42] If we place a fiber in a chamber and progressively eliminate nutrients from the surrounding medium, axonal function in the short run proceeds normally as long as oxygen is supplied, carbon dioxide is eliminated (pH maintained), and a minimal amount of extracellular calcium is present. Along the nerve fiber amino acids and glucose are not apparently needed, since they arrive from the cell body along with mitochondria for energy generation.

Let us then look first at the available information on these features of the lamina's vascular supply in glaucoma. Unfortunately almost nothing is known about carbon dioxide and ionic concentration. Oxygen levels are very difficult to measure, even in experimental animals. Ernest's and Potts' most recent attempts[12] indicate that the oxygen level is autoregulated in monkey eyes. Although this may not be true of older human beings with chronic glaucoma, at least the nerve head at elevated IOP is not prone to anoxia when its normal functions are intact. An indirect way of judging the role of anoxia is to increase tissue oxygen level substantially and in this way attempt to prevent axonal injury. Minckler, Bunt, and Johanson[32] saw no protective effect from 100% oxygen, and we detected no benefit from 100% oxygen at 3 atmospheres (hyperbaric) pressure.[42] In our experiment tissue oxygen level was likely to be 20 times normal. Retinal protein synthesis occurred even without detectable retinal blood flow by angiography, suggesting inner retinal nutrition by the choroid under these conditions. Yet in neither experiment could it be certain that there was a normal oxygen level at the scleral lamina. Whereas the data suggest that anoxia is not involved, the conclusive demonstration of this point awaits a satisfactory measurement of tissue oxygen concentration.

If we have not yet shown an axonal injury that is pathognomonic for anoxia, and if we have no direct evidence for an abnormality in vascular supply, then any other evidence for or against this mechanism of glaucoma damage is by its very nature indirect. Nonetheless we have several such indirect pieces of evidence to consider; some have been cited for many years, and others represent newer data.

First, vascular function might be abnormal if the vessels themselves were injured or damaged by the glaucoma process. Some previous reports suggested that the capillaries of the human nerve head are selectively lost in glaucoma.[8,14] Most eyes examined in these studies were blind or nearly so, and detailed histories are not provided in the report of Cristini,[8] in which a light microscopic method was used. My recent studies of human eyes and experimental glaucoma studies in monkeys contradict these previous reports.[37,39,43,45] It is important to stress that none of these studies measured blood flow; their purpose was to count the number of capillaries. Furthermore, it is difficult to quantify the capillaries in the human nerve head given variable degrees of autolysis. There was no attempt to quantify the findings in the previous reports.

My human specimens represent a wide range of damage. The number of capillaries appeared not to have declined compared to similarly prepared normal eyes (Fig. 8-5). It was particularly impressive to see capillaries remaining throughout the scleral lamina even in advanced damage specimens. I thought, however, that a quantitative study was required to aid in answering this question. Therefore, chronic optic nerve damage was produced in monkey eyes, and in each animal the area of the tissue occupied by capillary lumens was directly measured and compared to the normal capillary area under standard conditions. The result was clear and conclusive—the percentage of tissue that was made up of capillaries remained remarkably constant in early or late glaucoma

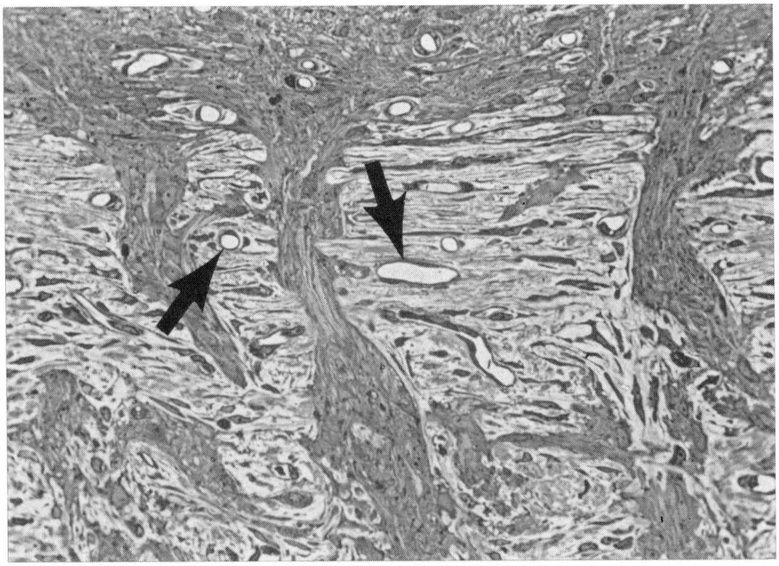

Fig. 8-5. This light micrograph shows scleral lamina cribosa region of nerve head with advanced glaucoma damage. Nerve bundles are replaced by glial cells (vertical, darker material in *columns*). Light tissue is collagenous connective tissue of lamina, and open circles indicated by *arrows* are capillaries. Note that there are many small blood vessels seen in this section. In controlled study of primate eyes using material similar to this, percentage of tissue made up of capillaries was the same in glaucomatous and normal eyes. (×150, paraphenylenediamine.)

damage. As added proof, capillaries disappear from the nerve head as nerve fibers disappear, at just the rate necessary to maintain the usual ratio of capillaries to tissue. Generally the loss of capillaries and nerve fibers seemed to occur at the same time; otherwise, we would have observed an abnormal ratio at some stages of damage. Further evidence for the lack of preferential loss of capillaries is the failure of chronic IOP elevation to lead to detectable damage to capillaries by electron microscopy.[16,37,43] One study suggested that very high (greater than 100 mm Hg), acute IOP elevations might lead to leakage of labelled proteins from monkey nerve head vessels[46] There has been no similar demonstration in chronic, moderate IOP increase, and it is not clear that the apparent vascular leakage alone would indicate that the nutrition of axons is abnormal.

Our human and primate nerve heads then show that the percentage of tissue made up of capillaries remains stable as neural atrophy proceeds. This means that capillaries atrophy just as in other optic nerve atrophic processes. What happens to these vessels? One can conceive of the vessels of the nerve head as a continuous plexus of capillaries extending from the surface of the nerve head at the vitreous cavity into the retrobulbar nerve. The compression of the lamina and the loss of anterior neural tissue must cause increased force on capillaries attached to the retina at one end and the optic nerve at the other. In addition, with the loss of neural bundles between them, the capillaries are less well supported by surrounding tissue. As a result, capillaries might rupture their walls, causing hemorrhage (Fig. 8-6). If the most likely point of maximum stress were between the retinal edge of the disc rim and the anterior scleral lamina, then the hemorrhages would be flame shaped because of confinement between nerve fiber bundles. Such hemorrhages not only occur in glaucomatous discs, but are also associated with more rapid damage than that expected in an eye in which hemorrhage has not been observed.[10] The clinician must reevaluate the therapy in any glaucoma eye that has a disc hemorrhage.

However, the cause of the hemorrhage is a different matter. As suggested, it may occur as a result of neural atrophy, rim rearrangement, and stretch on the capillary plexus. Begg, Drance, and Sweeney[7] have speculated that the bleeding indicates ischemia of the nerve head. No direct evidence shows that spontaneous hemorrhage necessarily indicates a lack of sufficient vascular function. Spontaneous hemorrhages can occur because of nonischemic causes, such as minor trauma, elevated intravascular pressure, or abnormal capillary fragility. Without corroborative evidence it is an open question whether disc hemorrhage means insufficient blood supply. The analogy to anterior ischemic optic neuropathy was drawn in one report, but the differences between this event and disc hemorrhage in a glaucoma eye are manifold. The glaucoma eye with hemorrhage does not have disc swelling, often does not have an immediately definable new loss of field, and almost never suffers loss of visual acuity. Furthermore, the glaucoma patient in my experience is never symptomatic, in contrast to the ischemic neuropathy patients, who often are. A final problem with interpreting disc hemorrhage as an ischemic event related to the pathogenesis of damage is the site of damage being the scleral lamina. The capillaries there are surrounded by collagenous beams, and bleeding from them would not start and end up on the disc rim wall or the retinal edge of the disc. Thus, if hemorrhages seen on the disc rim are a reflection of poor vascular supply at the scleral lamina, they must be some indirect result of a deeper process.

We have examined two aspects of vascular function of the nerve head—evidence of actual loss of function (anoxia) and for loss of capillary number out of proportion to tissue loss—and have found little support for the concept that abnormalities in these elements occur in chronic glaucoma.

If blood flow to the scleral lamina were decreased by elevated IOP, we could assume that vascular dysfunction was an important part of glaucoma's pathogenesis. Of course, simply to say that blood flow decreases does not demonstrate that it decreases enough to damage nerve fibers. However, the demonstration of disturbed blood flow would provide substantial indirect evidence for possible ischemia. Unfortunately there is no reliable method at present for measuring blood flow in vivo in the human optic nerve head at the site of glaucoma damage. Fluorescein angiography shows blood vessels of the superficial nerve head, but capillaries of the scleral lamina are surrounded by collag-

A

B

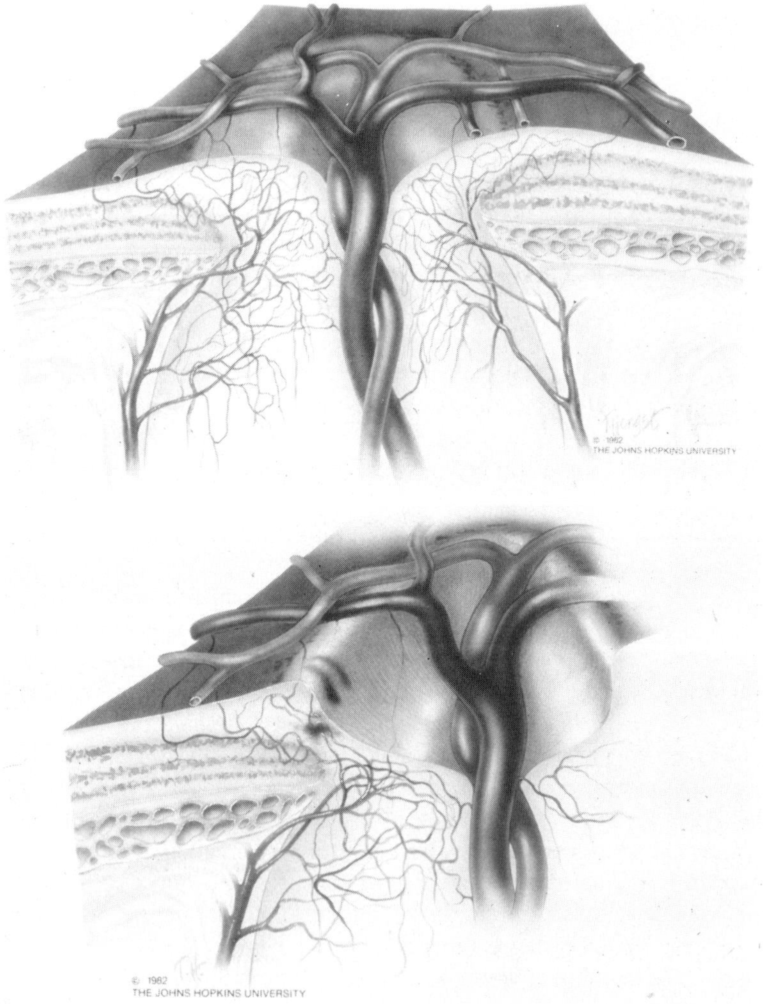

Fig. 8-6. These two photographs indicate schematically capillary plexus of optic nerve head in **A,** normal eye, and **B,** glaucoma-damaged eye. **B,** shows what might be effect on capillary plexus of continued loss of nerve rim tissue and backward compressive movement of lamina cribrosa. Capillaries are connected to retina *(above),* and this is immobile, but posterior tissue to which it is connected is moving backward. In addition, rim tissue that surrounds and supports capillaries has disappeared. At some point it is logical that some capillary under such stretch would rupture, and hemorrhage into the disc rim area would occur and be clinically visible *(below).*

enous tissue and are not detected in clinical angiography, except perhaps as a diffuse glow.[45] Fluorescein angiography is clearly not a method that quantitates blood flow. Whereas laser Doppler velocimetry and nuclear magnetic resonance techniques hold promise for noninvasive blood flow determinations in the future, they are not developed enough at present to provide information for this discussion.

Fluorescein angiography has provided interesting insights into the process of glaucomatous nerve damage, but the results have not been definitive and are open to diverse interpretation. Spaeth[56] demonstrated that glaucomatous discs have a slower filling time than normal discs. This is interesting, but it gives no direct information about the adequacy of nutrition of the nerve head. The appearance time of fluorescein depends on several factors, including the concentration and rate of injection.

Hayreh and Walker[23] and later Schwartz, Reiser, and Fishbein[51] pointed out that glaucomatous discs have areas with no detectable vessels by angiography. This was proposed as evidence for lack of adequate blood flow. Many examples of this phenomenon, referred to as "filling defects," are from eyes that clearly already have neuronal loss, judged by large cup/disc ratios and known field defects. As shown, at moderate and severe stages of disc damage the neuronal loss from the anterior disc is accompanied by a proportionate loss of capillaries. Much of the anterior disc tissue can be lost as the cup becomes larger. Since the vessels of the scleral lamina are not seen in angiography, the disc with moderate or severe cup enlargement will naturally have few detectable vessels. The appropriate question is, however, whether this is simply a result of the loss of tissue and not its cause. If eyes with small cup size and filling defects had a more rapid onset of nerve damage than similar eyes without such defects in prospective follow-up, then their etiologic significance would be enhanced. I am unaware of such data.

A final angiographic observation is that glaucomatous discs "leak" fluorescein more than do normal discs.[56] It has been suggested that this indicates a vascular abnormality. Leakage of fluorescein into the disc substance from the adjacent choroid via a physiologic lack of blood-brain barrier occurs in normal nerve heads and is well documented. The histology of the glaucomatous nerve head shows that the choroid is directly exposed to the vitreous cavity when the disc rim is narrowed, and excavation into the sub–Bruch's membrane area occurs. Thus the glaucoma nerve head has little intervening rim substance between choroid and vitreous with which to screen the physiologic fluorescein leak; and it is for this reason usually more apparent.

In summary, the observations of fluorescein angiography in human and primate glaucoma are interesting and understandable in the light of the histologic events but provide no direct support for the lack of adequate nutrition to axons.

The accumulating data on optic nerve head blood flow in animal eyes fail to support the idea that glaucoma damage results from poor vascular function. Some initial experiments in this area did suggest that blood vessels might be abnormal, however. Kalvin, Hamasaki, and Gass[26] caused extreme IOP elevations by alpha-chymotrypsin treatment, and injected intravascular India ink to delineate the blood vessels. They saw a difference between the apparent number of vessels compared to control eyes. The method was not a quantitative measurement of flow, and at least some of the animals had such severely increased IOP that retinal vascular occlusions had occurred before the injection studies. Other studies, using latex injections[13] and injections of nucleated red blood cells,[32] likewise suffered from the lack of quantitative method and used acute IOP elevations.

The injection of microspheres promised possible quantification of blood flow. An initial study by Alm and Bill[1] suggested that nerve head blood flow decreases with acute

IOP elevation, but a second study[17] indicated that scleral lamina flow was remarkably resistant to decrease in the face of IOP increases known to be acutely damaging to neurons.

Recently a new quantitative method has been applied in three laboratories to measure nerve head blood flow in animal eyes. The molecule iodoantipyrine is a small, inert tracer that easily crosses the blood-brain barrier. If it is made radioactive and injected into the venous blood, it rapidly enters the central nervous system extracellular space. Its amount in a frozen-section autoradiograph is an excellent measure of local blood flow at the time the circulation is stopped experimentally. Unlike microspheres, the injection itself never elevates systemic blood pressure. Using iodoantipyrine methods in the cat nerve head, Soosi and Anderson[54] found no decrease in scleral lamina flow when IOP was elevated to levels known to damage axons. We[25] studied monkey eyes using tritiated iodoantipyrine, detecting not only mass flow over the whole lamina, but flow in areas as small as individual nerve bundles. Despite looking at various zones of the nerve head with this sensitive method, we were unable to show a decrease in flow until the IOP reached the level of the diastolic blood pressure. Although flow decreases at such high IOP might be meaningful in acute glaucoma, there was no support for the idea that blood flow was affected by the IOP levels of chronic open-angle glaucoma. We are now engaged in a further study using iodoantipyrine blood flow measures in monkeys with chronic experimental glaucoma.

Soosi and Anderson,[55] in interpreting data from an experiment with acute experimental glaucoma in cat eyes, suggested that normal eyes can maintain adequate blood flow at the lamina but that glaucomatous eyes might not, perhaps as a result of the effect of circulating vasoconstrictors on the nerve head. However, Weinstein and others[58] reported that a potent vasoconstrictor, metaraminol, does not decrease blood flow in the cat nerve head. It will be ideal when in vivo human measurements are made, but the present laboratory data strongly point away from defective blood flow at the site of glaucoma damage as a causative factor.

To some readers this citation of animal experimentation may seem far removed from the clinical findings of human patients. But one must bear in mind that the monkey eyes studied in my laboratory had glaucomatous cupping and optic nerve damage similar to that seen in human histologic specimens. How then should one view the past summaries of clinical observations that seemed to support the notion that glaucoma damage depended on vascular insufficiency?

Among these is the occurrence of optic neuropathy simulating glaucoma in patients suffering an episode of sudden low blood pressure.[21] In perspective I find no contradiction between these observations and the lack of data supporting poor blood flow in typical open-angle glaucoma. These cases are atypical. We defined glaucomatous optic neuropathy as a slowly progressive disorder. The events described by Harrington were single events superimposed on a preexistent glaucomatous neuropathy. The initial fiber loss in these patients might or might not have occurred because of a vascular insufficiency. Simply because they seemed to suffer an ischemic event from dramatic hypotension does not demonstrate that their original damage occurred by this mechanism. It is widely accepted that sudden lack of blood flow causes a profound optic neuropathy (anterior ischemic optic neuropathy). However, this is an acute, symptomatic, one-time event associated with disc swelling. Also, we have now further evidence that the pattern of nerve fiber loss with this entity is quite different from that in human glaucoma,[40] despite similarities in field loss. The patient with hypotension or sudden decrease in nerve head blood flow whose previous glaucomatous field defect worsens could be the victim of two superimposed disease processes. The same could result if a glaucoma patient had diabetic neovascularization that damaged the retina contiguous with a previous field defect area. Few would assume that this indicates that glaucoma damage was a result of neovascularization.

Some glaucoma patients can suffer a profound drop in blood pressure without progressive field loss. This no more proves that the prior and later damage was not vascular than the isolated cases of the first type prove it is vascular. It may be dangerous for anyone to have the blood pressure suddenly lowered, and this is an important clinical point. Yet, the vast majority of glaucoma patients have no evidence of past shock, certainly not on an ongoing basis that would fit with a slowly progressive neuropathy. The relationship between blood pressure and glaucoma is far from clear, as demonstrated by an epidemiologist's review[30] of the literature that concludes: ''Although glaucoma field loss may be associated with either high or low levels of blood pressure, the evidence is not clear and these relationships need further evaluation.''

The fascinating subject of low-tension glaucoma is too complex to discuss in great detail here but represents another frequently cited example of clinical data believed by many to support vascular insufficiency as a mechanism of glaucoma damage. More than anything else, the existence of this group questions the relationship between elevated IOP and glaucoma damage. The argument then is made that if these patients have not been damaged by high IOP, than what could have done so? The ready conclusion is that the blood supply to their nerve head is deficient, but this is not directly supported by evidence; rather it is indirectly assumed to be true, since the IOP is not elevated. One interesting paradox about low-tension glaucoma is that all of the patients grouped under this diagnosis have by definition disc cup configurations and field defects similar, if not identical to, those of high-pressure glaucomatous eyes. How did the cup come to look this way?

I have examined one pair of eyes from such a patient with detailed clinical records, and the scleral lamina was compressed and distorted in a similar fashion to other eyes with histories of high IOP.[13] I might conclude that the lamina mystically took on this shape without the influence of elevated IOP, or I could suppose that the IOP was elevated at some point but was never recognized as such. If the latter is true, then low-tension glaucoma's mystery can only be solved by more extensive IOP monitoring. If the former is true, then the connective tissues of such patients duplicate the excavation of glaucomatous eyes at normal IOP. This would suggest that their nerve heads are built less strongly in some way. Our one specimen did seem different in architecture from many other eyes studied, but we need more such studies to solve this riddle.

A final observation in many articles on this subject is *cavernous optic atrophy*. Schnabel[50] reported that the optic nerve in a state of severe atrophy from glaucoma could be found to have spaces in the retrolaminar area filled with hyaluronidase-sensitive glycosaminoglycans. It was assumed that this was typical for glaucoma. Later similar pathology was reported in other optic atrophies.[18] Because of the similar appearance, some have inferred that the cause of the different atrophic processes must be the same. My study of more than 75 human glaucoma optic nerves revealed that cavernous degeneration is highly unusual in most open-angle glaucoma eyes. The only two such cases I found were from blind eyes with extremely high IOP. In primate eyes as well the entry of vitreous hyaluronate into the retrobulbar nerve only occurs with the highest attainable IOP,[26, 37] whereas in the chronic, moderate IOP elevation cases, neurons atrophy without detectable caverns. There is normally a movement of fluid through the extracellular space of the optic nerve, exchanging between the vitreous cavity and the cerebrospinal fluid space. The flow increases from vitreous to nerve if the IOP is elevated.[41] When there is a rapid loss of many nerve fibers, the sudden development of unoccupied space in the retrobulbar nerve would easily fill with fluid containing vitreous contents. This would likely occur to some degree in any rapid and profound optic atrophy, regardless of its cause. Acute or severe glaucoma would be common entities in which this would occur, since sudden axon loss is combined with the highest gradient of pressure forcing fluid from vitreous cavity to the nerve. Yet other disorders can share this common end pathway, accounting for the reported examples of nonglaucomatous cavernous degeneration. This does not demonstrate that the cause of the atrophy was the same in these conditions and in glaucoma.

SUMMARY

The past 10 years have brought many changes to our knowledge of the structure and function of the optic nerve head and its response in glaucoma. Physical changes in the established site of damage for axons, the scleral lamina cribrosa, occur at an early enough stage of neural loss that they must be considered part of the pathogenesis of glaucomatous optic neuropathy. The regional structure of the scleral lamina appears to match the pattern of regional nerve fiber loss in human glaucomatous optic nerves. Therefore, the characteristic field defects are in some sense a result of the relative strength of different laminar zones. It may be that the individual susceptibility to damage of each glaucomatous eye depends to some degree on the structural makeup of the nerve's head connective tissue. The histology of the glaucomatous nerve head in human and monkey eyes does not support the suggestions that capillary loss is disproportionately greater in glaucoma than in other optic neuropathies or that cavernous optic nerve degeneration is typical for most glaucomatous eyes. Experimental measurements of blood flow in the nerve head in monkeys with chronic glaucoma and in cats with acute IOP elevations show no blood flow decrease at IOP levels that damage neurons. Further study is needed to define the precise events of cellular injury in glaucoma and their cause.

The following research areas should be pursued vigorously to aid in further elucidation of glaucoma pathogenesis:

1. Development of a means to continuously monitor IOP.
2. Improved psychophysical tests to identify early glaucoma damage.
3. Development of better methods for the study of nerve head blood flow in vivo.
4. Epidemiologic study of factors modulating glaucoma damage.
5. Study of the actual efficacy of IOP lowering in preventing damage.
6. Further clinicopathologic correlations of human eyes to define the anatomic features responsible for individual susceptibility variation.

REFERENCES

1. Alm, A., and Bill, A.: Ocular and optic nerve blood flow at normal and increased intraocular pressures in monkeys (Macaca irus): a study with radioactively labelled microspheres including flow determination in brain and some other tissues, Exp. Eye Res. **15:**15, 1973.
2. Alterman, M., and Henkind, P.: Radial peripapillary capillaries of the retina. II. Possible role in Bjerrum scotoma, Bri. J. Ophthalmol. **52:**26, 1968.
3. Anderson, D.R.: Ultrastructure of human and monkey lamina crobrosa and optic nerve head, Arch. Ophthalmol. **82:**800, 1969.

4. Anderson, D.R.: Pathogenesis of glaucomatous cupping: a new hypothesis. In New Orleans Academy of Ophthalmology: Symposium on glaucoma. St. Louis, 1975, The C.V. Mosby Co.
5. Anderson, D.R., and Hendrickson, A.: Effect of intraocular pressure on rapid axoplasmic transport in monkey optic nerve, Invest. Ophthalmol. **13:**771, 1974.
6. Armaly, M.F.: Ocular pressure and visual fields. A ten-year follow-up study, Arch. Ophthalmol. **81:**25, 1969.
7. Begg, I.S., Drance, S.M., and Sweeney, V.P.: Ischaemic optic neuropathy in open-angle glaucoma, Br. J. Ophthalmol. **55:**73, 1971.
8. Cristini, G.: Common pathologic basis of the nervous ocular symptoms in chronic glaucoma: a preliminary note, Br. J. Ophthalmol. **35:**11, 1951.
9. Daicker, B.: Selektive atrophie der radialen peripapillaren Netzhautcapillaren und glaukomatose Gesichtsfelddefekte, Albrecht v. Graefes Arch. klin. exp. Ophthal. **195:**27, 1975.
10. Drance, S.M., and others: The importance of disc hemorrhage in the prognosis of chronic open-angle glaucoma, Arch. Ophthalmol. **95:**226, 1977.
11. Emery, J.M., and others: The lamina cribrosa in normal and glaucomatous human eyes, Trans. Am. Acad. Ophthalmol. Otolaryngol **78:**290, 1974.
12. Ernest, J.T.: Pathogenesis of glaucomatous optic nerve disease, Trans. Am. Ophthalmol. Soc. **73:**366, 1975.
13. Ernest, J.T., and Potts, A.M.: Pathophysiology of the distal portion of the optic nerve. II. Vascular relationships, Am. J. Ophthalmol. **66:**380, 1968.
14. Francois, J., and Neetens, A.: Vascularity of the eye and optic nerve in glaucoma, Arch. Ophthalmol. **71:**219, 1964.
15. Fuchs, E.: Uber die lamina cribrosa, Albrecht v. Graefes Arch. fur Ophthalmologie **91:**435, 1916.
16. Gaasterland, D., Tanishima, T., and Kuwabara, T.: Axoplasmic flow during chronic experimental glaucoma. I. Light and electron microscopic studies of the monkey optic nervehead during development of glaucomatous cupping. Invest. Ophthalmol. Vis. Sci. **17:**838, 1978.
17. Geijer, C., and Bill, A.: Effects of raised intraocular pressure on retinal, prelaminar, laminar, and retrolaminar optic nerve blood flow in monkeys, Invest. Ophthalmol. Vis. Sci. **18:**1030, 1979.
18. Giarelli, L., Melato, M., and Campos, E.: 14 cases of cavernous degeneration of the optic nerve, Ophthalmologica **174:**316, 1977.
19. Graham, P.A.: The definition of pre-glaucoma: a prospective study, Trans. Ophthalmol. Soc. U.K. **88:**153, 1968.
20. Grant, W.M.: Clinical measurements of aqueous outflow, Arch. Ophthalmol. **46:**113, 1951.
21. Harrington, D.O.: Pathogenesis of the glaucomatous visual field defect: individual variations in pressure sensitivity, In Newell, F.W., editor: Conference on glaucoma: transactions of the Fifth Josiah Macy Conference, New York, 1960, Josiah Macy Foundation.
22. Hayreh, S.S.: Pathogenesis of optic nerve damage and visual field defects. In Heilmann, K., and Richardson, K.T., editors: Glaucoma: conceptions of a disease, Philadelphia, 1978, W.B. Saunders Co.
23. Hayreh, S.S., and Walker, W.M.: Fluorescent fundus photography in glaucoma, Am. J. Ophthalmol. **63:**982, 1967.
24. Henkind, P., Leitman, M., and Weitzman, E.: The diurnal curve in man: new observations, Invest. Ophthalmol. **12:**705, 1973.
25. Hohman, R.M., Addicks, E.A., and Quigley, H.A.: Optic nerve and retinal blood flow measurement in experimental glaucoma using tritiated iodoantipyrine, Invest. Ophthalmol. Vis. Sci. **24**(suppl.):102, 1983.
26. Kalvin, N.H., Hamasaki, D.I., and Gass, J.D.M.: Experimental glaucoma in monkeys. II. Studies of intraocular vascularity during glaucoma, Arch. Ophthalmol. **76:**94, 1966.
27. Kirsch, R.E., and Anderson, D.R.: Identification of the glaucomatous disc, Trans. Am. Acad. Ophthalmol. Otolaryngol. **77:**143, 1973.
28. Kitazawa, Y., and Horie, T.: Diurnal variation of intraocular pressure in primary open-angle glaucoma, Am. J. Ophthalmol. **79:**557, 1975.
29. Kornzweig, A.L., Eliasoph, I., and Feldstein, M.: Selective atrophy of the radial peripapillary capillaries in chronic glaucoma, Arch. Ophthalmol. **80:**696, 1968.
30. Leske, C.: The epidemiology of open-angle glaucoma: a review, Am. J. Epidemiol. **118:**166, 1983.
31. Levy, N.S., Crapps, E.E., and Bonney, R.D.: Displacement of the optic nerve head: response to acute intraocular pressure elevation in primate eyes, Arch. Ophthalmol. **99:**2166, 1981.
32. Minckler, D.S., Bunt, A.H., and Johanson, G.W.: Orthograde and retrograde axoplasmic transport during acute ocular hypertension in the monkey, Invest. Ophthalmol. Vis. Sci. **16:**426, 1977.

33. Ochs, S.: Systems of material transport in nerve fibers (axoplasmic transport) related to nerve function and trophic control, Ann. N.Y. Acad. Sci. **228:**202, 1974.
34. Pederson, J.E., and Anderson, D.R.: The mode of progressive disc cupping in ocular hypertension and glaucoma, Arch. Ophthalmol. **98:**490, 1980.
35. Perkins, E.S.: The Bedford glaucoma survey. I. Long-term follow-up of borderline cases, Br. J. Ophthalmol. **57:**179, 1973.
36. Quigley, H.A., and Addicks, E.M.: Chronic experimental glaucoma in primates. I. Production of elevated intraocular pressure by injection of autologous red blood cells, Invest. Ophthalmol. Vis. Sci. **19:**126, 1980.
37. Quigley, H.A., and Addicks, E.M.: Chronic experimental glaucoma in primates. II. Effect of extended intraocular pressure on optic nerve head and axonal transport, Invest. Ophthalmol. Vis. Sci. **19:**137, 1980.
38. Quigley, H.A., and Addicks, E.M.: Regional differences in the structure of the lamina cribrosa and their relation to glaucomatous optic nerve damage, Arch. Ophthalmol. **99:**137, 1981.
39. Quigley, H.A., and Green, W.R.: The histology of human glaucoma cupping and optic nerve damage: clinicopathologic correlation in 21 eyes, Ophthalmology **10:**1803, 1979.
40. Quigley, H.A., Addicks, E.A., and Green, W.R.: Optic nerve damage in human glaucoma. III. Quantitative correlation of nerve fiber loss and visual field defect in glaucoma, ischemic neuropathy, papilledema, and toxic neuropathy, Arch. Ophthalmol. **100:**135, 1982.
41. Quigley, H.A., Guy, J., and Anderson, D.R.: Blockade of rapid axonal transport: effect of intraocular pressure elevation in primate optic nerve, Arch. Ophthalmol. **97:**525, 1979.
42. Quigley, H.A., and others: The mechanism of optic nerve damage in experimental acute intraocular pressure elevation, Invest. Ophthalmol. Vis. Sci. **19:**505, 1980.
43. Quigley, H.A., and others: Optic nerve damage in human glaucoma. II. The site of injury and susceptibility to damage, Arch. Opthalmol. **99:**635, 1981.
44. Quigley, H.A., and others: Morphologic changes in the lamina cribrosa correlated with neural loss in open-angle glaucoma, Am. J. Ophthalmol. **95:**673, 1983.
45. Quigley, H.A., and others: Blood vessels of the glaucomatous optic disk in experimental primate and human eyes, Invest. Ophthalmol. Vis. Sci. In press, 1984.
46. Radius, R.L., and Anderson, D.R.: Breakdown of the normal optic nerve head blood-brain barrier following acute elevation of intraocular pressure in experimental animals, Invest. Ophthalmol. Vis. Sci. **19:**244, 1980.
47. Radius, R.L., and Gonzales, M.: Anatomy of the lamina cribrosa in human eyes, Arch. Ophthalmol. **99:**2159, 1981.
48. Radius, R.L., Maumenee, A.E., and Green, W.R.: Pit-like changes of the optic nerve head in open-angle glaucoma, Br. J. Ophthalmol. **62:**389, 1978.
49. Robin, A.L., and others: An analysis of visual acuity, visual fields, and disk cupping in childhood glaucoma, Am. J. Ophthalmol. **88:**847, 1979.
50. Schnabel, J.: Die Entwicklungsgeschichte der glaukomatosen Exkavation, Zeitschr. Augenheilkd. **14:**1, 1905.
51. Schwartz, B., Reiser, J.C., and Fishbein, S.L.: Fluorescein angiographic defects of the optic disc in glaucoma, Arch. Ophthalmol. **85:**1961, 1977.
52. Shaffer, R.N.: The role of the astroglial cells in glaucomatous cupping, Doc. Ophthalmol. **26:**516, 1969.
53. Sjostrand, J., and others: Impairment of intraneural microcirculation, blood-nerve barrier and axonal transport in experimental nerve ischemia and compression. In Korr, I.M., editor; The neurobiologic mechanisms in manipulative therapy, New York, 1978, Plenum Publishing Corp.
54. Soosi, N., and Anderson, D.R.: Effect of elevated intraocular pressure on blood flow: occurrence in cat optic nerve head studied with iodoantipyrine I 125, Arch. Ophthalmol. **101:**98, 1983.
55. Sossi, N., and Anderson, D.R.: Blockage of axonal transport in optic nerve induced by elevation of intraocular pressure: effect of arterial hypertension induced by angiotensin I, Arch. Ophthalmol. **101:**94, 1983.
56. Spaeth, G.L.: The pathogenesis of nerve damage in glaucoma: contributions of fluorescein angiography, New York, 1977, Grune & Stratton, Inc.
57. Vrabec, F.: Glaucomatous cupping of the human optic disk: a neuro-histologic study, Albrecht v. Graefes Arch. klin. exp. Ophthal. **198:**223, 1976.
58. Weinstein, J.M., and others: Regional optic nerve blood flow and its autoregulation, Invest. Ophthalmol. Vis. Sci. **24:**1559, 1983.
59. Wilczek, M.: The lamina cribrosa and its nature, Br. J. Ophthalmol. **31:**551, 1947.

9

Nerve fiber loss and disparity of disc and field changes in glaucoma

Robert N. Shaffer

Thirty years ago Hans Goldmann stated that "blindness haunts people suffering from chronic glaucoma, not increased pressure." This is certainly true, but ophthalmologists remain concerned with intraocular pressure (IOP) because it is the one parameter that we know can be damaging and that we can control. How the optic nerve is damaged remains in doubt, and we do not yet understand certain factors.

THEORIES ON THE MECHANISM OF OPTIC NERVE DAMAGE

For the past 30 years the vascular theory of optic nerve damage has been dominant. It theorizes that optic disc ischemia results in the disc cupping and arcuate field defects typical of chronic glaucoma. However, it fails to explain the specificity of that damage.

More than 40 years ago, in my residency, we were told that the damage was caused by the nerves being kinked over the edge of the optic canal. This mechanical theory has been recently revived and supported by the exquisite anatomic studies of Maumenee, Quigley, Green, and Addicks.[11-14] They point out that the lamina cribrosa is bowed back in glaucoma, which could cause the superimposed sheets to slip, squeezing the nerve fibers as they pass through. They have demonstrated that the lamina has a weaker configuration at the upper and lower poles, a possible cause of the arcuate field changes.

Unfortunately, the findings of Schnabel,[15,16] Elschnig,[5] Fuchs,[6] and Goldmann[7] demonstrate that for a long period the lamina cribrosa does not participate in the glaucomatous excavation. Quigley's recent studies[12-14] confirm that backward bowing of the lamina is a relatively late finding. The increase in cupping and the compression of the inner lamellae could be based on the loss of neurons, since he has cases with confirmed 40% to 50% loss of nerve fibers with minimal or no field change. I have difficulty believing that rugged connective tissue sheets of collagenous, elastic, and astroglial fibers would yield under the minor 22 to 30 mm Hg pressures usually found in open-angle glaucoma. Inside a closed container pressure is exerted equally, so the innermost lamellae inside the eye must have equal pressure on all sides, making a movement in any direction impossible until the outer lamellae are pushed backward.

Johansson[10] recently carried out an interesting experiment on hooded male rats. These rats have only one layer of lamina cribrosa rather than the eight or nine sheets found in human beings. This largely precludes the possibility of a shearing effect on optic neurons when pressure is increased. Yet there was a 29% decrease in transport of horseradish peroxidase into the retina in vitro when pressures were increased to 29 mm Hg from the rat's normal pressure of 20 mm Hg. At IOPs of 50 mm Hg there was a 76% block in transport. Such findings cast doubt not only on the mechanical theory, but also on the vascular theory, since this experiment was conducted in vitro with no blood supply. The blockage seemed to result from direct pressure effect on the axons.

Since the small veins on the disc are under the influence of IOP and an abrupt drop to normal venous pressure outside the eye occurs, it seems logical that minimal shunting of blood away from the disc over a 10-year period by minor pressure elevations, along with possible breakdown of autoregulation, could lead to mild anoxia, mild blocking of axoplasmic flow, and progressive loss of neurons. Later a shift in the lamellae could aggravate the problem by squeezing the neurons.

All of us have seen cases of sudden advance of glaucomatous cupping and field loss when there has been a sudden drop in general blood pressure,[3,8] profound anemia, or severe illness.

Small splinter hemorrhages at the disc margin are known to have prognostic significance. Drance and Begg[4] first commented on this sign in 1970. Airaksinen and coworkers[1] stated that 34% of cases with such a hemorrhage later developed a field loss, although not necessarily in the area of the hemorrhage. Bengtsson and colleagues[2] noted disc hemorrhages over a period of years in 47% of 1511 glaucoma patients, whereas such hemorrhages were seen in only 0.5% of normal eyes.

The mechanical theorists suggest that the bleeding is the result of stretching of tiny vessels as the cup enlarges. However, I have seen patients with completely normal nerves and tiny physiologic cups develop a hemorrhage, followed by slight cupping and a corresponding relative arcuate scotoma. One patient had three observed episodes of bleeding at the lower temporal pole of the disc, with progressive excavation to the temporal rim and an accompanying dense upper arcuate field defect.

Spaeth[19] and Schwartz[17] have shown fluorescein angiographic changes in the disc vasculature, which become more marked with increased IOP. Heilmann[9] altered IOP and blood pressure by drugs. A relative scotoma was improved if the IOP was lowered and blood pressure stayed the same. When both were lowered, there was no improvement. If blockage of axoplasmic flow were completely mechanical, it should be unaffected by changes in blood pressure.[18]

Highly specialized, nondividing cells such as neurons must last a lifetime. Outfall of these neurons begins at the end of the growth period and is accelerated in the last decades of life. There is a 10% decrease in brain weight over a lifetime; an exaggerated loss is known as Alzheimer's disease.

Optic nerve fibers also drop out, depressing retinal function. A more rapid dropout occurs in glaucoma. Nerve fiber bundle defects can be demonstrated by color or flicker fusion long before defects can be shown by perimetry. Increased pressure certainly accelerates this loss. Quigley[13,14] has shown that 40% of the neurons can drop out without detectable field loss, although cupping would be present. Once cupping is present, there would be a reason for a shift in the lamellae and compression of specific neurons to account for arcuate scotomas.

More than 1 million neurons are estimated to be in each optic nerve. We normally are losing 5 to 6 thousand neurons per year; this is greatly exaggerated in glaucoma. It is possible that low-tension glaucoma could be considered an Alzheimer's disease of the optic nerve. Thus it is not surprising that ophthalmologists become discouraged at the slow loss of function in glaucomatous eyes despite their best efforts. We can probably slow down the abnormal loss of neurons, but we cannot prevent the normal attrition. Efforts must continue toward learning the factors that accelerate this loss. Elements of both the vascular and the mechanical theories are probably at work.

Of particular interest to the clinician is the specificity of neuron loss in glaucoma. Because of this specificity, in the large majority of cases an ophthalmologist should be able to look at a carefully performed qualitative visual field and know what damage the optic disc in that eye will show. Conversely, the clinician can carefully examine the optic disc and predict the probable field loss. If these two findings do not correspond, both examinations must be repeated. If there is still incongruity, the patient should remain in a questionable status for future evaluation. Examples of such lack of congruity follow.

REASONS FOR INCONGRUITIES OF DISC AND FIELD

Equipment and perimetrist

The tangent screen is still a commonly used method of perimetry; when carefully performed, it is an excellent method. In the average busy office standard lighting is rare, and meticulous quantitative technique is seldom used. Goldmann perimetry is a definite improvement, providing a standardized machine and method, but the technicians are often not well trained. The new automated perimeters do their own calibrating and eliminate perimetrist artifacts, except for errors in properly instructing and positioning the patient.

Example. A 55-year-old ocular hypertensive patient had IOPs ranging between 21 and 32 mm Hg in both eyes and had been followed for 3 years without change in his normal field or in optic nerves, which had a cup/disc ratio of 0.1.

One day an urgent call from his referring ophthalmologist stated that he had suddenly developed a double-arcuate ring scotoma in one eye. He was told to report immediately and to bring the field with him.

On arrival his Goldmann field certainly showed a dense double-arcuate scotoma between 10 and 20 degrees, with a peculiar bump to 30 degrees upper temporally. The Goldmann field was repeated, but no scotoma was found and the cup/disc ratio continued to be 0.1. It was determined that the new perimetrist at the referring physician's office had carefully mapped out the correcting lens rim, complete with the finger holder in the upper temporal area.

Patient

The patient is always a variable. With an unreliable patient, the automated perimeter produces more artifacts than a trained technician. A smaller pupil than appeared at previous perimetry or clouding of the media, such as cataract, depresses fields and exaggerates existing defects. Glasses' frames, eyebrows, and lids can interfere with the upper visual field. Improper placement or an incorrect power of correcting lens, including mascara on the lens, can alter a field. Patient's responses can also be misleading—the clinician must continue to be suspicious if a field defect is not matched by a corresponding change in the optic disc.

Example. A 28-year-old patient had had IOPs ranging between 20 and 35 mm Hg for the past 5 years. Her mother and a sister had glaucoma. Intensive medication failed to control the pressure, and fields had slipped down to the central 6 degrees. Two filtering operations in one eye and one in the other had also failed to control IOP.

On consultation she was found to have vision of 20/20, tension of 28 mm Hg, and open angles in both eyes. Goldmann fields showed bilateral constrictions to the central 6 degrees. However, optic discs had good neural rims, with a cup/disc ratio of 0.5. The patient moved about the office without difficulty. A tangent field at 1 and 2 M was done, and the field defect remained the same at both distances. The constricted field was caused by hysteria; the patient had undergone three unnecessary operations. The diagnosis of hysteria can be made using the tangent screen but is impossible on Goldmann-type perimeters.

Disc and retinal pathology

Disc and retinal pathology can produce field defects identical in appearance to those produced by glaucoma. If ocular hypertension is also present, the ophthalmologist can easily be misled.

Example. An airline pilot with ocular hypertension was recently found to have an arcuate scotoma. If its cause was glaucoma, he would be grounded. There was no cupping. He was found to have bilateral drusen of the discs, most marked in the area coinciding with the scotoma. Of course, such lesions can progress, and he must continue to be monitored.

Pericentral scotomas can be produced by many abnormalities around the disc, such as optic pits, colobomas, medullated nerve fibers, juxtapapillary choroiditic scars, myopic degenerative changes, and posterior staphylomas.

Occlusion of retinal vessels or their branches, cerebrovascular accidents or tumors, particularly meningiomas near the chiasm, can be misleading, especially if superimposed on a preexisting glaucomatous defect.

A particularly interesting monocular glaucoma with a peripheral field defect can be produced by a small localized tear and detachment of the retina. Often there is a faint flare, which leads to a misdiagnosis of iritic secondary glaucoma. The peripheral detachment is frequently difficult to see, especially through small pupils. Its diagnosis and successful treatment results in a complete normalization of IOP. The clue to this diagnosis is the presence of a peripheral field defect in an eye with a perfectly normal optic nerve.

In all of these cases the key is careful, accurate ophthalmoscopy and perimetry, with findings in consistent agreement. The rule governing congruity of disc and field is as follows:

1. With a normal disc and an abnormal field, recheck both disc and field.
2. With an abnormal disc and a normal field, recheck both disc and field.
3. With incongruity of either disc or field, recheck both, then thoroughly examine entire retina and visual system.
4. With incongruity of findings, always keep rechecking.

REFERENCES

1. Airaksinen, P.J., and others: Optic disc hemorrhages: analysis of stereo photographs and clinical data of 112 patients, Arch. Ophthalmol. **99:**1795, 1981.
2. Bengtsson, B., and others: Disc hemorrhage and glaucoma, Acta Ophthalmol. **5:**1, 1981.
3. Drance, S.M.: Some studies on the relationship of haemodynamics and ocular pressure in open-angle glaucoma, Trans. Ophthalmol. Soc. U.K. **88:**633, 1969.
4. Drance, S.M., and Begg, I.S.: Sector Hemorrhage—a probable acute ischemic disc change in chronic simple glaucoma, Can. J. Ophthalmol. **5:**137, 1970.
5. Elschnig, A.: Uber physiologische, atropische und glaukomatose Exkavation, Ber Deutsch Ophthal. Gesellsch. **34:**2, 1907.

6. Fuchs, E.: Uber die Lamina cribrosa, von Graefes Arch. f. Ophthal. **91:**435, 1916.
7. Goldmann, H.: The glaucoma problem. In Newell, F.W., editor: Glaucoma, Transactions of the Second Conference, Dec. 3-5, 1956, New York, 1957, Josiah Macy Jr. Foundation.
8. Harrington, D.O.: Pathogenesis of the glaucomatous visual field defects: individual variations in pressure sensitivity. In Newell, F.W., editor: Glaucoma, Transactions of the Fifth Conference, March 6-9, 1960, New York, 1961, Josiah Macy Jr. Foundation.
9. Heilmann, K.: Progression and regression of visual field defects. In Heilmann, K., and Richardson, K., editors: Glaucoma, Stuttgart, 1978, Georg Thieme Publishers.
10. Johansson, J-O.: Inhibition of retrograde axoplasmic transport in rat optic nerve by increased IOP in vitro, Invest. Ophthalmol. Vis. Sci. **24**(12):1552, 1983.
11. Maumenee, A.E.: Causes of optic nerve damage in glaucoma, Ophthalmology **90**(7):741, 1983.
12. Quigley, H.A., and Green, W.R.: The histology of human glaucoma cupping and optic nerve damage: clinicopathologic correlation in 21 eyes, Ophthalmology **86**(10):1803, 1979.
13. Quigley, H.A., Addicks, E.M., and Green, W.R.: Optic nerve damage in human glaucoma. III. Quantitative correlation of nerve fiber loss and visual field defect in glaucoma, ischemic neuropathy, papilledema, and toxic neuropathy, Arch. Ophthalmol. **100**(1):135, 1982.
14. Quigley, H.A., and others: Optic nerve damage in human glaucoma. II. The site of injury and susceptibility to damage, Arch. Ophthalmol. **99**(4):635, 1981.
15. Schnabel, J.: Entwicklungsgeschichte der glaukomatosen Exkavation, Ztschr. f. Augen. **14:**1, 1905.
16. Schnabel, J.: Klinische Daten zur Entwicklungsgeschichte der glaukomatosen Exkavation, Ztschr. f. Augen. **19:**335, 1908.
17. Schwartz, B., Rieser, J.C., and Fishbein, S.L.: Fluorescein angiographic defects of the optic disc in glaucoma, Arch. Ophthalmol. **95**(11):1961, 1977.
18. Sossi, N., and Anderson, D.R.: Blockage of axonal transport in optic nerve induced by elevation of intraocular pressure, Arch. Ophthalmol. **101:**94, 1983.
19. Spaeth, G.L.: Fluorescein angiography: its contributions towards understanding the mechanisms of visual loss in glaucoma, Trans. Am. Ophthalmol. Soc. **73:**491, 1976.

10

Complications of laser trabeculoplasty

James B. Wise

Discussions of laser trabeculoplasty complications nearly always focus on relatively short-term phenomena, such as iritis or pressure rises,[8-10,13] occurring in the first few hours or weeks after the procedure. However, the most important complication of laser trabeculoplasty is the same as the most important complication of both medical and surgical therapy of glaucoma—failure to lower the intraocular pressure (IOP) far enough to prevent further field loss.[2,11] It is frequently not appreciated how low the pressure must be to protect severely damaged discs.

In their discussion of blindness from glaucoma, Grant and Burke[3] showed that patients who had visual field defects both above and below when first started on therapy would go blind unless their pressure were kept in the low teens (boxed material below). Even if the patients had field loss only above or below, they could have field loss at a pressure of 20 mm Hg. Abedin, Simmons, and Grant[1] found that a pressure of 12 mm Hg or less was required to stop progressive visual field loss in patients with extreme cupping of the optic nerve. Quigley[7] has shown that even at the onset of field loss, 50% of the nerve fibers can be missing, and that with very modest degrees of measurable field loss, nerve fiber loss in the range of 70% to 80% can be present.

The severe distortion of the lamina cribrosa in far-advanced glaucoma cupping produces so much obstruction of axoplasmic flow that only pressures near hypotony are low enough to allow partial reversal of the cupping and release of the pressure on the squeezed and distorted axons. Even when the pressure has been markedly lowered by the use of laser trabeculoplasty, the physician must make sure that the pressure achieved is actually low enough to be safe for the degree of cupping present in the treated eye. Careful serial disc observations and visual field measurement should be made to confirm

Long-time relationships of stage, tension, and visual field loss

I Abnormal disc, normal fields: loss common at high-20 to mid-20 tension.
II Field defect above or below: loss common at mid-20 to 20 tension.
III Field defect above and below: loss common at high-teens tension.

From Grant, W.M., and Burke, J.F.: Why do some people go blind from glaucoma? Ophthalmology **89:**991, 1982, with permission.

that adequate pressure lowering is present. Although no arbitrary figures apply to all cases, I have found the degree of cupping to be strongly indicative of the "safe" IOP (Table 10-1).

Another major complication of glaucoma therapy both before and after laser trabeculoplasty is failure to detect progressive angle closure. If laser treatment is squeezed into a narrow angle in a eye with a relative pupillary block, resulting mild iritis can accentuate the pupillary block, closing the angle further and causing extensive peripheral anterior synechiae. Because pupillary block is so often progressive, I strongly advise that eyes with significant pupillary block, even if the angle is still open, have a laser iridectomy performed. This can be done alone, or combined with a limited trabeculoplasty. The remainder of the trabeculoplasty can be performed a month later. The chipping technique of laser iridectomy (boxed material below) simply evaporates a line of iris without producing extensive burning or damage to the rest of the iris. This method produces little or no increase in iritis and pressure rise over a trabeculoplasty alone. In my referral practice of glaucoma, an astonishing percentage of patients have at least partial angle closure. In 1983, 355 new eyes were treated with laser trabeculoplasty. Of these, 111 had simultaneous laser iridectomy at the time the first half of the trabeculoplasty was performed. This constitutes 31% of the total number of eyes receiving trabeculoplasty. Overall, 35% of the eyes had laser iridectomy before, during, or after the

Table 10-1. Suggested "safe" levels of IOP for various amounts of cupping

Cup/disc ratio	*IOP (mm Hg)*
To 0.5	Under 23
0.5-0.7	Under 20
0.7-0.8	Under 16
0.9 or more	Under 13
Any cup to rim	Under 15

Laser iridectomy technique

1. Always use Abraham iridectomy lens.
2. Almost never use "stretch burns."
3. Use only the 50 μ spot.
4. Use 0.05 second for blue or light-brown iris.
5. Use 0.02 second for dark-brown, thick iris.
6. Pick a thin area in peripheral superior iris.
7. Focus precisely each time.
8. Use enough power to give cutting effect.
9. Usual power is 800 to 1500 mW true output.
10. Cut a line parallel to limbus, across iris fibers.
11. Keep chipping until stroma and pigment are gone.
12. Note that usually 150 to 300 shots are required.
13. Make a clean, 300 μ diameter hole.

laser trabeculoplasty (Table 10-2), emphasizing the prevalence of creeping angle closure in patients with medically controlled "open-angle" glaucoma.

Black patients are particularly likely to develop plateau iris and peripheral angle closure in association with pupillary block, yet maintain a deep chamber centrally. These eyes will develop extensive peripheral synechiae if trabeculoplasty alone is performed. Because such eyes are rather susceptible to inflammation, they should have laser iridectomy as a separate procedure, followed by two-stage laser trabeculoplasty beginning 1 or 2 weeks after the iridectomy. Any other course in these deeply pigmented eyes with plateau irides is very prone to give extensive peripheral anterior synechiae. Simply flattening the peripheral iris with 200 μ laser burns (laser peripheral iridoplasty) is not recommended, as the pupillary block remains and will ultimately force the iris forward again. Because patients cannot be examined on a daily or weekly basis, I believe any eye requiring trabeculoplasty for medically uncontrolled open-angle glaucoma that also shows significant peripheral bulging of the iris should have a small laser iridectomy done at the same time. This adds little, if any, danger to the procedure and over the years will prevent many late complications from angle closure.

The short-term and intermediate-term complications of trabeculoplasty can be divided into those caused by poor technique and those that are apparently inherent risks of the procedure. Technical errors include (1) ocular ischemia from giving subconjunctival anesthetic containing epinephrine; (2) complications of retrobulbar anesthesia, which is never necessary for trabeculoplasty; (3) errors in spot size and power setting leading to overtreatment or undertreatment; (4) errors in spot placement leading to endothelial damage from anterior placement and cyclitis, pain, hemorrhage, and synechiae from posterior placement; and (5) failure to adequately follow the patient and detect such complications as postsurgical pressure rises and steroid glaucoma.

There are certain minor complications inherent in trabeculoplasty. Mild iritis is common but is usually barely detectable if the number of laser burns is limited to 50 or 60 at one session. As noted, performance of a small laser iridectomy by the chipping technique appears to give no increase in iritis. Corneal burns can occur and take two forms. Small epithelial burns tend to develop in the region of corneal iron lines, such as the Hudson-Stähli line. These burns clear in a day or two without any residual scarring. I have seen two cases with endothelial corneal burns. In each case the endothelium was pigmented, in one eye from argyrosis and in the other from corneal blood staining. Faint signs of the endothelial burns were visible years later, but no corneal decompensation occurred in these two cases. In perhaps 2% of eyes treated with laser trabeculoplasty, an ooze of blood will appear from an impact site in the trabecular meshwork, nearly always from a heavily pigmented area between 11 and 1 o'clock. These can be

Table 10-2. Association between laser trabeculoplasty (LTP) and laser iridectomy (LI)—1983 study

LTP/LI	*Number*	*Percentage*
Total eyes with LTP	355	100
LI before LTP	11	3.1
LI during LTP	111	31.3
LI after LTP	2	0.6
Total LI with LTP	124	35

stopped with a 200 μ, 0.2 second burn of low power, but they will also stop rather quickly if the contact lens is removed, releasing the compression of the episcleral circulation. A rare nervous patient may become syncopal, with typical findings of nausea, weakness, and slow pulse. This is easily controlled by placing the patient on the floor with the legs elevated and then giving 0.4 mg of intravenous atropine. In a few minutes the attack will be over and treatment can be resumed.

Another common occurence is failure to obtain an immediate reduction of IOP. Many eyes treated with laser trabeculoplasty will show little or no decrease in pressure in the first week or two and then a marked decrease about 3 or 4 weeks after surgery. The patient should be warned of this phenomen to prevent undue anxiety.

Pressure rises after laser trabeculoplasty have received wide publicity. They can be divided into four categories: immediate, intermediate, late, and very late. Immediate pressure rises occur within 1 to 8 hours after laser trabeculoplasty and on the average peak at 6 to 8 mm Hg[5,13] but sometimes can be as much as 20 mm Hg above the baseline pressure. These pressure rises are influenced by the number of laser burns[12] and are more common and greater in magnitude with the use of 100 burns compared to 50 burns per session.[8] They are not influenced by subconjunctival dexamethasone given immediately after the trabeculoplasty but are considerably reduced by placing an ice bag over the eye for 15 minutes before and 3 hours after the treatment. Use of the ice bag is recommended for patients who have severe disc damage; oral glycerol may also be given. Except for possible danger to very compromised discs, these rises are of little importance and do not influence the ultimate result of the treatment.

Intermediate-term pressure rises occur from 1 to 21 days after laser treatment and can sometimes reach very high levels, especially in patients treated with 100 or more laser burns in a single session.[6,9,10,14]

Case report. A 77-year-old, blue-eyed man had glaucoma for 20 years, with a pressure in the left eye of 43 mm Hg on therapy with epinephrine, timolol, pilocarpine, and acetazolamide. He received 112 laser burns of 50 μ each at 0.1 second and 1300 mW, spaced 360 degrees. The next day the eye was markedly injected, and the pressure was 55 mm Hg. The pressure progressively rose to a level of 65 mm Hg at 5 days despite all treatment. A successful trabeculectomy was performed, with long-term control of the pressure at a level of 13 mm Hg. The patient's other eye also had a pressure varying from 30 to 42 mm Hg on similar therapy, with a cup/disc ratio of 0.7. It was treated with 35 laser burns in 120 degrees of the angle and showed a short-term rise to 42 mm Hg, responsive to increased medical therapy. Ten days later a second 120 degrees of angle was treated with another 35 burns, and no pressure rise occurred. One week later the pressure was 13 mm Hg. It remained at this level for 3 years without further laser treatment, with timolol therapy alone.

Using the initial technique of laser trabeculoplasty,[15,16] 366 eyes have been treated with 90 or more burns in a single session. Of these, 19 (5.2%) eyes developed a pressure rise of 10 mm Hg or more above the baseline in the period 1 to 21 days after surgery. In five eyes (1.4%) the pressure could not be controlled, and filtering surgery was required. In more than 1000 eyes subsequently treated with 70 or fewer laser burns in a single session, none have required filtering surgery for acute pressure rises. These rises were clearly inflammatory, as the eyes were obviously red, and they often respond to subconjunctival dexamethasone. Histologically lymphocytes, macrophages, activated trabecular endothelial cells, and tissue debris were present.[4]

A pressure rise greater than 10 mm Hg above the baseline reduces the prognosis

(Table 10-3). The probable mechanism is adhesion of the inflamed trabecular layers, worsened by direct compression by the elevated pressure. Avoiding these pressure rises improves the prognosis, as seen in the case report. Thomas, Simmons, and Belcher[9] divide laser trabeculoplasty into two sessions by placing 50 burns into 180 degrees of the angle, then placing 50 burns into the other 180 degrees 1 month later. The two-session procedure produces much lower pressure rises (Table 10-4), with equally good control of the glaucoma, and it is now the most widely used version of the procedure.

Late pressure rises (1 to 3 months) after an initial good result usually mean failure of therapy. Typically they are seen when unusual or poor prognosis cases (juvenile, aphakic, uveitic) have been treated. The initial drop is probably caused by temporary trabeculopuncture. When the punctures close, the basic trabecular insufficiency is evident. Additional trabeculoplasty has always failed in my experience, and some other procedure should be used.

Very late rises (after 6 months) are usually seen when inadequate trabeculoplasty, using 80 or fewer burns of true 50 μ size, has been done. When the rise occurs, it represents recurrent trabecular collapse. Late retreatment does not appear to be additive with the first treatment. Additional treatment with 70 to 80 burns in a single session should be given, and the patient should understand that surgery will be done if the pressure does not decrease promptly. In about one half of such cases, the repeat trabeculoplasty will allow control to be regained.

Table 10-3. Results in 37 eyes having postlaser pressure rises >10 mm Hg above prelaser pressure

Average highest IOP	44.5 mm Hg
Range of highs	29-68 mm Hg
Later filters	13/37 (35%)
IOP <21 mm Hg at 1 year	18/37 (48.6%)
IOP <21 mm Hg at 2 years	11/28 (39.3%)

Table 10-4. Comparison of 100 burns in one session with two sessions of 50 burns each

	One session	*Two sessions*
Number of eyes	139	102
Percentage control	84.9%	86.3%
IOP rise >5 mm Hg	14.4%	8.8%
IOP rise >10 mm Hg	9.4%	2.9%

From Thomas, J.V., Simmons, R.J., and Belcher, C.D., III: Argon laser trabeculoplasty in the presurgical glaucoma patient, Ophthalmology **89:**187, 1982, with permission.

REFERENCES

1. Abedin, S., Simmons, R.J., and Grant, W.M.: Progressive low-tension glaucoma: treatment to stop glaucomatous cupping and field loss when these progress despite normal intraocular pressure, Ophthalmology **89:**1, 1982.
2. Cairns, J.E.: The case for early surgery in primary open-angle glaucoma, Glaucoma **4:**7, 1982.
3. Grant, W.M., and Burke, J.F.: Why do some people go blind from glaucoma? Ophthalmology **89:**991, 1982.
4. Greenidge, K.C., and others: Acute intraocular pressure elevation after argon laser trabeculoplasty and iridectomy: a clinicopathological study, Ophthalmic Surg. **15:**105, 1984.
5. Hoskins, H.D., and others: Complications of laser trabeculoplasty, Ophthalmology **90:**796, 1983.
6. Levy, N.S., and Bonney, R.C.: Argon laser therapy in advanced open-angle glaucoma, Glaucoma **4:**25, 1982.
7. Quigley, H.A., Addicks, E.M., and Green, W.R.: Optic nerve damage in human glaucoma. III. Quantitative correlation of nerve fiber loss and visual field defect in glaucoma, ischemic neuropathy, papilledema, and toxic neuropathy, Arch. Ophthalmol. **100:**135, 1982.
8. Schwartz L.W., and others: Variation of techniques on the results of argon laser trabeculoplasty, Ophthalmology **90:**781, 1983.
9. Thomas, J.V., Simmons, R.J., and Belcher, C.D., III: Argon laser trabeculoplasty in the presurgical glaucoma patient, Ophthalmology **89:**187, 1982.
10. Thomas, J.V., Simmons, R.J., and Belcher, C.D., III: Complications of argon laser trabeculoplasty, Glaucoma **4:**50, 1982.
11. Watson, P.G., and Grierson, I.: The place of trabeculectomy in the treatment of glaucoma, Ophthalmology **88:**175, 1981.
12. Weinreb R.N., and others: Influence of the number of laser burns on the early results of argon laser trabeculoplasty, Am. J. Ophthalmol. **95:**287, 1983.
13. Weinreb, R.N., and others: Immediate intraocular pressure response to argon laser trabeculoplasty, Am. J. Ophthalmol. **95:**279, 1983.
14. Wilensky, J.T., and Jampol, I.M.: Laser therapy for open angle glaucoma, Ophthalmology **88:**213, 1981.
15. Wise, J.B.: Glaucoma treatment by trabecular tightening with the argon laser, Int. Ophthalmol. Clin. **21**(1):69, 1981.
16. Wise, J.B., and Witter, S.L.: Argon laser therapy for open-angle glaucoma: a pilot study, Arch. Ophthalmol. **97:**319, 1979.

11

Laser treatment of macular disease: patient and laser selection

Robert C. Watzke

SELECTION OF PATIENTS

Modern treatment of macular disease involves the detection of subretinal neovascular membranes from whatever cause and their eradication by properly selected and applied laser photocoagulation. The causes of subretinal neovascular membranes are numerous:

Disciform macular degeneration
Histoplasmosis
Angioid streaks
Choroidal rupture
Myopia
Heredodegenerative diseases
Optic nerve head drusen
Benign choroidal tumor
Inflammation
Postphotocoagulation
Idiopathic causes

Such a membrane can be recognized, however, by four characteristics: (1) serous retinal detachment, (2) grayish yellow subretinal exudates, (3) intraretinal or subretinal hemorrhage, and (4) lipid exudates.

Symptoms of blurred vision, metamorphopsia, and distortion are caused by a serous detachment of the retina that involves the fovea. The most common cause of a serous macular retinal detachment is a subretinal neovascular membrane. Patients with such symptoms must be carefully examined for this by the best possible method of examination: a careful slitlamp biomicroscopic examination of the macula with a flat contact lens. Examination by direct ophthalmoscopy or Hruby lens is not enough. It is unnecessary, expensive, and unjustified to order a fluorescein angiogram in such patients without a prior contact lens and biomicroscopic examination. Fluorescein angiograms should not be ordered as a screening device, but only if there is a reasonable expectation of finding treatable macular disease.

The most common cause of subretinal neovascular membranes is aging macular degeneration, the most reliable sign of which is drusen. It is convenient to classify drusen into three types: hyalin, soft, and regressing (calcified).

Hyalin drusen are small, round, yellow excrescences of Bruch's membrane; they are

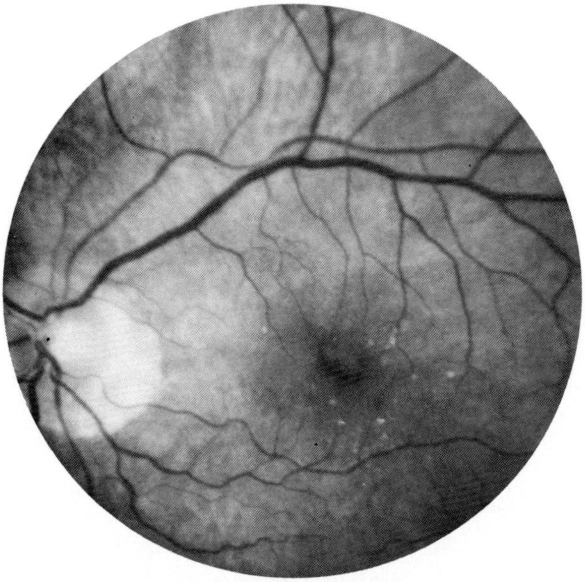

Fig. 11-1. Hyaline drusen in 77-year-old man. There is pigment epithelial atrophy of fovea. Vision is 20/40.

regular in size and outline. They are usually not associated with surrounding atrophy of the retinal pigment epithelium, photoreceptor degeneration, or subretinal neovascular membranes (Fig. 11-1).[3] They are quite common, and their presence alone does not justify the diagnosis of aging macular degeneration or indicate a poor prognosis for central vision.

Soft drusen are larger, irregularly shaped, yellow plaques of material under the retinal pigment epithelium (Fig. 11-2). This material has been characterized as electron-dense debris from malfunctioning retinal pigment epithelial cells.[3] The debris collects between the basement membrane of the retinal pigment epithelium and the collagen layer of Bruch's membrane. Clinically, soft drusen are pleomorphic in size, shape, and number; are often confluent; and change in appearance over time. The adjacent pigment epithelium is abnormal. Subretinal neovascular membranes frequently are associated with soft drusen.[4] Soft drusen resemble pigment epithelial detachments, except that pigment epithelial detachments are usually larger and more regular and have a more liquid material within them. Both have similar fluorescein characteristics, but pigment epithelial detachments stain more intensely and hyperfluoresce for a longer period, probably because fluorescein seeps into the serous fluid more rapidly. Soft drusen are of extreme clinical importance, since older patients with them are at a high risk of losing central vision and of developing subretinal neovascular membranes.

Regressing or calcified drusen appear as glittering yellow crystals within a halo of scarred and atrophic pigment epithelium (Fig. 11-3). Eyes with such drusen usually have poor vision and have little risk of occult subretinal neovascular membranes.

It is evident that patients with soft drusen should be counseled about the symptoms of serous detachment, given a means of recognizing such symptoms, and directed to see an ophthalmologist soon if such symptoms appear. The Amsler grid is the most useful method for such self-examination. Since subretinal membranes may rapidly become

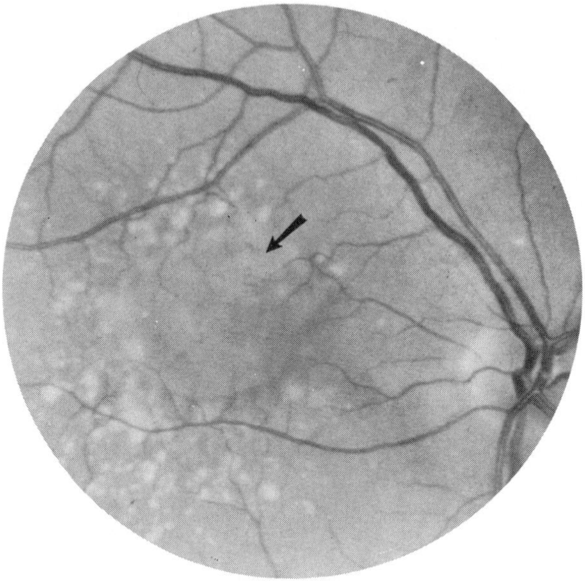

Fig. 11-2. Soft drusen and pigment epithelial *(arrow)* detachment in a 66-year-old woman. Vision is 20/400.

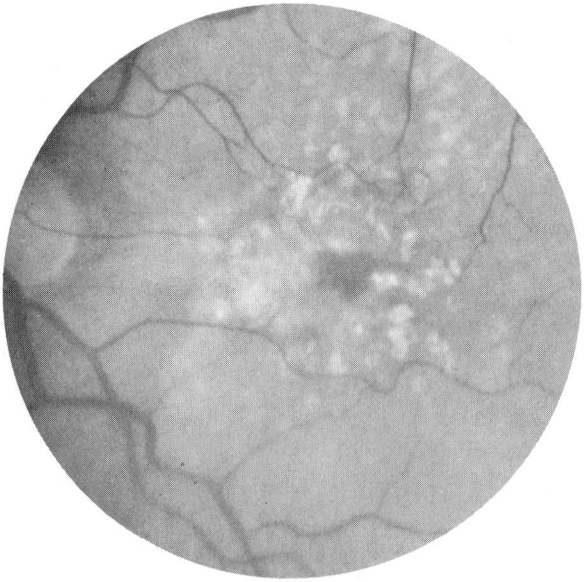

Fig. 11-3. Regressing or calcified drusen and advanced pigment epithelial atrophy in 70-year-old woman. Vision is very poor.

untreatable after they once become symptomatic and detectable, patients should be evaluated and treated soon after becoming symptomatic.

Once a subretinal membrane is suspected, a fluorescein angiogram is done to confirm its presence, location, and extent. The fluorescein characteristics of such a membrane consist of a lacelike frond of new vessels beneath an atrophic pigment epithelium, from which fluorescein leaks into the subretinal space (Fig. 11-4).

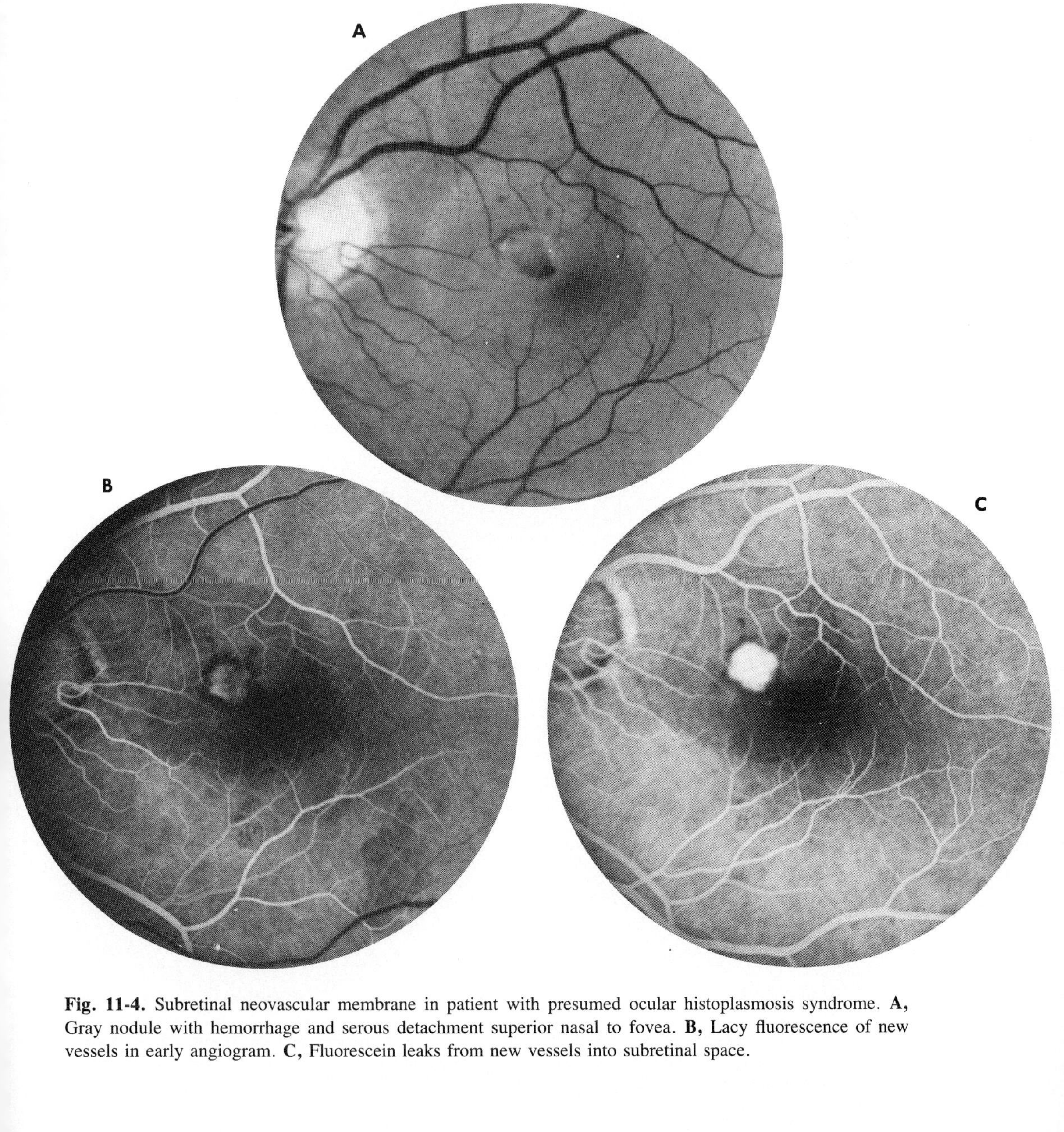

Fig. 11-4. Subretinal neovascular membrane in patient with presumed ocular histoplasmosis syndrome. **A,** Gray nodule with hemorrhage and serous detachment superior nasal to fovea. **B,** Lacy fluorescence of new vessels in early angiogram. **C,** Fluorescein leaks from new vessels into subretinal space.

However, many neovascular membranes are more difficult to see because of hyperfluorescence from adjacent drusen and atrophic retinal pigment epithelium and screening by hypertrophic retinal pigment epithelium or subretinal hemorrhage. Neovascular tissue may only be inferred as present by clues such as increasing hyperfluorescence and staining of a localized area under a serous retinal detachment (Fig. 11-5). Laser treatment of such membranes is probably justified, but the physician cannot expect results as good

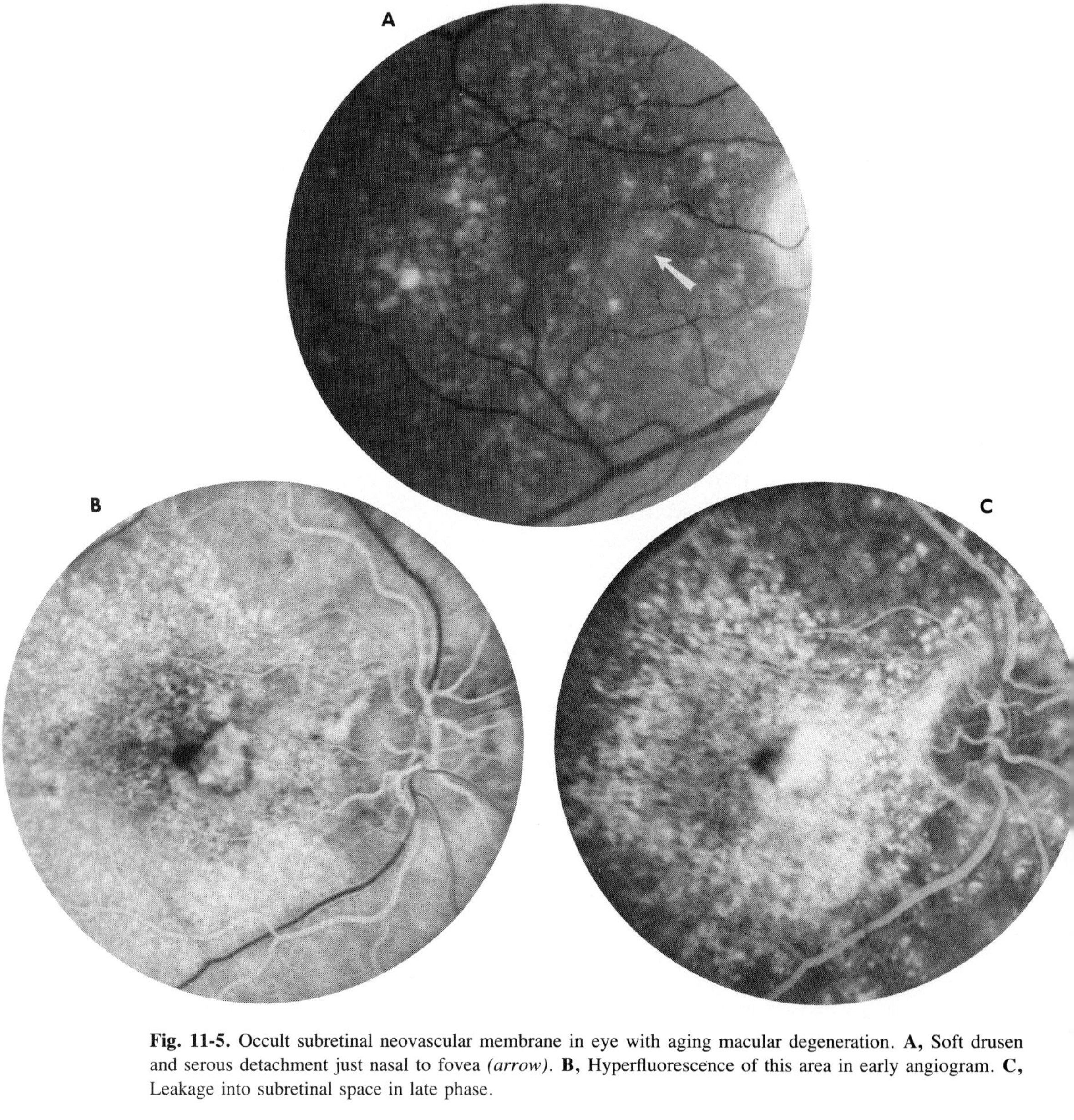

Fig. 11-5. Occult subretinal neovascular membrane in eye with aging macular degeneration. **A,** Soft drusen and serous detachment just nasal to fovea *(arrow)*. **B,** Hyperfluorescence of this area in early angiogram. **C,** Leakage into subretinal space in late phase.

as those obtained in the Macular Photocoagulation Study, in which only clearly recognizable membranes were treated.[1]

Finally the edge of the neovascular membrane, including surrounding blood and hyperpigmentation, should be evaluated in relation to the center of the foveal avascular zone. A membrane whose foveal edge is 200 μ or more may be treated with argon blue-green photocoagulation. If treatment is properly done, results similar to those of the Macular Photocoagulation Study may be expected.

The best way to estimate this critical distance is to take the best early film of a recent angiogram, estimate the center of the foveal avascular zone by bisecting the distance from several perifoveal capillaries, and then measuring from such a center to the nearest edge of blocked fluorescence of the subretinal neovascular membrane (Fig. 11-6).* Since the width of the average retinal vein at the disc is 125 μ, the clinician can use the reticle in a 6× magnifier to estimate 200 μ (approximately 1½ vein widths) and measure accordingly.† It is inaccurate to use fixation photography or estimate the center of the fovea from color photographs.

Laser photocoagulation must be reserved for treatment of neovascular membranes that are reasonably certain to be present and whose extent and outline are not obscured

*This method has been devised and used by the Reading Center, Macular Photocoagulation Study.

†Available from Edmunds Scientific Co., 101 E. Gloucester Pike, Barrington, NJ 08007. Order E41,055 plus metric scale reticle E30,323 at $49.95 plus postage.

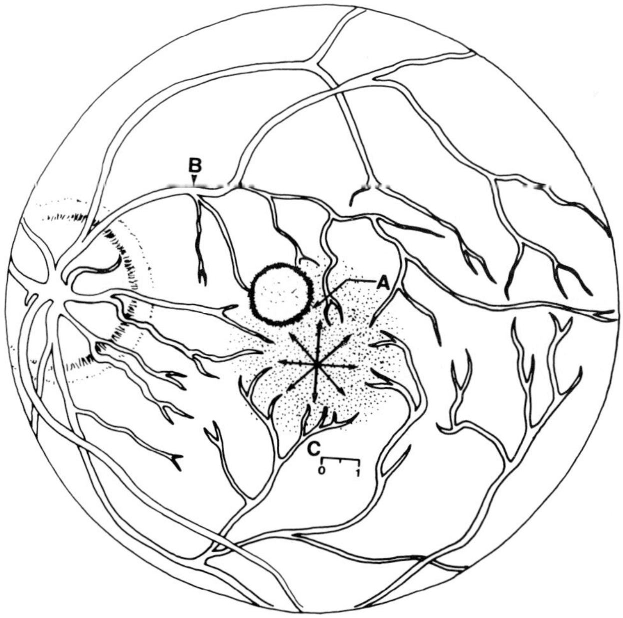

Fig. 11-6. Estimation of distance of foveal edge of subretinal membrane to center of fovea. (Subretinal neovascular membrane from patient described in Fig. 11-4.) **A,** Measurements are taken from outer edge of zone of blocked fluorescence. **B,** Width of vein at disc averages 125 μ. **C,** if distance from zone of blocked fluorescence to center of fovea measures more than 6 segments on reticle scale of 6X magnifier, membrane is treatable with argon blue-green photocoagulation. This membrane measures 10 segments.

by hyperfluorescence from drusen, scarred retinal pigment epithelium, or blood. If in doubt, it is best to follow the patient closely rather than photocoagulate an area in the hope that treatment will "do some good." Results of such treatment are poor, and patients are prone to blame the treatment for loss of central vision.

SELECTION OF LASER

The selection of the appropriate laser depends on both proved and speculative clinical advantages of different laser wavelengths. Practically speaking, the clinician may use argon blue-green, argon green, or krypton red for photocoagulation (see boxed material).

Argon blue-green (488.0 nm plus 514.5 nm) has the outstanding advantage of being proved effective.[1] Its disadvantage is absorption by macular xanthophyll pigment, so it cannot be used within the foveal avascular zone.[2] These wavelengths are well absorbed by melanin and hemoglobin. Although it is usually said to cause more damage to the inner retina and overlying blood vessels than krypton red (647.1 nm), this advantage is of little clinical significance, since both wavelengths will produce paracentral scotomas anyway. Furthermore, argon blue-green is well absorbed by neovascular tissue, which is the target of macular photocoagulation therapy.

In a recent experimental study argon blue-green, as well as krypton red, has been shown to penetrate superficial retinal hemorrhage and produce outer retinal and pigment epithelial burns.[5] Thick intraretinal or preretinal hemorrhage precludes any type of laser photocoagulation, since the location and extent of a neovascular membrane is not visible.

Considerations in laser selection

Argon blue-green

Proved effective by controlled trial
Absorption by hemoglobin and melanin

Argon green

Unproved for treatment by clinical trial
Absorption by hemoglobin and melanin

Krypton red
Advantages

Nonabsorption by xanthophyll
Penetrates vitreous hemorrhage
Penetrates nuclear sclerotic cataract
Less inner retinal burn; less retinal vasculitis
Penetrates superficial retinal hemorrhage to produce outer retinal burn

Disadvantages

Unproved by controlled clinical trial
Less absorption by hemoglobin; less effective in vessel closure?

Since argon blue-green has been proved effective by a controlled clinical trial, it should be used whenever possible instead of using an unproved wavelength because of a speculative advantage.

Argon green (514.5 nm) has the disadvantage of being unproved as treatment when compared to argon blue-green. However, in view of its absorption spectrum by melanin and hemoglobin, compared to argon blue, it seems reasonable to consider it equally effective. Since there is only slight absorption by xanthophyll of argon green, the ophthalmologist can treat lesions inside the foveal avascular zone with less danger of excessive spread and heat damage.

Krypton red is still unproved for treatment of subretinal neovascular membranes, and its popularity depends on apparent clinical advantages.[6,7] It is selectively absorbed by melanin, and thus even moderately intense krypton photocoagulation burns will produce only outer retinal choriocapillaris and pigment epithelial burns.[2] Yet it is not absorbed well by hemoglobin and does not destroy neovascular tissue directly. It will penetrate a thin intraretinal or preretinal hemorrhage to produce scars with less damage to the inner retina than if argon is used. However, argon blue-green photocoagulation can penetrate such retinal hemorrhages and produce outer retinal burns as well, depending on the intensity of the treatment and the thickness of the hemorrhage.[5]

Krypton red photocoagulation usually produces less inner retinal edema and retinal vasculitis, so fluorescein angiography can be done within 24 hours after photocoagulation. Whether this is necessary remains to be proved. It is not absorbed by xanthophyll and can be used safely within the foveal avascular zone. A high recurrence rate of krypton red–treated membranes has been noted, which has led to increasingly intense treatment and earlier and more frequent posttreatment angiograms.[6,7] In short, krypton red treatment of subretinal neovascular membranes is still unproved and experimental.

REFERENCES

1. Macular Photocoagulation Study Group: Argon laser photocoagulation for senile macular degeneration: results of a randomized clinical trial, Arch. Ophthalmol. **100:**912, 1982.
2. Marshall, J., and Bird, A.C.: A comparative histopathological study of argon and krypton laser irradiations of the human retina, Br. J. Ophthalmol. **63:**657, 1979.
3. Sarks, S.H.: Drusen and their relationship to senile macular degeneration, Aust. J. Ophthalmol. **8:**117, 1980.
4. Sarks, S.H., and others: Softening of drusen and subretinal neovascularization, Trans. Ophthalmol. Soc. U.K. **100:**414, 1980.
5. Shortt, S.G., and Folk, J.C.: Penetration of argon and krypton laser through blood, scientific poster, American Academy of Ophthalmology Annual Meeting, Oct. 30-Nov. 3, 1983, Chicago, Ill.
6. Singerman, L.J.: Red krypton laser therapy of macular and retinal vascular diseases, Retina **2:**15, 1982.
7. Yannuzzi, L.A., and Shakin, J.L.: Krypton red laser photocoagulation of the ocular fundus, Retina **2:**1, 1982.

12

Transscleral laser cyclocoagulation

Hugh Beckman

The surgical treatment of glaucoma is generally directed at effecting an increase in aqueous outflow. This is primarily accomplished by filtering surgery or more recently laser procedures such as argon laser trabeculoplasty. There are, however, cases that are unresponsive to these modalities, in which either their ineffectiveness has been proved or an attempt at further surgery is deemed imprudent or dangerous. In an effort to manage these eyes, which most notably falls into the neovascular glaucoma, glaucoma in aphakia, and secondary glaucoma groups, noninvasive ciliodestructive procedures have been devised. Vogt[5] described cyclodiathermy with electrocautery in 1936. This was replaced by cyclocryotherapy, first described by Bietti[3] in 1950, which has been the most common ciliodestructive procedure for more than a decade. Recently Coleman[4] has described the use of therapeutic ultrasound to create ciliodestructive lesions for the purpose of reducing intraocular pressure (IOP).

In 1972 we reported on the use of a specially designed ruby laser (Fig. 12-1) to perform transscleral ruby laser irradiation of the ciliary body in the treatment of intractable glaucoma.[2] This was followed shortly by a similar report on the use of glass:neodymium (nd) laser energy for the same purpose.[1] Over the years we have found the laser to be a safer, more effective modality with less patient morbidity than cyclocryotherapy, but the unavailability of the necessary special equipment prevented the technique from finding widespread acceptance in ophthalmology.

Noting the dissemination of high-powered ophthalmic nd:YAG lasers in the last 2 years, we hoped that this laser used in the thermal (ms pulse) mode might duplicate the success of our prior work. To prepare for this, we removed the ruby rod from our solid-state ruby laser, inserted the nd:glass rod, and once more began performing nd:glass transscleral cyclocoagulation. Having assured ourselves of the prospects for success, we then began some 8 months ago using the LASAG MR-2 in thermal mode to evaluate its relative efficacy for transscleral laser cyclocoagulation.

All treatments with all three modalities were performed using 32 impacts of laser energy circumlimbally through intact conjunctiva and sclera 3.5 mm posterior to the limbus. The initial ruby series was performed using 7.5 joules (J) per lesion, with the second series using 6.0 J per lesion. The original neodymium series was performed using what we thought was 6.5 J per lesion. On recalibration of the instrument at a later date, it became apparent that we were actually using closer to 7 or 8 J of neodymium energy per lesion. Since we believed that the degree of pressure control was poor at this level, the more recent nd:glass series was performed at 14.5 J/mm^2/lesion. Both

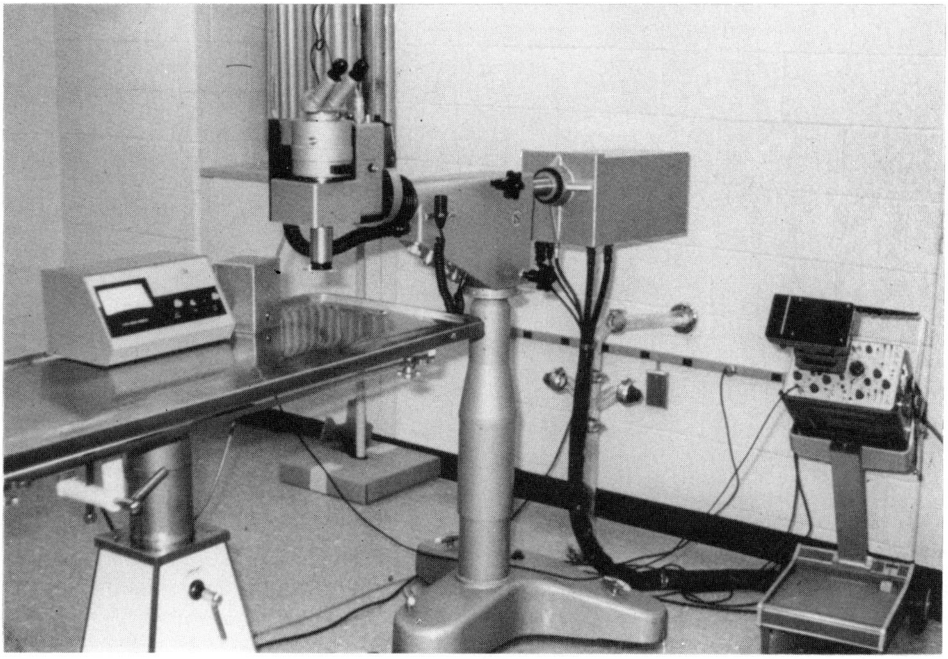

Fig. 12-1. Ruby laser.

Table 12-1. Summary of parameters in transscleral laser therapy series

Parameter	*Ruby*	*Nd:glass*	*Nd:YAG*
Power	6.0 J	14.0 J	8.5 J
Lesions	32	32	32
Distance from limbus	3.5 mm	3.5 mm	3.5 mm
Depth of focus	8 mm	8 mm	1 mm
Focused	On surface	On surface	3.6 mm beyond surface
Spot size	1 mm	1 mm	0.9 mm

nd:glass and ruby series had 6 ms pulses. The non-Q-switched nd:YAG laser at full multimode output yields 8 J/mm^2 when the laser beam is defocused into the ciliary body 3 mm with the retrofocusing device. A 10 ms pulse is used. A summary of parameters appears in Table 12-1. All eyes received 3 cc of 1.5% mepivacaine with hyaluronidase as a retrobulbar injection; without it, the procedure would be painful. Immediately after treatment, a rosary of conjunctival burns (Fig. 12-2) is seen about the limbus. The lesions are more pronounced with nd:glass, since the absorption by the conjunctiva is greater. To date the lesions created with nd:YAG have been smaller, probably because of retrofocusing and the shorter focal spot. There is wide variation in the postoperative pain, with many patients having none at all. Most have 1 to 2 hours of moderate discomfort, with occasional severe pain lasting overnight but seldom longer than 24 hours. The pressure generally falls from 24 to 48 hours after the procedure, with the low point of pressure appearing about 2 weeks after therapy at the height of the intraocular reac-

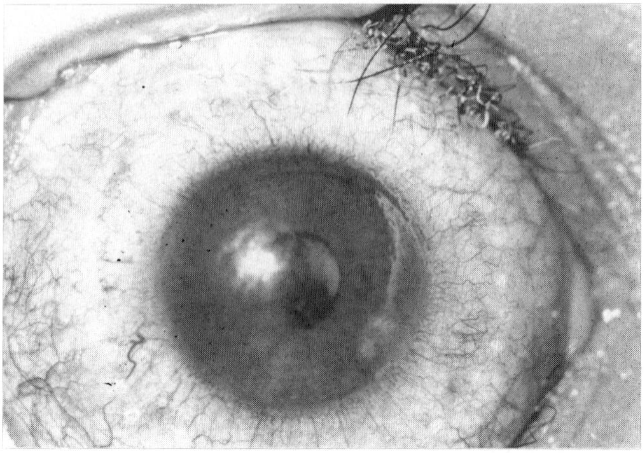

Fig. 12-2. Rosary of burns from ruby laser.

tion. The eye then begins to whiten rather quickly, with most eyes losing their injection by 1 month. In many cases, particularly those of neovascular glaucoma, a 2+ to 3+ flare persists for many months after the procedure.

RESULTS

We have defined success as an IOP not greater than 22 mm Hg and not less than 5 mm Hg. We use the 22 mm Hg figure, since it is generally acceptable for preservation of visual function in glaucomatous eyes. The lower 5 mm Hg limit is an arbitrary figure, below which many believe the hypotony present might be harmful to an eye. Many of the eyes with pressures greater than 22 mm Hg were painfree and white, and the patients were grateful for preservation of their globe. Many eyes with pressures less than 5 mm Hg also had no problems, and the diagnosis of phthisis was made only when actual shrinking or chronic inflammation accompanied the low IOP. No cases of phthisis occurred with IOPs greater than 5 mm Hg. Only three enucleations were performed in the entire series.

The majority of cases over the years were severe, intractable glaucomas that had been treated with multiple surgeries; the diagnosis was often obscured. They have been categorized as best as possible by primary diagnosis, as seen in Table 12-2. The best and most consistent results were in the eyes having the diagnosis of primary open-angle glaucoma in aphakia. Of 40 total eyes treated, 85% had successful control of pressure. The worst prognosis for success was in the largest group treated—neovascular glaucoma—in which 94 of 176 eyes were termed successful by these strict criteria. The average success rate of the whole group was 53%, with the worst in the original 7.5 J ruby and 7.5 J nd:glass series. As seen in Table 12-3, the reason for the lack of success was different with these two modalities. The two ruby series had too high a percentage of hypotony and phthisis (24%), whereas the neodymium series had more inadequate control of IOP (47% and 33%). The figures somewhat reversed in series when the ruby energy was decreased to 6.0 J, and the neodymium energy was changed to 14.0 J. That is, the incidence of hypotonous and phthisical eyes decreased with the lower-energy ruby laser series, and to date the incidence of successful pressure control has increased

Table 12-2. Primary diagnoses in transscleral laser therapy series (success criteria: IOP < 22 mm Hg; > 5 mm Hg)

	Ruby 7.5 J		*Ruby 6.0 J*		*Neodymium 7.0 J*		*Neodymium 14.0 J*		*Nd:YAG 8.0 J*		*Total*	
Type	*No.*	*Success*	*No.*	*Success*	*No.*	*Success*	*No.*	*Success*	*No.*	*Success*	*No.*	*Success*
Neovascular	77	38 (49%)	58	34 (59%)	14	5 (36%)	20	11 (55%)	7	6 (86%)	176	94 (53%)
Poag aphakic	13	11 (85%)	24	21 (99%)	2	1 (50%)	1	1 (100%)	—	—	40	34 (85%)
Poag phakic	8	5 (62%)	5	3 (60%)	—	—	1	1 (100%)	1	1 (100%)	15	10 (67%)
Secondary	11	8 (73%)	19	13 (68%)	3	2 (66%)	5	2 (40%)	4	2 (50%)	42	27 (64%)
Traumatic	9	4 (44%)	12	10 (83%)	—	—	1	—	—	—	22	14 (64%)
Congenital	4	2 (50%)	1	1 (100%)	—	—	—	—	1	1 (100%)	6	4 (67%)
TOTAL	122	68 (56%)	119	82 (69%)	19	8 (42%)	28	17 (61%)	13	10 (77%)	301	183 (61%)

Table 12-3. Reasons for failure in transscleral laser therapy series (success criteria: IOP < 22 mm Hg; > 5 mm Hg)

	Number	*Success*	*< 22 mm Hg*	*> 5 mm Hg*
Combined ruby	241	150 (62%)	34 (14%)	57 (24%)
7.5 J nd:glass	19	8 (42%)	9 (47%)	2 (11%)
14.0 J nd:glass	30	17 (57%)	10 (33%)	3 (10%)

in the higher-energy nd:glass and better-focused YAG series. The average of 53% success is still better than any long-series cyclocryotherapy report. The results in secondary glaucoma, in which 42 cases were treated, showed reasonable consistency, with 64% of patients having successful control of pressure. In the phakic open-angle, traumatic, and congenital glaucoma groups with much smaller numbers, success percentage rates ran in the middle-sixties.

Complications in the ruby series included 12 hyphemas, 11 of which were in the neovascular glaucoma group, 8 band keratopathies, all in patients who had had multiple prior surgical procedures, one cystoid macular edema, one anterior segment eschemia with plastic iritis and secondary cataract, and two subchoroidal effusions. By far the most common and severe complication was phthisis, which occurred in 13 or 11% of the 7.5 J series and two or 2% of the 6.0 J ruby series. Two cases of phthisis occurred in the combined neodymium series. A complication unique to the nd:glass group was the formation of corneal dellen in three cases as a result of conjunctival edema. This was probably caused by increased conjunctival absorption of 1.06 μ energy by the conjunctiva. To date no severe complications have taken place in the YAG series, with the exception of one plastic iritis. Dellen have not yet been a problem with this modality.

As shown in Table 12-4, 81% of the 16 eyes with visual acuity of 20/200 or better retained their visual acuity after treatment with 7.5 J ruby laser energy. The loss was not related to the treatment in two of the three eyes that lost acuity. In the 6.0 J ruby series 12 of the 20 with good acuity retained their acuity. Of the eight with decreased acuity, five resulted from complications of the treatment, such as bullous keratopathy, cystoid macular edema, and one case of cataract formation following anterior chamber ischemia. Thus far, in the 14.0 J nd:glass series, all five patients with preoperative 20/200 acuity have retained it, as have all three of the YAG-treated patients.

The lessened postoperative pain and morbidity associated with laser cyclocoagulation would by itself make it preferable to cyclocryotherapy in the treatment of those conditions requiring ciliodestructive procedures. The ability to reproducibly vary the amount of energy used for treatment enables a much more controlled treatment, and the degree of success would indicate it to be more efficacious in treating these same modalities. I hope the availability of thermal-mode nd:YAG equipment will make this type of treatment available to ophthalmologists everywhere, as well as allowing other investigators to refine the parameters for treatment.

Table 12-4. Acuity retained by those with better than 20/200 in transscleral laser therapy series

	Number	*Retained*	*Nontreatment related loss*
7.5 J ruby	16	13 (81%)	2/3
6.0 J ruby	20	12 (60%)	3/8
7.5 J nd:glass	0	—	—
14 J nd:glass	5	5 (100%)	—
8 J nd:YAG	3	3 (100%)	—

REFERENCES

1. Beckman, H., and Sugar, H.S.: Neodymium laser cyclocoagulation, Arch. Ophthalmol. **90:**27, 1973.
2. Beckman, H., and others: Transscleral ruby laser irradiation of the ciliary body in the treatment of intractable glaucoma, Trans. Am. Acad. Ophthalmol. Otolaryngol. **76:**423, 1972.
3. Bietti, G.: Surgical intervention on the ciliary body, J.A.M.A. **142:**889, 1950.
4. Coleman, J.: Personal communication, American Academy of Ophthalmology, November 1983.
5. Vogt, A.: Versuche zue intraokularen druckherabsetzung mittelst diathermie schadigung des corpus ciliare, Klin. Monatsbl. Augenheilkd. **97:**67, 1936.

13

Usual and unusual uses of the laser in glaucoma

Richard J. Simmons
James A. Savage*
C. Davis Belcher III*
John V. Thomas*

The closed-eye techniques made possible by argon laser photosurgical beams are revolutionizing the management of a wide variety of anterior segment disorders. Argon laser trabeculoplasty, in the treatment of various open-angle glaucomas, has become the next therapeutic step following medical therapy, lessening the frequency with which conventional glaucoma surgery is needed.

Laser iridectomy (iridotomy) is a safe, effective procedure that has rapidly replaced the standard surgical procedure in almost all instances in which the creation of a full-thickness iris hole is desired. Avoiding standard surgical intervention prevents such complications as hemorrhage, infection, wound leak, flat anterior chamber, and associated problems related to anesthesia and hospitalization. For these reasons, laser iridectomy has rapidly achieved a major place in ophthalmic surgical armamentarium.

These two important subjects are covered at length in Chapters 14 and 23 and are not discussed further here.

This chapter is devoted to the many additional roles that can be found for the laser in the treatment of glaucoma and some associated problems of the anterior segment of the eye (see boxed material on p. 155). Although these methods are needed less frequently and have been less well appreciated than laser trabeculoplasty and laser iridectomy, in many instances excellent results can be obtained using these outpatient photosurgical techniques.

LASER IRIDOPLASTY

Laser energy applied to the iris can alter its configuration in the treatment of various anterior segment conditions. These general techniques are called laser iridoplasty. When the iridoplasty treatment is applied to the peripheral iris, *laser gonioplasty* is the term we prefer. When the iridoplasty treatment is applied to the iris adjacent to the pupil, we prefer to call the procedure *laser pupilloplasty,* when we wish to change the shape of a pupil such as a updrawn pupil; or *laser photomydriasis* when we wish to dilate a round but excessively miotic pupil.

---

*M.D.s, Glaucoma Consultation Service, Massachusetts Eye and Ear Infirmary, Harvard Medical School and the New England Glaucoma Research Foundation, Boston, Mass.

Anterior segment uses of the laser in glaucoma

Laser trabeculoplasty
Laser iridectomy
Laser iridoplasty
A. Peripheral iris: gonioplasty
B. Central iris
  1. Photomydriasis
  2. Laser pupilloplasty
Laser for intraepithelial cysts of the iris and ciliary body
Laser to ciliary processes for malignant glaucoma
Laser opening of closed glaucoma filtration fistulas
A. Argon
B. Neodymium:YAG
Laser suture-cutting following trabeculectomy and other filtering operations
Cyclophotocoagulation: laser to ciliary processes
Laser to anterior segment neovascularization: goniophotocoagulation and pananterior segment ablation of new vessels
Laser for wound neovascularization with recurrent hemorrhage and glaucoma
Laser in the diagnosis and treatment of epithelial invasion of the anterior chamber
Laser for hypotony caused by cyclodialysis

Peripheral iris: laser gonioplasty

Laser photocoagulation to treat the peripheral iris—gonioplasty—causes contracture of the anterior iris stroma[35,37,46] (Fig. 13-1). Laser gonioplasty is useful in decreasing peripheral iris convexity, widening narrow angles, breaking "fresh" peripheral anterior synechias, and reopening closed cyclodialysis clefts (see boxed material on p. 157).

In open-angle glaucoma

Laser gonioplasty can allow accurate laser trabeculoplasty in eyes where peripheral iris convexity prevents accurate visualization of the chamber-angle landmarks and application of laser burns.[37] Usually 1 to 3 applications per clock hour are sufficient. Rather than the conventional laser settings for gonioplasty given in the boxed material, is it often convenient to use the same settings as the trabeculoplasty (50 μ spot size, 1000 mW power, 0.1 second per application) and apply oblique burns to the peripheral iris roll as needed. The laser can be slightly defocused, giving a larger spot if the tissue reaction is excessive. In this manner the surgeon does not have to continually change the laser settings during the procedure.

In angle-closure glaucoma

Primary angle-closure. In primary acute angle closure, argon laser gonioplasty can be used before laser iridectomy as a means of opening part of the angle to lower intraocular pressure (IOP), decrease corneal edema, and allow the surgeon to perform a successful iridectomy.[26] Gonioplasty also retracts the iris from the cornea, reducing or eliminating endothelial burns that may occur during laser iridectomy, preventing deliv-

A B C

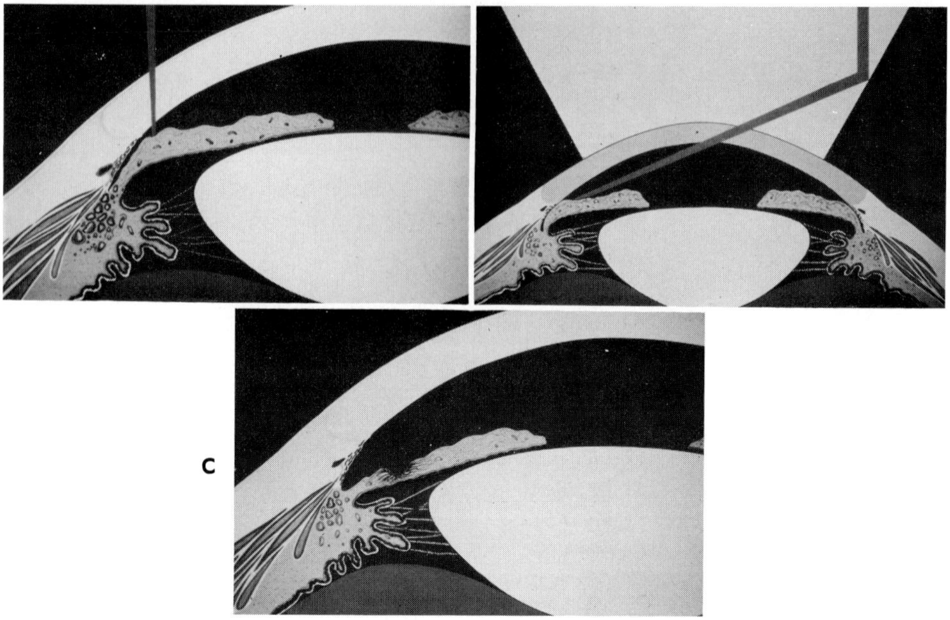

Fig. 13-1. A, Diagram of laser gonioplasty treatment directly through peripheral cornea; **B,** indirectly through mirrored goniolens; and **C,** diagram of desired depth of lesion from laser gonioplasty. (From Belcher, C.D., Thomas, J.V., and Simmons, R.J., editors: Photocoagulation in glaucoma and anterior segment disease, Baltimore, 1984, Williams & Wilkins, pp. 124-125.)

ery of adequate power to the iris to penetrate the iris successfully. In addition, after a successful laser iridectomy has been performed, the iris may remain in apposition to the trabecular meshwork because of early, weakly bonded peripheral anterior synechiae. The angle, however, may not be irreversibly closed with synechiae. In many cases laser gonioplasty will retract the iris from the meshwork and open the angle. When much of the angle's circumference can be opened in such a fashion, filtration surgery can be avoided. The laser surgeon must be persistent and, if necessary, repeat the treatment in 24 to 48 hours as the cornea clears.

In cases of subacute or chronic angle closure and of open-angle glaucoma in the presence of very narrow angles in which some closure is suspected, gonioplasty can be used to decrease iris convexity to widen or open the angle. Although this technique can be helpful when successful laser iridectomy is not possible, gonioplasty does not replace iridectomy as treatment for pupillary block or for frank angle closure in these cases. Conventional laser gonioplasty settings are used (see boxed material), with 2 to 5 applications per clock hour. It is advisable to treat one quadrant per session, with follow-up every month for 3 months, then every 3 to 6 months thereafter. Recommended testing during the follow-up period includes gonioscopy and tonometry. An optional test that can be clinically useful is goniophotography, which can serve as a comparison at future examinations.

Plateau iris. Plateau iris derives its name from eyes that have the configuration of normal axial depth of the anterior chamber with an extremely narrow chamber angle,

Laser gonioplasty

Indications for use

Open angle-glaucoma—adjunct to argon laser trabeculoplasty
Angle-closure glaucoma

A. Primary
   1. Acute—selected cases only in conjunction with laser iridectomy
   2. Subacute—selected uses only
   3. Chronic—selected uses only
   4. Combined-mechanism open-angle glaucoma/angle closure
   5. Plateau iris
   6. Nanophthalmos
B. Others
   1. Peripheral anterior synechiae
      a. Pseudophakic and aphakic pupillary block
      b. Uveitis
      c. Neovascular glaucoma
   2. Patient unsuitable for successful laser iridectomy
      a. Uncooperative
      b. Corneal edema
      c. Other

Cyclodialysis cleft

A. Reopening a closed cyclodialysis cleft
B. Pretreatment of iris before cyclodialysis surgery

Technique

Protocol	Outpatient Topical anesthesia (occasionally retrobulbar) Usually use goniolens
Laser settings	Spot size: 200 to 500 μ (start at 200 and increase if necessary) Power: 50 to 400 mW (start low and increase) Time: 0.2 seconds per application initially and increase to 0.5 seconds if needed Number of applications: three to 12 evenly spaced burns per clock hour (the number varies according to the task)
Desired effect	Use the lowest possible energy settings to produce a moderate stromal burn with contracture of stroma and flattening of the immediately adjacent iris. Avoid extreme contracture, explosion, pigment dispersion, and distortion of the pupil.

which is liable to closure (Fig. 13-2). In such eyes, since pupillary block is not the major factor leading to angle closure, iridectomy may fail to break an attack or visibly widen the angle.[57] Prone darkroom provocative testing is often insufficient to produce angle closure in these eyes, and mydriatic provocative testing (with a combination cycloplegic/direct sympathomimetic agent) is more likely to identify plateau iris eyes that are susceptible to closure. In such predisposed eyes we prefer to use the term *plateau iris configuration* for those that have plateau iris but do not have a closable angle, and the term *plateau iris syndrome* for those eyes in which the angle will close despite successful iridectomy.

Although pilocarpine can be employed on a continuing basis for the treatment of plateau iris syndrome, gonioplasty is a useful technique for widening the angle to reduce the likelihood of angle closure, which usually permanently eliminates the plateau configuration and the danger of closure. The technique we prefer to employ is to use the settings in the boxed material. The patient is followed with periodic gonioscopy and the treatment is repeated as necessary.

Nanophthalmos. Nanophthalmos is a serious and important entity characterized by eyes in which the globe and anterior segment are very small (average axial length: 17 mm, with ocular volume two-thirds normal), but the lens is of normal size and volume.[4,16,32,47] As a result, a greater proportion of the anterior segment is occupied by the lens, which crowds the anterior chamber and causes an extremely narrow angle (Fig. 13-3). As one would expect, these eyes are usually, but not always, markedly hyperopic (+7 D or more). The patient has the characteristic facies of narrow palpebral fissures, small corneal diameters, and aphakic-like spectacles on a phakic eye. These eyes also have thick sclera, which is thought to contribute to increased resistance to outflow through the vortex veins.[16] Because of this or other yet to be identified factors, nanoph-

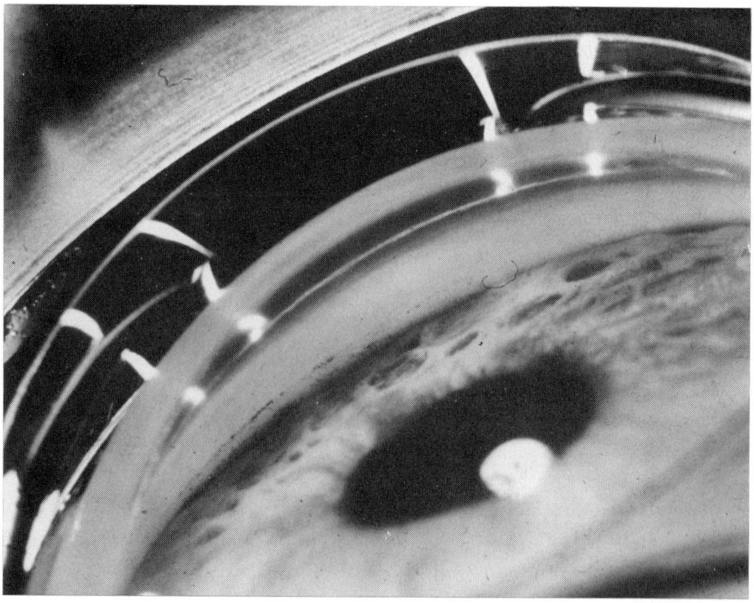

Fig. 13-2. Gonioscopic view of plateau iris. Angle is exceedingly narrow, whereas flat iris plane is present with very little iris convexity.

thalmic eyes have a tendency toward significant uveal effusion, which compounds the problem of already narrowed angles. These eyes have a propensity to angle closure, especially with advancing age. The uveal effusions are of particular concern during intraocular surgery and have led to disastrous complications. Intraoperative loss of these eyes is not unusual. Because patients with these eyes are such poor surgical candidates, noninvasive laser techniques that treat the propensity of these eyes to angle closure are logical and desirable.

Nanophthalmic eyes should be followed closely for signs of progressive narrowing of the angle. In the event that the angle does narrow and partial closure is threatened, laser iridectomy, if it can be achieved, is done as primary therapy. Gonioplasty is then used to treat subsequent narrowing. These eyes should be followed with gonioscopy every 3 months, since the status of the angle has been noted to fluctuate considerably, perhaps as a result of intermittent choroidal effusions. Whereas we often employ any form of gonioscopy, including Koeppe gonioscopy, to evaluate the width and potential for closure of the anterior chamber angle, in eyes such as these with particularly small anterior segments, evaluation of the chamber angle width may be more accurate with the Goldmann lens, since the anterior segment may be distorted by the adult Koeppe lens in such cases.

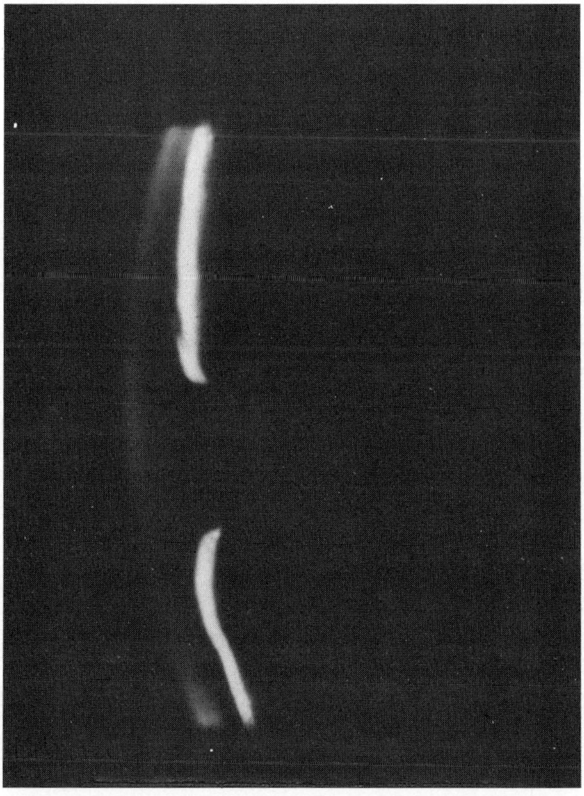

Fig. 13-3. Slitlamp photograph of eye with nanophthalmos, demonstrating marked iris convexity and shallowness of anterior chamber.

Singh and co-workers[47] reported on the use of gonioplasty in 12 of a series of 32 eyes with nanophthalmos. In 11 of the 12 (91.6%), the angle visibly widened, and the vision was stable or improved. In all 12 the tension was improved. Follow-up ranged from 15 to 62 months, with an average of 36.4.

Other uses

Burns placed at the base of iris tissue, which is in apposition to the trabecular meshwork, can open the angle and break "fresh" peripheral anterior synechiae.[46] This technique is routinely employed, for instance, following laser iridectomy in which peripheral anterior synechiae persist, since some such synechiae are reversible when gonioplasty is used to stretch the iris root away from the trabecular meshwork. Conventional laser settings (see boxed material) are recommended, with the application of 3 to 12 spots per clock hour of angle. The pupil should be constricted with frequent pilocarpine, such as 4% solution every 15 minutes, with six administrations, before the laser session.

In addition to those synechiae resulting from primary angle-closure, gonioplasty can be used with laser iridectomy for those synechiae that result from aphakic and pseudophakic pupillary block[27] (Fig. 13-4). In some cases of neovascular glaucoma gonioplasty can be used to break peripheral anterior synechiae and widen the angle to permit the treatment of new vessels (see section on goniophotocoagulation and pananterior segment ablation of new vessels). In addition, retraction of the peripheral iris may inhibit the ability of the fibrovascular membrane to close the angle, for example, while the surgeon is using goniophotocoagulation, awaiting the effect of panretinal photocoagulation.

Some have suggested gonioplasty be used to reopen closed cyclodialyses and to pretreat the iris in preparation for cyclodialysis surgery,[3] although the first suggestion has been unsuccessful when we have employed it in a few cases.

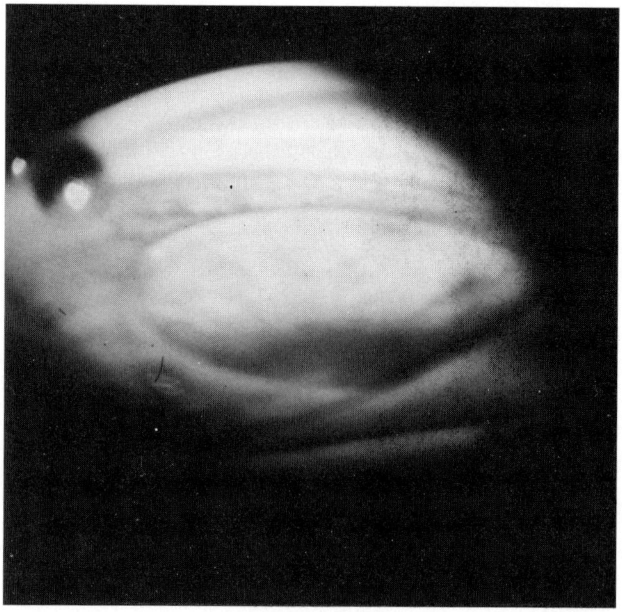

Fig. 13-4. Gonioscopic view of chamber angle in which laser gonioplasty was used to open angle by eliminating peripheral anterior synechiae caused by pseudophakic pupillary block.

Contraindications and disadvantages

A hazy cornea is a relative contraindication to gonioplasty, depending on the ability to deliver laser energy. Gonioplasty is contraindicated as sole treatment in cases of extensive pupillary block, such as true primary angle-closure glaucoma. Iridectomy remains the treatment for pupillary block. In eyes with extreme amounts of iris atrophy, gonioplasty has a decreased effect and may be less effective. The complications of gonioplasty are minor:

Pigment dispersion (minimal)
Failure to widen or open the angle
Pupillary distortion
Mild iritis

Although gonioplasty is a valuable tool in selected cases, its effect may be transient. Because of this, these patients must be followed closely, and repeated laser sessions may be necessary.

Central iris: laser pupilloplasty and photomydriasis

Laser treatment to the pupillary margin can reshape or enlarge the pupillary opening.[14,20,52] This technique may be used in aphakic eyes, in which visual impairment exists caused by a hammock or updrawn pupil, or in phakic eyes, in which vision is impaired by a miotic pupil resulting from medical glaucoma therapy, especially if a cataract is present. In cases of subluxated lenses pupilloplasty can be used to facilitate vision through an aphakic portion of the pupil or through a more central portion of the lens, whichever seems most appropriate for the particular case. In the presence of lens remnants following extracapsular cataract extraction, the iris can be altered to allow vision through an unobstructed portion of the pupil. The double-ring technique advocated by L'Esperance and James[20] is described as follows:

Protocol	Prelaser evaluation of visual acuity and visual field before and after dilation Iris transillumination to identify any areas of iris atrophy where the treatment will have little or no effect Topical anesthesia usually suffices Aim beam away from macula Multiple applications made in two rings in a contiguous fashion directed to the region of the iris sphincter Minimal dispersion of pigment and plasmoid aqueous production is the desired end point, not a severe explosion If retreatment is necessary, the double-ring technique could be used again with the same laser parameters but with the pupil dilated.
Laser settings[14,20]	Inner ring: Spot size: 200 μ Power: 250 to 600 mW Time: 0.2 seconds per application Outer ring: Spot size: 500 μ Power: 350 to 600 mW Time: 0.2 seconds per application
Postlaser regimen	Topical steroids every 2 hours for 48 hours, then four times a day for 5 days Carbonic anhydrase inhibitors as necessary Phenylephrine 2.5% three times a day for 2 weeks Discontinue miotics and start timolol if possible Mild analgesics as necessary Check IOP in 1 to 2 hours and again in 24 hours

In certain aphakic eyes with updrawn pupils, in which damage to the crystalline lens need not be a concern the neodymium (Nd):YAG laser will provide gratifying visual results by extending the pupil inferiorly by creating a Nd:YAG sphincterotomy toward the desired visual axis.[52] Our typical Nd:YAG laser settings for this technique are 3.5 to 5.0 mj per shot, 1 to 5 shots per burst, usually 4 rapid-fire bursts, repeated 2 to 4 times, through a contact lens. The risk of this procedure in phakic eyes is as yet uncertain.

A

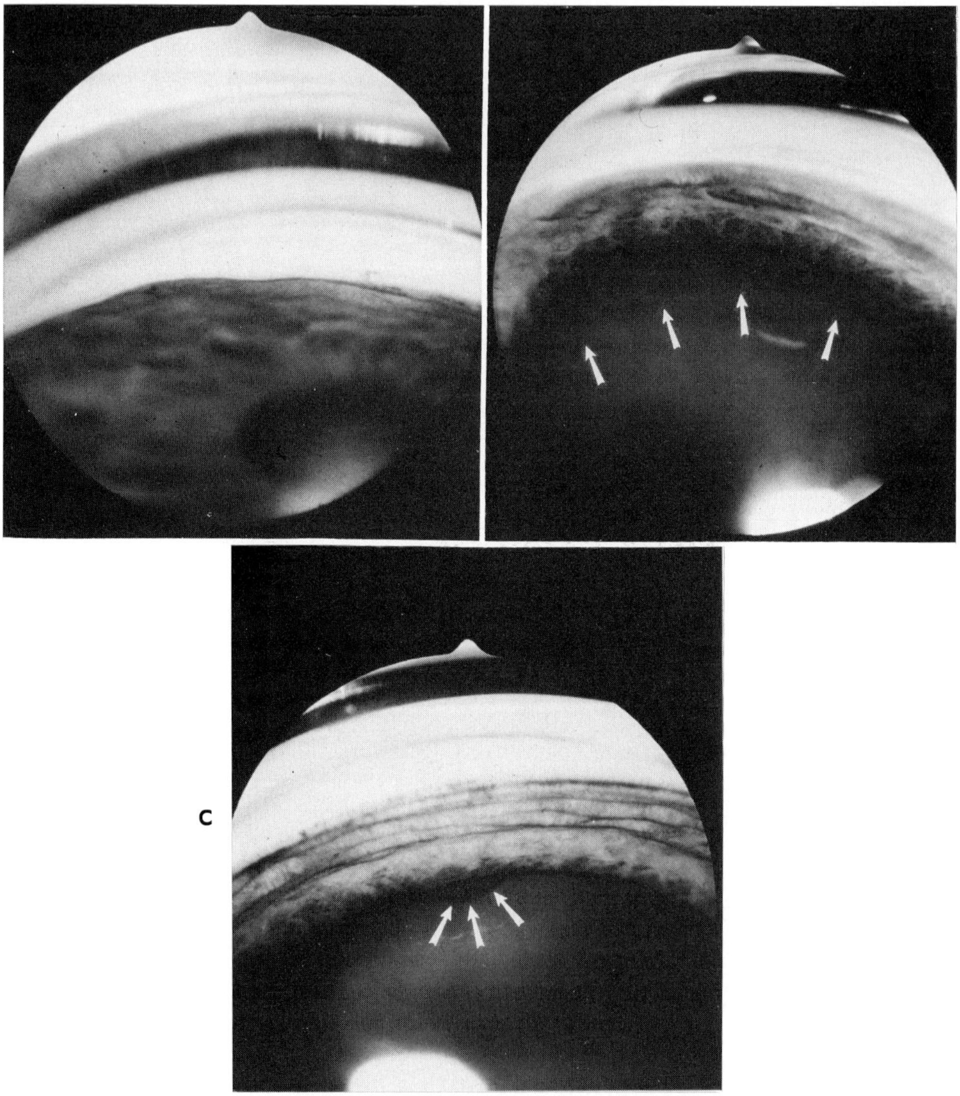

B

C

Fig. 13-5. A, Gonioscopic view of intraepithelial cyst of ciliary body with irregular closure of chamber angle. **B,** Same patient with dilated pupil, which shows broad outline of cyst *(arrows).* **C,** Following treatment with argon laser, cyst is greatly reduced in size *(arrowheads),* and angle is open. (**B** from Belcher, C.D., Thomas, J.V., and Simmons, R.J., editors: Photocoagulation in glaucoma and anterior segment disease, Baltimore, 1984, Williams & Wilkins, p. 142.)

LASER FOR INTRAEPITHELIAL CYSTS OF THE IRIS AND CILIARY BODY

Fluid-filled cysts can sometimes spontaneously form in the potential space between the epithelial layers of the iris or ciliary body.[7] Because of their location, these usually escape diagnosis. They are usually first noticed as a localized bulge in the iris that irregularly narrows and in some cases closes the angle[8] (Fig. 13-5). When large, these are sometimes visible with the slitlamp at the pupil. Although these cysts usually go undetected, they occasionally enlarge and cause chronic angle-closure glaucoma, obstruction of the pupillary visual axis, corneal decompensation by pressing the iris against the endothelium, or an inflammatory reaction in the anterior chamber. In these instances treatment is indicated, and the argon laser is the method of choice.

The technique for argon laser treatment of spontaneous intraepithelial cysts of the iris and ciliary body is outlined as follows[2]:

Protocol	Outpatient
	Topical anesthesia
	Goldmann lens
	Dilated pupil (with large cyst: laser first, then dilate, to avoid precipitating angle closure)
	Topical steroids following laser treatment
Laser settings	Spot size: 50 to 100 μ
	Power: 150 to 300 mW
	Time: 0.2 seconds per application
	Number of applications: usually less than 10
Desired effect	Immediate collapse of cyst

Postoperatively debris in the anterior chamber is common for approximately 24 hours. Although inflammation is usually minimal following this treatment, an antiinflammatory medication is usually prescribed. For eyes in which treatment has been done because of angle closure caused by the cyst, pilocarpine drops are used four times a day for up to a week to help open the angle. Gonioplasty to try to reverse early peripheral anterior synechiae may be attempted, if these are present. After the immediate postlaser period, the patient is followed with periodic (every 3 to 6 months) gonioscopy to evaluate the anterior segment for cyst recurrence as well as for the formation of new cysts.

Complications are usually transient and not particularly bothersome. Iritis and/or elevation of IOP may occur. The cysts often recur or new cysts form, and patients frequently require further laser treatment. Careful follow-up is therefore needed.

LASER TO CILIARY PROCESSES FOR MALIGNANT GLAUCOMA

Laser to the ciliary processes has been reported by Herschler and others as a safe, simple, and effective treatment for malignant glaucoma.[13,18,60] In eyes that have been unresponsive to medical therapy, we have been successful in two cases and unsuccessful in several others with the laser in treating malignant glaucoma. However, when the ciliary processes are visible and the correct diagnosis has been made, laser treatment is simple and should be tried. In many cases, however, the ciliary processes are not clearly enough seen to permit visualization and access with the laser.

The treatment of malignant glaucoma begins with proper diagnosis by ruling out the other causes of postoperative flat anterior chamber: choroidal separation, pupillary block, and suprachoroidal hemorrhage.[31,39,41] Intensive medical therapy is then initiated and consists of mydriatic-cycloplegic drops, carbonic anhydrase inhibitors, and hyperosmotic agents. If this regimen is unsuccessful after 4 or 5 days and the media are sufficiently clear, laser therapy should be tried. This may be done with topical anesthesia. A topical hyperosmotic agent such as glycerin may be required to clear the cornea for visibility of the structures to be treated. The Goldmann lens is usually required to visualize and treat the ciliary processes, and according to Herschler's findings, only two to four need be treated. Laser settings are as follows: 100 to 200 μ spot size, 300 to 1000 mW power, 0.1 second per application, and 30 to 50 applications. Slight deepening of the anterior chamber may be noted immediately after treatment, and this continues over the next several days. Other than failure to achieve control of the malignant glaucoma, we have insufficient experience with this technique to identify what complications, if any, are associated with its employment.

If laser therapy fails or laser use on the ciliary processes is not possible because of unclear media, then Chandler's deep vitreous surgery procedure should be employed.[6,39,41] This operation may occasionally need to be repeated. Rarely, even this fails; vitrectomy, cryosurgery or lens extraction can then be considered.

The successful treatment of malignant glaucoma with the laser should not imply that the exact etiology of this condition is known. The successfully treated patients reported by Herschler were continued on medical therapy after the laser session; thus one cannot say that the prolonged medical therapy was not responsible for the successful outcome.[33] Because of its simplicity and apparent safety, however, we believe that the laser therapy recommended by Herschler should be tried in these cases.

LASER OPENING OF CLOSED GLAUCOMA FILTRATION FISTULAS

Glaucoma filtration surgery can fail because of occlusion of the fistula at one of various sites.[10,22] For those cases in which the fistula becomes occluded "internally" at its inner opening to the anterior chamber, laser therapy can be an excellent technique to noninvasively restore filtration. This "internal" obstruction occasionally takes the form of a pigmented membrane, and several reports of successful treatment of these with the argon laser have been published. Laser settings varied from 50 to 100 μ spot size, 800 to 2000 mW power, 0.1 to 1.0 second per application, and "several" to 200 applications.[54-56]

Because of the interaction between argon laser light and tissue, this technique is not effective when the fistula is occluded by a nonpigmented or transparent membrane. Also, if the filtration bleb has never functioned, this technique is not likely to produce filtration.[39] If, as is often the case, the obstruction to filtration is "external," at the scleral or episcleral level, argon laser is not recommended. Some have wondered about the use of argon laser for transconjunctival treatment of fibrous "caps" over filtration sites, but we find that the conjunctiva is usually insufficiently transparent and the obstruction site insufficiently pigmented to advise this approach.

For cases in which "internal" obstruction to filtration takes the form of a clear or nonpigmented membrane, the Nd:YAG laser can be used with a goniolens to attempt to restore flow of aqueous through the fistula, with laser settings of 5 to 8 mj energy; one pulse/burst, increasing to nine; and 50 to 300 applications.

LASER SUTURE CUTTING FOLLOWING TRABECULECTOMY AND OTHER FILTERING OPERATIONS

The argon laser can be used to modify aqueous runoff following glaucoma filtration surgery by using the laser to cut sutures at the filter site[36] (Fig. 13-6). Trabeculectomy and other "guarded" filtration procedures have the advantage that a flat anterior chamber with its attendant sequellae is less likely than with conventional full-thickness filtration procedures such as Scheie cautery, posterior lip sclerectomy, and trephining. Excess aqueous runoff is inhibited by the ''guarded'' fistula, which is created by the scleral flap or suture(s) and prevents the cycle of flat anterior chamber, hypotony, and ciliochoroidal detachment.[30] However, we believe that lower postoperative IOP, better filtration blebs, and fewer late failures of filtration occur with full-thickness procedures when special measures have been taken during the immediate postoperative period to temporarily impede excess runoff of aqueous with the glaucoma shell tampon.[28,30,34,40]

Without question, situations exist in which excessively low postoperative pressures do not appear to be needed; in such cases trabeculectomy is the most appropriate procedure. However, in our view the surgeon should not be wedded to a single operation, but rather should have a variety of operations in the surgical armamentarium to be tailored to the particular case.[30]

Occasionally, during the immediate or early postoperative period following trabeculectomy or combined trabeculectomy/cataract extraction, the resistance to outflow is too great, and the pressure can rise to high levels. In this instance the fistula site can be opened with the argon laser by transconjunctivally cutting the black 10-0 nylon suture or sutures holding the scleral flap. To maximally visualize the suture, the central unmirrored portion of the Zeiss compression goniolens is placed against the conjunctival surface. If the bleb tissue is unusually opaque or if subconjunctival blood is present, the suture may not be sufficiently visible to treat, but usually the overlying tissue is clear enough when compressed with the Zeiss lens. Several drops of topical proparacaine anesthesia is sufficient for this procedure. Test shots with the laser at a distant conjunc-

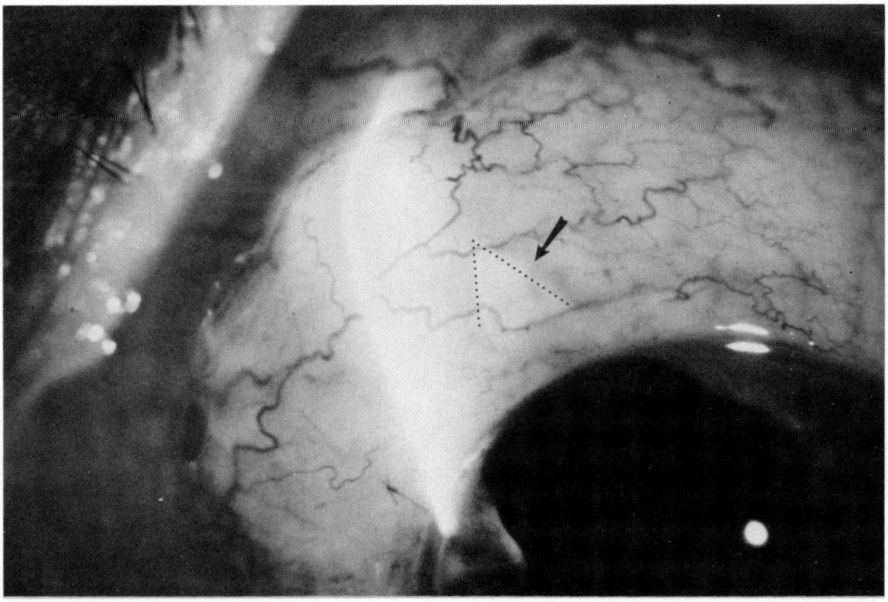

Fig. 13-6. Slitlamp photo following laser suture cutting of 10-0 nylon suture at apex of triangular scleral trabeculectomy flap. Note abundant filtration and triangular scleral flap reflected forward against inner conjunctiva *(arrow)*.

tival site are desirable before aiming at the suture to avoid excessive power. Laser settings for this technique are 100 μ spot size, 400 mW power, 0.2 second per application, and 2 to 4 applications per suture. The IOP should be closely monitored for several hours following the session to observe for pressure decrease, shallowing of the anterior chamber, and obvious increase in filtration. If the anterior chamber should shallow following the laser session, this is treated in the same manner as any postoperative case with cycloplegics, decreased activity, and the glaucoma shell tampon. If inadequate increase in flow is achieved, digital pressure can be employed at the slitlamp by the ophthalmologist to initiate increased flow through the trabeculectomy.

Suture tamponade-laser technique

In addition to the postoperative modification of trabeculectomy, we have developed a different technique to give a new "hybrid" operation. We call this the "suture tamponade-laser" technique, in which sutures are used to tamponade flow through a full-thickness thermal sclerostomy.[36] The procedure has characteristics of filtration midway between those of trabeculectomy and full-thickness operations and benefits similar to those of the glaucoma shell tamponade technique: control over aqueous outflow after surgery with attendant control over the anterior chamber depth and hypotony.[28,30,34,40] Yet we retain the benefit of very low resultant pressures needed for some advanced open-angle glaucoma patients and for low-tension glaucoma patients in whom a subnormal tension is chosen as a desirable level.[1] The technique consists of a 4 mm thermal sclerostomy at the usual site, slightly shelved at 75 to 80 degrees so the sutures can bite the anterior edge. Three to four 10-0 nylon sutures are deeply placed, tightened, and tied to give runoff similar to that of a trabeculectomy. This runoff is judged by filling the anterior chamber with balanced salt solution through a paracentesis wound made at the beginning of the procedure and touching the posterior lip of the filtration site with a cellulose sponge. During the immediate postoperative period the resistance to outflow can be "titrated" by cutting sutures with the argon laser transconjunctivally through a Zeiss compression goniolens to blanch conjunctival vessels. If the view is insufficiently clear transconjunctivally to permit this route for the laser, the argon or Nd:YAG laser can be used with a mirrored lens via the anterior chamber to cut the sutures. If any sutures are cut, those at the ends of the sclerostomy are done first to give the smallest, most controlled increments in increased flow. If at any time aqueous runoff is excessive and leads to a shallow or flat anterior chamber, the glaucoma shell tampon can be used to restore depth by temporary inhibition of the undesired runoff until the eye is stable.

The aqueous outflow characteristics at the trabeculectomy scleral flap site are permanently determined by the nature of its closure at the time of surgery. The important advantage of the suture tamponade-laser technique over trabeculectomy is that the resistance to aqueous outflow is temporary and present early when the eye is unstable, and it can be reduced in a controlled fashion after the eye stabilizes. The advantage of the suture tamponade-laser technique over full-thickness glaucoma filtration operations performed without the use of the shell tampon is that filtration offers no control over excessive postoperative aqueous runoff, which can lead to hypotony, flat anterior chamber, and ciliochoroidal detachment. Although our technique and shell tamponade are similar in that both allow the surgeon to control postoperative aqueous runoff and decrease resistance when the eye is stable and aqueous production has returned to normal, the suture tamponade-laser technique has the advantages of being a simpler and an external device, with its very special dressing techniques, is not required postoperatively.

CYCLOPHOTOCOAGULATION: LASER TO CILIARY PROCESSES

In certain difficult glaucoma cases a variable number of ciliary processes may be visible through iris colobomas or around atrophic iris with the goniolens. In some of these patients the application of laser to the ciliary processes can result in lower IOP, perhaps a result of the same mechanism as cyclocryotherapy.[18,19,24,51,62] The technique employed has varied from observer to observer, as have the results. We have occasionally seen lowering of IOP, but this has been difficult to predict. Since the usual situation is a very desperate case, we consider this technique as one to be tried before more destructive procedures such as cyclocryotherapy, which may increase the likelihood of severe complications such as phthisis bulbi and cystoid macular edema. Laser to the ciliary processes may be useful in cases of traumatic glaucoma, glaucoma in aphakia, and glaucoma following surgery for epithelial downgrowth. The use of laser to the ciliary processes in the management of malignant glaucoma has been described and is discussed separately in a previous section.

To reasonably expect success, a sufficient number of ciliary processes must be visible for the transpupillary treatment. Lee believes that a minimum of 16 ciliary processes must be visible to justify the employment of this treatment, according to the following parameters:

Protocol[51]	Prelaser mydriasis Topical anesthesia May require extreme gaze for visualization Goniolens (Goldmann three-mirror, Lee goniolens, or Ricky cyclolens) Avoid capillaries Postlaser cycloplegics and topical steriods Follow-up at 1, 3, and 6 weeks; retreat same processes at 4 to 6 weeks if necessary.
Laser settings*	Spot size: 50 to 100 μ Power: 600 to 1000 mW Time: 0.1 to 0.2 second per application Number of applications: variable, depending on the number of ciliary processes (usually 3 to 5 spots per ciliary process)
Desired response	Concave, craterlike burn on the tip of the ciliary process with production of a gas bubble; undesirable whitish discoloration of the ciliary process is caused by insufficient power settings and can result in inability to deliver laser light with subsequent applications

LASER TO ANTERIOR SEGMENT NEOVASCULARIZATION: GONIOPHOTOCOAGULATION AND PANANTERIOR SEGMENT ABLATION OF NEW VESSELS

The direct application of laser energy to new vessels in the chamber angle can be a useful adjunct in the management of rubeosis and neovascular glaucoma associated with diabetic oculopathy, central retinal vein occlusion or other causes of progressive anterior segment neovascularization.[11,38,42-45] Simmons first employed goniophotocoagulation in 1973 in an attempt to eliminate new vessels in the anterior segment and prevent or diminish synechial angle closure while awaiting the beneficial effect of panretinal pho-

*NOTE: various investigators have used laser settings different from these. These represent those settings used in the largest and most successful clinical series to date.[19]

tocoagulation in cases of central retinal vein occlusion and diabetic oculopathy.[17,21] In some cases, neither goniophotocoagulation or panretinal photocoagulation alone are sufficient, but both used in concert can alter the progressive downhill course of many such desperate eyes.

In selected cases of neovascular glaucoma, goniophotocoagulation can be of particular value. High risk cases, such as those following central retinal vein occlusion can demonstrate a rapid, relentless course toward synechial closure with rubeosis. In these cases, the angle can permanently close while one awaits the effect of panretinal photocoagulation to decrease the stimulus for neovascular proliferation. In this circumstance, goniophotocoagulation, with its immediate effect, can be applied to eliminate new vessels on the iris and in the angle so that the angle remains open until the stimulus for new vessel growth abates.

Other high-risk situations include (1) eyes with massive anterior segment neovascularization when first seen, with the angle almost totally open; (2) eyes in which neovascularization progresses despite initial laser therapy to the anterior or posterior segment or both; (3) eyes in which neovascularization progresses despite full panretinal photocoagulation; (4) eyes with proliferative diabetic retinopathy undergoing cataract extraction; and (5) eyes with anterior segment neovascularization requiring glaucoma surgery.[11] These situations, in which a good chance exists for progression to severe neovascularization and total closure of the angle, are the major indications for vigorous repeated goniophotocoagulation. In contrast, certain low-risk cases exist in which the stimulus for progression of anterior segment neovascularization is low or diminishing; in these cases and *only* in these cases, goniophotocoagulation as sole therapy may be sufficient to control the progression of the disease.

Our technique for goniophotocoagulation is summarized as follows:

Protocol	Outpatient
	Topical anesthesia (occasionally retrobulbar)
	Combine with panretinal photocoagulation whenever possible, since this is needed to decrease or eliminate stimulus to growth of more new vessels
Laser settings	Spot size: 100 to 200 μ
	Power: 150 to 800 mW
	Time: 0.2 second per application
	Number of applications: variable, usually fewer than 300 for patient comfort
Desired effect	Immediate destruction of the vessels
	Vessels are initially treated at the scleral spur using the mirrored goniolens and posteriorly over iris root. Eventually, over several sessions, all anterior segment neovascular vessels are obliterated in the angle and on the iris.
	Use the minimim energy setting required to blanch the vessel (lower settings are required on the iris surface because of adjacent pigment).
	Initially the patient may need repeated reevaluation each 2 or 4 days, since when such vessels line an open angle, total angle-closure can occur within days.

Vessels are treated sufficiently to cause contracture, blanching, and obliteration of the neovascularization. Treatment is done in multiple sessions a few days apart to minimize inflammation, bleeding, and discomfort. The initial session is directed at the angle and peripheral iris, through the mirrored portion of the goniolens (Fig. 13-7). These sessions

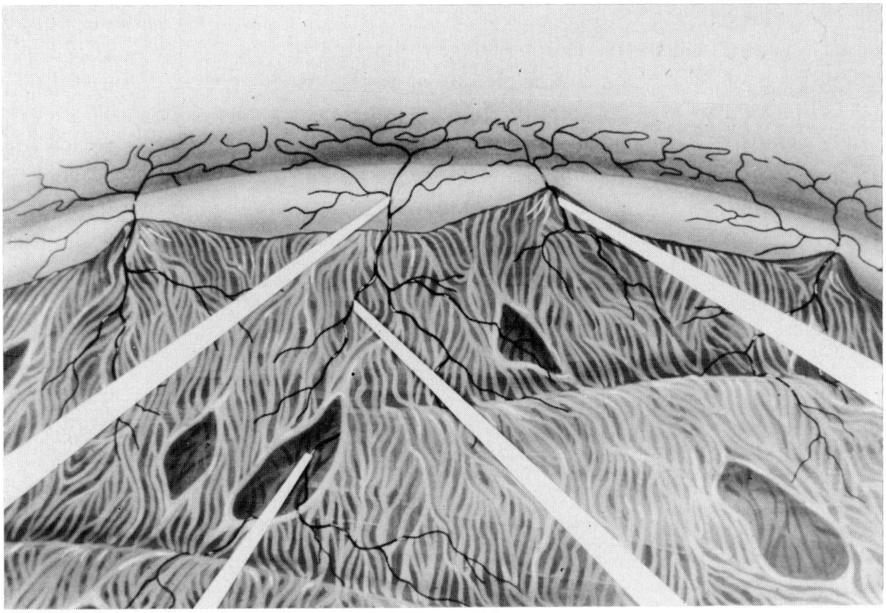

Fig. 13-7. Drawing of examples of laser applications in goniophotocoagulation used for immediate control of anterior segment neovascularization in conjunction, when possible, with panretinal photocoagulation. In series of sessions all neovascular vessels will be treated and retreated until they cease to recur or until angle closes despite all treatment. (From Simmons, R.J., Dueker, D.K., and Deppermann, S.R.: Role of anterior segment laser photocoagulation in prophylaxis and treatment of neovascular glaucoma. In New Orleans Academy of Ophthalmology: Symposium on glaucoma, St. Louis, 1981, The C.V. Mosby Co., pp. 396.)

can be rather long and, for patient comfort, we usually use 300 or less applications of laser per session. Successive sessions are carried centrally toward the pupil through the central, unmirrored portion of the goniolens. Initially, at intervals of 3 to 7 days, the eye should be reexamined and additional laser applied. After 2 to 4 weeks, if control of the anterior segment neovascularization is improving, subsequent treatment can be at progressively longer intervals, such as 7 to 14 days. If after 2 to 4 weeks, in spite of all anterior segment and posterior segment treatment the neovascularization has progressed to full closure of the angle, other therapy such as surgery will usually be required.

All of the complications of goniophotocoagulation have been transient. The only significant complication appears to be gross hyphema (3.4% of cases), which clears in 2 to 3 weeks. Microscopic hyphema is more commonly encountered (20%) but is not a problem.[44] Patient discomfort during the treatment session is frequently moderate but can be more severe. Topical proparacaine may be supplemented with topical cocaine, and the surgeon rarely requires the use of a retrobulbar anesthetic.

LASER FOR WOUND NEOVASCULARIZATION WITH RECURRENT HEMORRHAGE AND GLAUCOMA

Not uncommonly vessels may grow in surgical wounds or perforation sites into the anterior chamber. The vessel extension is most likely in wounds at the limbus, such as cataract sections in which the overlying episclera serves as a source of vessels.[38,49,58,59]

Watzke has reported the incidence of such new vessels in cataract wounds as 12%.[59] These vessels can bleed and cause a transient blurring of vision, for which the patient may even give a history identical to amaurosis fugax. In one patient we saw an extensive carotid vascular workup take place because of such a classic history. The patient was even having episodes of bleeding from new vessels in a previous cataract wound; by the time he was seen in the office after each episode, the blood had already cleared (Fig. 13-8). In addition to the visual complaints, elevated IOP can also result from the episodes of bleeding. The key to making this diagnosis is a high index of suspicion, which prompts the ophthalmologist to perform gonioscopy. Also, during gonioscopy bleeding from the offending vessels often occurs.[38]

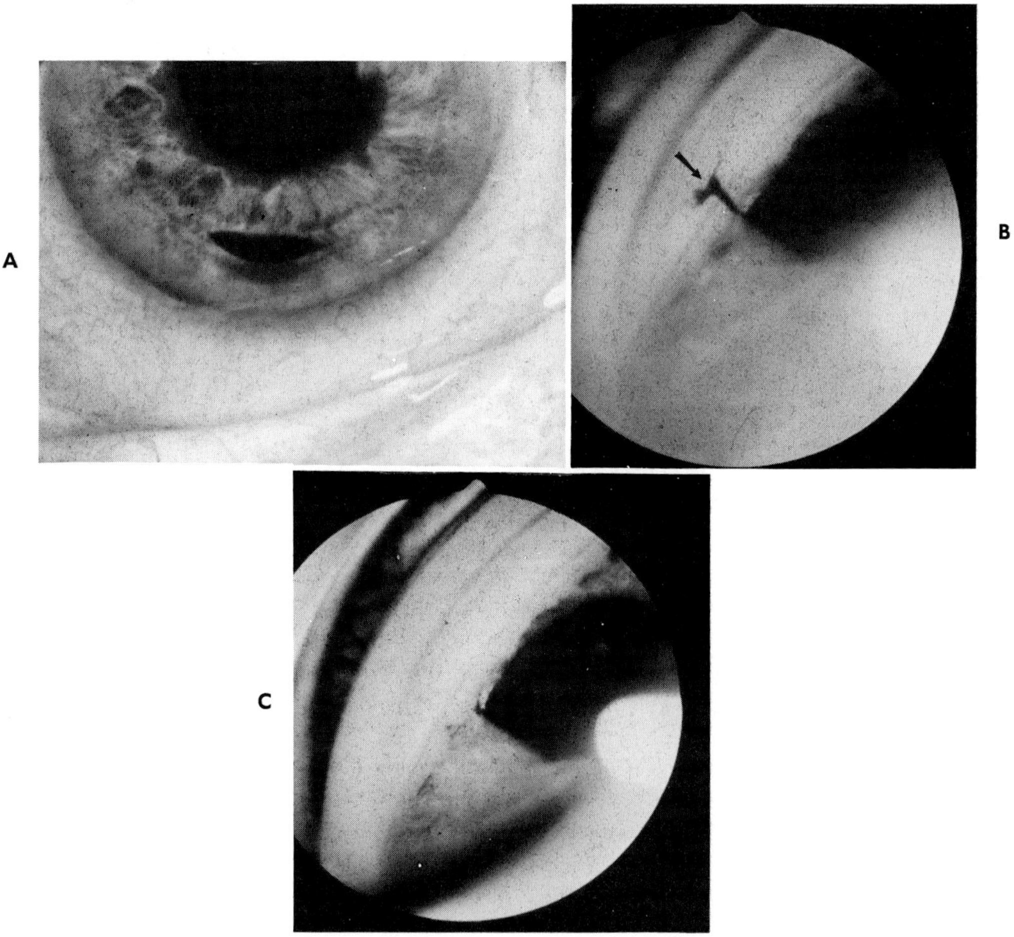

Fig. 13-8. A, Recurrent glaucoma in patient years after cataract surgery, with no apparent cause, until ultimately small hyphema was discovered. **B,** Gonioscopy in same patient revealed a neovascular tuft *(arrow)* at the site of wound closure from the cataract operation. **C,** Following treatment with the argon laser, the tuft is no longer visible, and patient has had no further episodes of glaucoma or hyphema. (**A** from Belcher, C.D., Thomas, J.V., and Simmons, R.J., editors: Photocoagulation in glaucoma and anterior segment disease, Baltimore, 1984, Williams & Wilkins, p. 216.)

Topical anesthesia with proparacaine is generally sufficient for these cases but occasionally retrobulbar anesthesia is required. The Goldmann or similar mirrored lens is used to visualize and treat the vessels, which may appear as discrete vessels or as a reddish patch in the wound area. The vessels are treated directly with the following settings: 100 μ spot size, 200 to 400 mW power, and 0.2 to 0.5 second per application. The power may be increased to blanch the vessels. Repeated sessions may be necessary for recurrent hemorrhage. Cryotherapy at the limbus[58,59] and direct surgical treatment[49,50] are other, more invasive techniques that have been advocated for repeated, uncontrolled hemorrhage.

LASER IN DIAGNOSIS AND TREATMENT OF EPITHELIAL INVASION OF ANTERIOR CHAMBER

Following perforating trauma, surgical or otherwise, to the anterior segment, epithelial invasion of the anterior segment may occur and take one of three forms. The first, pearl tumor of the iris, results from the implantation of a hair follicle or other fragment of skin onto the iris. It is not connected to the perforating wound, is usually a relatively benign condition, and does not require the laser in its treatment.

The other forms of epithelial invasion are the result of epithelial cells extending through a wound, most commonly after nonsurgical trauma or cataract surgery with incomplete wound closure. These invading epithelial cells can take the form of an advancing sheet of cells called epithelial downgrowth or may form cysts called epithelial inclusion cysts. In both these conditions, particularly with downgrowth, glaucoma can commonly result.

Epithelial downgrowth

The role of the laser in the management of epithelial downgrowth is diagnostic, except when glaucoma persists following radical excision of the invading tissue; in these cases the laser is applied to the ciliary processes for pressure control (see previous section on cyclophotocoagulation).

In cases of suspected epithelial downgrowth or when the cytologic diagnosis has been made by examination of sediment from an anterior chamber tap,[29] argon laser can be used to outline the extent of the proliferating sheet of tissue on the iris surface,[48,53] according to the following technique:

Protocol	Done at least 24 hours before surgery because of resultant anterior segment inflammation
	Topical anesthesia
	Goldmann contact lens
	Topical steroid prescribed following laser
Laser settings	Spot size: 500 μ
	Power: 100 to 200 mW
	Time: 0.2 second per application
	Number of applications: varies according to the number required to outline the extent of downgrowth

This is done to define the extent of planned excisional surgery and cryotherapy, as described by Stark, Michels, and Maumenee.[48] When a laser burn is applied to an area where the iris is covered by the epithelial sheet, a white spot is produced, compared to the dark spot obtained on normal iris tissue. The exact location of the edge of the

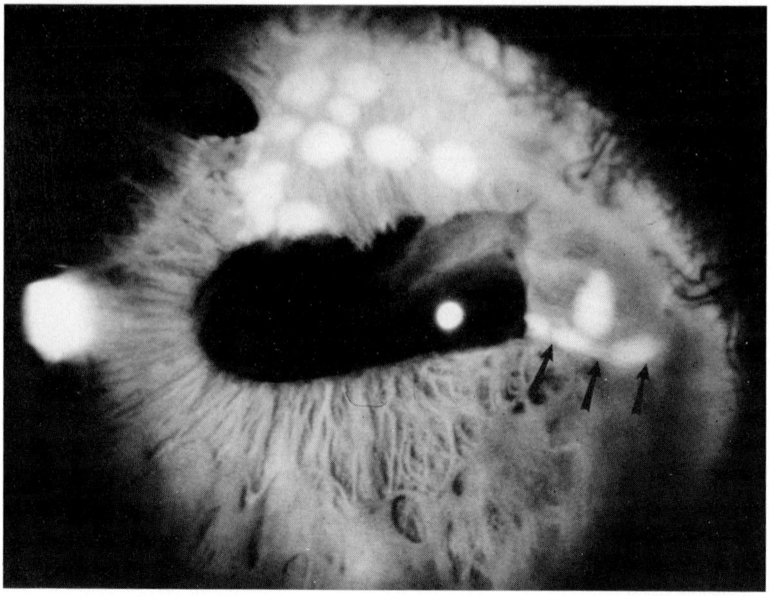

Fig. 13-9. Use of argon laser to outline extent of epithelial downgrowth 10 months following uncomplicated intracapsular cataract extraction. Note sharp border of sheet of epithelial cells made visible by laser applications *(arrows)*.

downgrowth can be defined in this manner, which helps to plan the extent of surgery (Fig. 13-9).

Epithelial inclusion cysts

Epithelial invasion of the anterior chamber is most likely to take the form of a grayish, translucent cyst that is connected to the point of entry. Some of these grow little or not at all, even for decades, and need only be observed periodically for growth or associated inflammation. Other cysts may grow to such an extent that angle-closure and glaucoma result. Others may obstruct the visual axis. At the first sign of growth, glaucoma, decreased vision, or iridocyclitis, treatment is indicated. The argon laser can be used in their treatment.[20,53] It is generally preferrable to aspirate the cyst contents through its base prior to treatment with the laser, especially for large cysts. However, in some cases, small cysts can be successfully treated with the laser without prior aspiration of the cyst contents. The technique follows:

1. Laser following aspiration of cyst contents

Protocol	Pigmentation of at least a portion of the wall required
	Topical anesthesia with proparacaine and cocaine
	Can be done in the office if sterility and patient cooperation are assured
	Cyst contents aspirated with sharp 27-gauge needle via its base at the limbus to collapse the cyst; its walls must remain intact.
	Laser with a Goldmann lens, which is especially useful if the cyst extends into the angle
	Topical cycloplegics are prescribed after surgery.
	Repeat treatment may be necessary and effective.

Laser settings — Spot size: 200 μ
Power: 200 mW; after the initial laser application, the tissue is treated with powers up to 500 to 1000 mW to thermally destroy all epithelial cells.
Time: 0.2 second per application

2. Laser without aspiration of cyst contents (can be tried for very small cysts with sufficient pigmentation)

Protocol — Posterior wall of cyst is coagulated first in a confluent applications of laser shots. The anterior wall is then treated in similar fashion.
The laser burns may cause the release of pigment, debris, and proteinaceous material into the anterior chamber, which decreases visibility and may necessitate postponement of further therapy for 3 to 7 days.
Topical cycloplegics are prescribed after surgery.
Collapse of cyst is not immediate and may take several days.
Repeat treatment may be necessary and effective.

The best results from laser are generally obtained with smaller cysts. For these methods to work, pigment must be present on at least some of the cyst wall to absorb the laser energy. Should laser therapy not be possible or if it is employed but fails, other therapies are available, such as xenon arc photocoagulation,[9,25] aspiration of the cyst followed by diathermy, surgical removal,[5] and others. Care must be taken with any direct manipulation of an epithelial implantation cyst, since conversion to epithelial downgrowth, and the following frequently devastating complications can occur:

Transient iritis
Transient elevation of IOP
Corneal opacities
Hemorrhage, if iris vessels are present in the cyst walls
Conversion of cyst to epithelial downgrowth, resulting from puncture during needle aspiration of cyst contents or any other direct manipulation

LASER FOR HYPOTONY CAUSED BY CYCLODIALYSIS

In cases where a traumatic, inadvertent, or intentional cyclodialysis results in hypotony, corneal folds, macular edema, and decreased visual acuity, the laser has been employed to limit dialysis function and raise the IOP. Other treatments have been recommended in the past, such as silicone-rod scleral buckling, surgical incarceration of the iris and/or ciliary body in a limbal wound, application of topical steroids, walling off of the cyclodialysis with diathermy,[23] or the use of a McCannell suture to close the cleft. Employing an argon laser for this condition represents a less invasive alternative and should be tried when clarity of media permits its use.

The settings that have been reported[12,15] for successful results are 100 to 200 μ spot size, 350 to 800 mW power, 0.1 second per application, and approximately 100 to 200 applications, which vary with the size of the dialysis. Numerous laser applications are made into the depths of the dialysis through a goniolens.[37] In cases of extreme hypotony corneal folds may prevent adequate visualization of the angle for the treatment. Although the desired site of treatment is in the depths of the cleft, we believe that in eyes where a desired cyclodialysis is present and argon laser trabeculoplasty is being performed, the trabecular meshwork in the immediate vicinity of the cleft should be avoided, since this might have some deleterious effect on the function of the cleft.

During the 2 days following laser therapy, the eye must be observed closely for rapid, substantial increases in IOP that require medical therapy. Such pressure elevations are of particular concern in patients with advanced glaucoma and susceptible optic nerves that cannot tolerate acute pressure rises without significant visual field damage. Usually, with increased medical therapy, the pressure can be brought back into the 13 to 19 mm Hg range.

The mechanism whereby this treatment alters the function of cyclodialyses is unknown. No reports of postlaser gonioscopy that describe actual closure of the cleft exist, although it is possible that closure occurs at a site out of the goniolens' view. It may be that increased inflammation and altered aqueous composition as a result of the laser treatment are responsible for the increased pressure. An interesting finding in the cases when, before successful laser treatment, the visual acuity was decreased from retinal edema, the vision returned to remarkably improved levels following elevation of the IOP. This type of macular edema seems to carry an entirely different prognosis than other types of postoperative macular edema, such as the cystoid macular edema encountered after cataract surgery, in that it appears to be reversible even after years of hypotony.

SUMMARY

The use of outpatient photosurgical laser procedures is now common in the management of glaucoma. In addition to argon laser trabeculoplasty and laser iridectomy, there exists a spectrum of anterior segment problems amenable to laser techniques, as reviewed in this chapter.

Argon laser photocoagulators and nd:YAG photodisruptors represent a very important step toward safer and more effective treatment of problems of the eye's anterior segment.

REFERENCES

1. Abedin, S., Simmons, R.J., and Grant, W.M.: Progressive low-tension glaucoma: treatment to stop glaucomatous cupping and field loss when these progress despite normal intraocular pressure, Ophthalmology **89:**1, 1982.
2. Belcher, C.D.: Laser therapy for intraepithelial cysts of the iris and ciliary body. In Belcher, C.D., Thomas, J.V., and Simmons, R.J., editors: Photocoagulation in glaucoma and anterior segment disease, Baltimore, 1984, Williams & Wilkins.
3. Braconier, H., and Dueker, D.K.: Personal communication.
4. Brockhurst, R.J.: Nanophthalmos with uveal effusion: a new clinical entity, Arch. Ophthalmol. **93:**1289, 1975.
5. Bruner, W.E., and others: Management of epithelial cysts of the anterior chamber, Ophthalmic Surg. **12:**279, 1981.
6. Chandler, P.A.: A new operation for malignant glaucoma: a preliminary report, Trans. Am. Ophthalmol. Soc. **62:**408, 1964.
7. Chandler, P.A., and Braconier, H.E.: Spontaneous intraepithelial cysts of the iris and ciliary body with glaucoma, Am. J. Ophthalmol. **45:**4, 1958.
8. Chandler, P.A., and Grant, W.M.: Lectures on glaucoma, Philadelphia, 1965, Lea & Febiger.
9. Cleasby, G.W.: Photocoagulation of iris-ciliary body epithelial cysts, Trans. Am. Acad. Ophthalmol. Otolaryngol. **75:**638, 1971.
10. De Blasio, P., and Simmons, R.J.: Unpublished data.
11. Depperman, S.R.: Goniophotocoagulation. In Belcher, C.D., Thomas, J.V., and Simmons, R.J., editors: Photocoagulation in glaucoma and anterior segment disease. Baltimore, 1984, Williams & Wilkins.
12. Harbin, T.S.: Treatment of cyclodialysis clefts with argon laser photocoagulation, Ophthalmology **89:**1082, 1982.
13. Herschler, J.: Laser shrinkage of the ciliary processes: a treatment for malignant (ciliary block) glaucoma, Ophthalmology **87:**1155, 1980.

14. James, W.A., and others: Argon laser photomydriasis, Am. J. Ophthalmol. **81:**62, 1976.
15. Joondeph, H.C.: Management of postoperative and posttraumatic cyclodialysis clefts with argon laser photocoagulation, Ophthalmic Surg. **11**(3):186, 1980.
16. Kimbrough, R.L., and others: Angle closure glaucoma in nanophthalmos, Am. J. Ophthalmol. **88**(3):572, 1979.
17. Krill, A.E., Archer, D., and Newell, F.W.: Photocoagulation in complications secondary to branch vein occlusion, Arch. Ophthalmol. **85**(1):48, 1971.
18. Lee, P.F.: Argon laser photocoagulation of the ciliary processes in cases of aphakic glaucoma, Arch. Ophthalmol. **97:**2135, 1979.
19. Lee, P.F., and Pomerantzeff, O.: Transpupillary cyclophotocoagulation of rabbit eyes, Am. J. Ophthalmol. **71:**911, 1971.
20. L'Esperance, F.A., and James, W.A.: Argon laser photocoagulation of iris abnormalities, Trans. Am. Acad. Ophthalmol. Otolaryngol. **79:**321, 1975.
21. Little, L., Rosenthal, A., and Dellaporta, A.: The effect of pan-retinal photocoagulation on rubeosis iridis, Am. J. Ophthalmol. **81**(6):804, 1976.
22. Maumenee, A.E.: External filtering operations for glaucoma: the mechanism of function and failure, Trans. Am. Ophthalmol. Soc. **58:**319, 1960.
23. Maumenee, A.E., and Stark, W.J.: Management of persistent hypotony after planned or inadvertent cyclodialysis, Am. J. Ophthalmol. **71:**320, 1971.
24. Merritt, J.C.: Transpupillary photocoagulation of the ciliary processes, Ann. Ophthalmol. **8:**32, 1976.
25. Okun, E., and Mandell, A.: Photocoagulation as a treatment of epithelial implantation cysts following cataract surgery, Trans. Am. Ophthalmol. Soc. **72:**170, 1974.
26. Ritch, R.: Argon laser treatment for medically unresponsive attacks of angle-closure glaucoma, Am. J. Ophthalmol. **94:**197, 1982.
27. Shrader, C.E., and others: Pupillary and iridovitreal block in pseudophakic eyes. (Submitted for publication.)
28. Simmons, R.J.: Discussion of trabeculectomy and shell tamponade techniques, Br. J. Ophthalmol. **56**(3):305, 1972.
29. Simmons, R.J.: Free cells in the aqueous and their possible importance in glaucoma. In Merte, H.J., editor: Doc. Ophthalmol. Proc. **16,** 1974.
30. Simmons, R.J.: Filtering operations. In Chandler, P.A., and Grant, W.M., editors: Glaucoma, Philadelphia, 1979, Lea & Febiger.
31. Simmons, R.J.: Malignant glaucoma. In Chandler, P.A., and Grant, W.M., editors: Glaucoma, Philadelphia, 1979, Lea & Febiger.
32. Simmons, R.J.: Nanophthalmos: diagnosis and treatment. In Chandler, P.A., and Grant, W.M., editors: Glaucoma, Philadelphia, 1979, Lea & Febiger.
33. Simmons, R.J.: Discussion of Herschler, J.: Laser shrinkage of ciliary processes: a treatment for malignant (ciliary block) glaucoma, Ophthalmology **87:**1158, 1980.
34. Simmons, R.J., and Kimbrough, R.L.: Shell tamponade in filtering surgery for glaucoma, Ophthalmic Surg. **10**(9):17, 1979.
35. Simmons, R.J., and Kolker, A.: Laser goniocoagulation. Presented at the annual meeting of the American Academy of Ophthalmology, November 1979, San Francisco.
36. Simmons, R.J., and Savage, J.A.: Unpublished data.
37. Simmons, R.J., and Simmons, R.B.: Gonioplasty. In Belcher, C.D., Thomas, J.V., and Simmons, R.J., editors: Photocoagulation in glaucoma and anterior segment disease, Baltimore, 1984, Williams & Wilkins.
38. Simmons, R.J., and Simmons, R.B.: Laser vascular ablation in the anterior segment. In Belcher, C.D., Thomas, J.V., and Simmons, R.J., editors: Photocoagulation in glaucoma and anterior segment disease, Baltimore, 1984, Williams & Wilkins.
39. Simmons, R.J., and Simmons, R.B.: Other glaucoma uses of photocoagulation: techniques of photosclerostomy and treatment of malignant glaucoma. In Belcher, C.D., Thomas, J.V., and Simmons, R.J., editors: Photocoagulation in glaucoma anterior segment disease, Baltimore, 1984, Williams & Wilkins.
40. Simmons, R.J., and Singh, O.S.: The shell tamponade technique in glaucoma surgery. In New Orleans Academy of Ophthalmology: Symposium on glaucoma, St. Louis, 1981, The C.V. Mosby Co.
41. Simmons, R.J., and Thomas, J.V.: Malignant glaucoma. In Ritch, R., and Shields, M.B., editors: The secondary glaucomas, St. Louis, 1982, The C.V. Mosby Co.
42. Simmons, R.J., Deppermann, S.R., and Dueker, D.K.: Laser prophylaxis of neovascular glaucoma: by

goniophotocoagulation alone or in combination with pantetinal photocoagulation, Doc. Ophthalmol. Proc. Series. **22:**203, 1980.
43. Simmons, R.J., Deppermann, S.R., and Dueker, D.K.: The role of goniophotocoagulation in neovascularization of the anterior chamber angle, Ophthalmology **87:**79, 1980.
44. Simmons, R.J., Dueker, D.K., and Depperman, S.R.: Role of anterior segment laser photocoagulation in prophylaxis and treatment of neovascular glaucoma. In New Orleans Academy of Ophthalmology: Symposium on glaucoma, St. Louis, 1981, The C.V. Mosby Co.
45. Simmons, R.J., Dueker, D.K., and Kimbrough, R.L.: Goniophotocoagulation for neovascular glaucoma, Trans. Am. Ophthalmol. Otolaryngol. **83:**80, 1977.
46. Simmons, R.J., and others: Laser gonioplasty for special problems in angle-closure glaucoma. In Transactions of the New Orleans Academy of Ophthalmology: Symposium on glaucoma, St. Louis, 1981, The C.V. Mosby Co.
47. Singh, O.S., and others: Nanophthalmos: a perspective on identification and therapy, Ophthalmology **89:**9, 1982.
48. Stark, W.J., Michels, R.G., and Maumenee, A.E.: Surgical management of epithelial ingrowth, Am. J. Ophthalmol. **85:**772, 1978.
49. Swan, K.C.: Hyphema due to wound vascularization after cataract extraction, Arch. Ophthalmol. **89:**87, 1973.
50. Swan, K.C.: Late hyphema due to wound vascularization, Trans. Am. Acad. Ophthalmol. Otolaryngol. **81:**138-44, 1976.
51. Thomas, J.V.: Photocoagulation of the ciliary processes. In Belcher, C.D., Thomas, J.V., and Simmons, R.J., editors: Photocoagulation in glaucoma and anterior segment disease, Baltimore, 1984, Williams & Wilkins.
52. Thomas, J.V.: Pupilloplasty and photomydriasis. In Belcher, C.D., Thomas, J.V., and Simmons, R.J., editors: Photocoagulation in glaucoma and anterior segment disease, Baltimore, 1984, Williams & Wilkins.
53. Thomas, J.V., Ledrer, C.M., and Simmons, R.J.: Photocoagulation for epithelial ingrowth and cysts of the anterior chamber. In Belcher, C.D., Thomas, J.V., and Simmons, R.J., editors: Photocoagulation in glaucoma and anterior segment disease, Baltimore, 1984, Williams & Wilkins.
54. Ticho, U., and Ivry, M.: Reopening of occluded filtering blebs by argon laser photocoagulation, Am. J. Ophthalmol. **84:**413, 1977.
55. Ticho, U., and Zauberman, H.: Argon laser application to the angle structures in the glaucomas, Arch. Ophthalmol. **94:**61, 1976.
56. Van Buskirk, E.M.: Reopening filtration sites with the argon laser, Am. J. Ophthalmol. **94:**1, 1982.
57. Wand, M., and others: Plateau iris syndrome, Trans. Am. Acad. Ophthalmol. Otolaryngol. **83:**122, 1977.
58. Watzke, R.C.: Intraocular hemorrhage from wound vascularization following cataract surgery, Trans. Am. Ophthalmol. Soc. **72:**242, 1974.
59. Watzke, R.C.: Intraocular hemorrhage from vascularization of the cataract incision, Ophthalmology **87:**19, 1980.
60. Weber, P.A., and others: Argon laser treatment of the ciliary processes in aphakic glaucoma with flat anterior chamber, Am. J. Ophthalmol. **97:**82, 1984.
61. Zimmerman, T., Worthen, D.M., and Wickham, G.: Argon laser photocoagulation of the ciliary processes and pigmented pupillary membranes in man, Invest. Ophthalmol. **12:**622, 1973.

14

Laser iridotomy

Hugh Beckman

Meyer-Schwickerath[4] in 1956 described iridotomies in aphakic eyes that were created with the xenon arc photocoagulator for the treatment of pupil-block glaucoma. Because of the excessive heat dissipation created by the high-energy, low-powered system, adjacent structures of the eye were adversely affected by the treatment, and a high incidence of cataract formation in phakic eyes precluded the popularity of the technique.

In 1968 I modified a commercial solid-state ruby laser, wedded it to a Zeiss OPMI-II operating microscope, and began experimentation to produce single-pulse iridectomies that remained reliably patent. Since peripheral iridectomy ab externo is a relatively inocuous, extremely reliable procedure, I have always believed that laser iridectomy should be at least as easy and reliable.

In 1971 Perkins[5] reported partially penetrating iridotomies performed with a low-powered ruby laser and thought that aqueous percolated through the iridotomies, although direct communication with the posterior chamber was not achieved. In that same year my co-workers and I[2] reported on the successful treatment of pupil-block glaucoma with penetrating ruby laser iridectomies at power levels of 4.5 mm/cm^2. Given a hazel eye with moderate pigmentation, a brown eye, or a dark-brown eye, I could create an iridectomy each time with a single pulse, and since the iridectomies were rather large, their reliability for maintained patency was greater than 95%. Because of the poor absorption of ruby wavelength (6943 Angstrom) by nonpigmented iris stroma, there was inadequate absorption by blue irides for iridectomy formation. Neodymium: glass (1.06 μ energy) in long-pulse mode (6 ms) delivered with the same instrument resulted in excessive corneal burns because of absorption by the cornea of the 1.06 μ, with little hole formation occurring, even in heavily pigmented irides.

In 1973 Sugar and I[2] reported our inability to produce long-pulsed neodymium (nd) iridectomies and reported the first successful argon laser iris penetration,[2] but we believed at that time that the power levels of the argon lasers available were insufficient to produce iridectomies that would remain reliably patent. Let me emphasize again that the iridectomy should be both easy to create and must remain patent. I believe that the patency of the hole is the result of the interplay of two factors: (1) the size of the hole—the larger the hole, the less the ability of body reparative processes to fill it; and (2) the amount of tissue damage created around the hole during the performance of the laser iridectomy—the greater the inflammation created in the tissue immediately surrounding the hole, the greater the inflammatory response that occurs and the greater the chance of the hole being filled in by melalanocytes or fibroblasts. The original argon iridotomies were filling in at the rate of 30%.

The work of Abraham and Miller[1] and Pollack and Patz[6] was received skeptically by the ophthalmic community, and it was only with the development of the Abraham lens, which increased the power density of the marginal argon laser to the point where techniques for the ''occasional laser iridotomist'' could be well taught, that Ritch[7] popularized the technique. These original techniques yielded tiny holes referred to as argon laser microiridotomies. The Abraham lens reduced the 50 μ spot size to 30 μ, and although it gave the surgeon a much higher percentage of technical success in performing the iridotomy, in my hands the patency failed at a rate of 25%. I began augmenting my argon iridotomies with ruby to enlarge the size and succeeded in dropping my closure rate to 17%. Since the world was not yet ready for an ophthalmic solid-state laser, and since there was obviously no need to teach ophthalmologists how to use equipment that they did not have available, I dedicated my efforts toward what I described as the formation of the ''perfect argon laser iridotomy.'' By perfect, I meant that it should be (1) easy to teach, (2) easy to learn to use with a high degree of technical success, and (3) remain reliably patent.

An analysis of my own data (Table 14-1) showed a definite trend for the viability of patency to be directly proportional to the size of the iridotomy created. Thus large, 1 mm or greater ruby iridotomies stayed open better than the ruby-augmented argon iridotomies, which in turn stayed open better than the 50 μ early iridotomies performed with the Abraham lens. Over time I worked to develop a technique that would yield about a 200 μ iridotomy with a minimal of surrounding tissue damage. The object is to drill a 200 μ cylinder without having to enlarge it. To do this, I select a homogeneous area of iris, since I believe this tissue mass augments the buildup of heat in the base of the crater, resulting in a more reliable vaporization. A bubble forms in this crater (Fig. 14-1), and the work of Schirmer[9] would indicate that this bubble serves as an additional focusing lens, increasing the power density. It also serves to trap the heat of laser absorption within the crater, thus increasing vaporization efficiency (Fig. 14-2). Using a 200 μ spot with 600 to 1000 mW and an exposure time of 0.5 second, a crater can be formed in any colored iris with minimal carbonization and a minimal heat-effected zone surrounding the crater. Parameters for this are shown in Table 14-2. The base of the crater is then etched away using a 50 μ spot beam until the pigment epithelium is exposed. One must be careful to avoid lasering the side walls of the crater, as this puckers in adjacent iris. The pigment epithelium is then vaporized away. Using this technique, I can achieve a patent laser iridectomy in almost 100% of eyes on the first try, and after the iridotomy they remain patent in 95% of the cases.

Table 14-1. Failure of patency rates for different lasers

Laser	*Number*	*Repeats*	*% Reliably patent*
Ruby	92	5	95
50 W argon	89	27	70
Argon-ruby	30	5	83
50 W argon (lens)	47	12	75
100 W argon (lens)	38	7	82
200 W argon (lens)	106	8	92
YAG	9	0	100

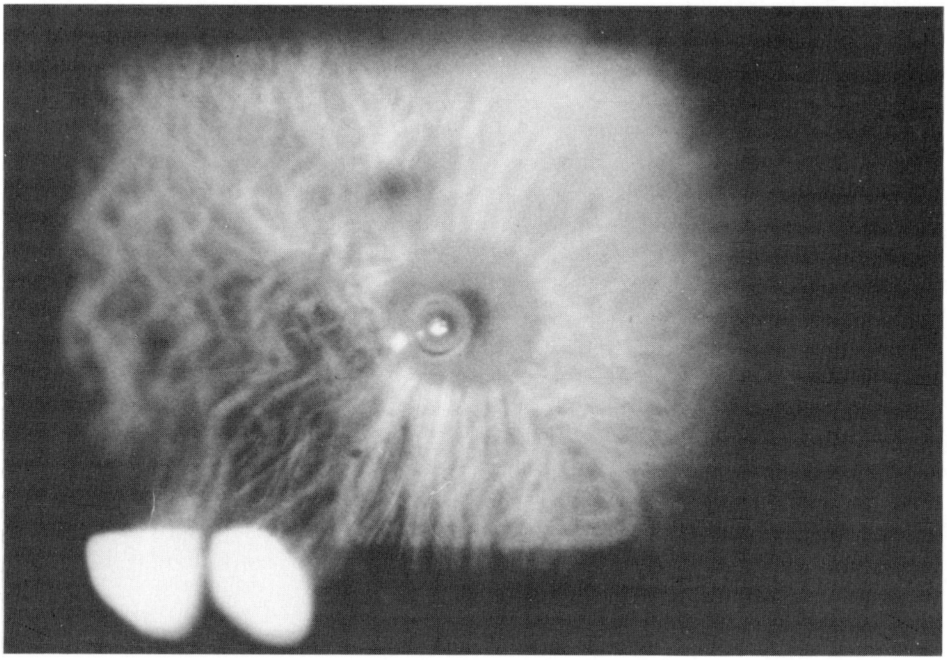

Fig. 14-1. Bubble in crater during iridotomy.

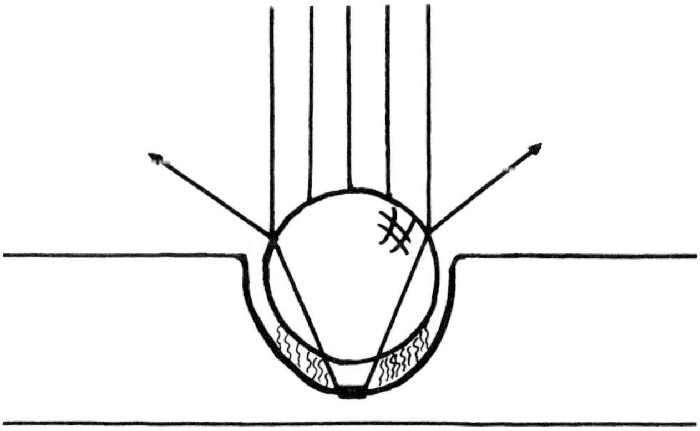

Fig. 14-2. Bubble increases power density and traps heat.

Table 14-2. Parameters for crater formation in irides during iridotomy

Iris	*Spot* (μ)	*Power*	*Time (second)*
Blue	200	1.0 W	1.0
Hazel	200	1.0 W	1.0
Brown	200	600 mW	1.0
Dark brown	200	600 mW	0.5

The two problems—formation of the iridotomy and the maintenance of patency—are discussed separately.

PROBLEMS IN IRIDOTOMY FORMATION

1. *Visualization.* To do the type of clean surgery necessary, the ophthalmologist must be able to visualize the target area. Corneal opacity, lack of contrast, or clouding of the cornea in shallow chambers by corneal denaturization resulting from heat rising from the crater all are obstacles to visualization. Therefore, the darker the iris and the shallower the chamber, the less of a peripheral attempt is used in attempting the iridotomy.

2. *Movement of patient or eyes.* Patient trembling, uncooperativeness, or reflex movements make it difficult to place the energy within the target or keep the energy on the target site long enough to effect vaporization. Retrobulbar anesthesia may be necessary in extreme cases.

3. *Difficulties with tissue precluding end-stage thermal effect (vaporization) to occur.* Examples of this are seen in epithelial downgrowth, in which popcorning of the epithelium covering the iris precludes vaporization; and iridoschisis, in which a thick, optically transparent stroma acts as a heat sink, precluding vaporization levels.

CASES IN WHICH FACTORS LEAD TO INCREASED PATENCY FAILURE

1. *Preexisting inflammation,* such as occurs in iritis or iridocyclitis.

2. *Presence of vitreous* up to or in the hole, such as occurs in flat anterior chamber syndrome (malignant glaucoma, internal iris prolapse, oversized anterior chamber lens–induced vitreous-forward syndrome). Vitreous or an aqueous-vitreous mixture seems to act as a scaffold for migration of pigmented iris into the hole, with frequent early closure occurring.

Following cataract surgery, particularly with insertion of anterior chamber intraocular lenses, the chamber may collapse with the iris bowing forward. If no optically patent iridectomy is seen, there is reasonable chance that a single iridotomy may break the pupil block, allowing the iris to fall backward and the anterior chamber to form. In those cases in which an optically patent iridectomy is already present, the prognosis for laser iridotomy is considerably less. Vitreous, probably mixed with aqueous, is permeating forward, and this viscous substance may be present in the anterior chamber. This is evidenced by debris remaining suspended during iridotomy formation in the mixture rather than flowing away, as when aqueous percolates through the wound. Multiple iridotomies occasionally succeed in relieving such situations, but more often, after an initial deepening of the anterior chamber, there is subsequent failure as the viscous mixture plugs the holes and pigment migrates into the crater. These cases usually require pars plana aspiration of vitreous for resolution of the process.

3. Rare cases in which patients may be on *medications* such as levodopa, which have melanocyte-stimulating effects, bringing unwanted melanocytes into the iridotomy and facilitating their closure.

Iridectomy formation in all of these problem cases would be facilitated by a laser that works faster and cooler and creates less inflammation. For this reason I believe that we are now seeing the beginning of a return to the solid-state pulsed laser iridotomy. Since long-pulsed ruby (ms) is ineffective on light irides, the use of Q-switched neodymium:YAG, Q-switched erbium-YLF, and Q-switched ruby lasers is evolving. The most available of these at this time are the neodymium:YAG lasers—in the past year I have performed one-shot iridotomies at first on problem cases (epithelial downgrowth, iridoschisis, chronic iritis) with universal success and with 100% maintenance of patency.

Recently encouraged by the results of Spaeth and Schwartz[10] with neodymium:YAG and Robin and Pollack[8] with Q-switched ruby lasers, I have performed nine YAG iridectomies on phakic patients using the LASAG MR-2 laser. The laser has been set for an energy level of 10 mJ, a pulse train of 5, with the YAG laser retrofocused 0.4 mm behind the helium-neon spot, which is focused on the anterior surface of the iris. The iridotomy was achieved in all nine cases in a single pulse, and all have remained patent. Minimal bleeding at the iridotomy site has been reported, but without clinical significance. Transient pressure rises occur, as with many laser iridotomies. No capsular rupture has been reported, but one should keep the iridotomy approach very peripheral. I believe that the ability of the YAG laser to create a relatively cold (low inflammation) iridotomy independent of patient cooperativeness will result in its more common use for noninvasive iridotomy formation in those centers in which suitable equipment is available.

REFERENCES

1. Abraham, R.K., and Miller, G.L.: Outpatient argon laser iridectomy for angle-closure glaucoma: a two-year study, Trans. Am. Acad. Ophthalmol. Otolaryngol. **79:**529, 1975.
2. Beckman, H., and Sugar, H.S.: Laser iridectomy therapy of glaucoma, Arch. Ophthalmol. **90:**453, 1973.
3. Beckman, H., and others: Laser iridectomies, Am. J. Ophthalmol. **72:**393, 1971.
4. Meyer-Schwickerath, G.: Erfahrungen mit der lichtkoagulation der metzhaut und der iris, Doc. Ophthalmol. **10:**91, 1956.
5. Perkins, E.S.: Laser iridotomy for secondary glaucoma, Trans. Ophthalmol. Soc. U.K. **91:**777, 1971.
6. Pollack, I.P., and Patz, A.: Argon laser iridotomy: an experimental and clinical study, Ophthalmic Surg. **7:**22, 1976.
7. Ritch, R.: The treatment of chronic angle-closure glaucoma. (editorial), Ann. Ophthalmol. **13:**21, 1981.
8. Robin, A., and Pollack, I.: Q-switched ruby laser iridotomies. Paper presented at Fifth International Congress of Lasers in Surgery and Medicine, Detroit, 1983.
9. Shirmer, K.: Personal communication.
10. Spaeth, G., and Schwartz, L.: Q-switched YAG:neodymium iridotomy. Paper presented Fifth International Congress of Laser Surgery and Medicine, Detroit, 1983.

15

New laser systems and their potential clinical usefulness

Francis A. L'Esperance, Jr.

During the last decade the krypton laser has become commercially available, the carbon dioxide laser has moved from the experimental to the clinical phase in the treatment spectrum, the dye laser has been introduced as a multiple-color laser with enormous potential in the field of photodynamic therapy, the Q-switched or mode-locked neodymium:YAG laser has been introduced for photodisruption of transparent intraocular tissues, and even the argon laser has been reevaluated to determine potential tissue responses to the green or blue wavelengths. The pioneering ingenuity of many investigators to manipulate existing lasers to control glaucoma, to substitute laser procedures for former surgical operations, and to become expert in the use of the advanced technologic precision inherent in ophthalmic lasers has been significant. This chapter's purpose is to introduce several new laser and delivery systems that should have considerable potential in the therapy of ocular diseases because of their specific wavelength, high power output, or unique photobiologic action.

FREQUENCY-DOUBLED NEODYMIUM:YAG LASER

Instrumentation

The clinical use of the frequency-doubled neodymium (Nd):YAG (yttrium-aluminum-garnet) laser as a source for the photocoagulation of ocular tissue was first achieved clinically in human beings in 1970 (Fig. 15-1). Specifically, this highly collimated, intense, monochromatic beam was employed successfully to therapeutically photocoagulate various chorioretinal abnormalities in seven patients[4] (Fig. 15-2).

At that time the frequency-doubled Nd:YAG laser was loaned to our laboratory by Medical Lasers, Inc., in Burlington, Mass. and consisted of the following parts: (1) a dual elliptic gold-plated cavity; (2) two 3000 W tungsten quartz halogen incandenscent lamps; (3) a 3 × 75 mm yttrium-aluminum-garnet host doped with triple-ionized neodymium; (4) two dielectrically coated mirrors; and (5) a barium sodium niobate crystal in a temperature-controlled oven.

The fundamental output of the Nd:YAG laser is at 1064 nm. By adding the nonlinear crystal in the resonant cavity between the Nd:YAG crystal and the output mirror, the second harmonic is obtained as a bright green beam at 532 nm (Fig. 15-3). The output is obtained through the front mirror, which is dielectrically coated for maximum reflectance at 1064 nm and maximal transmittance of 532 nm.

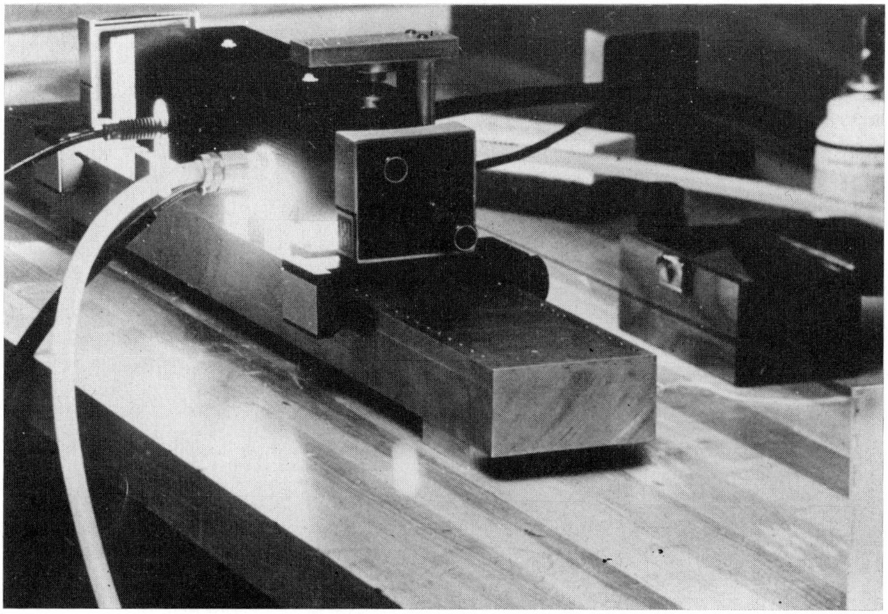

Fig. 15-1. Prototype version of the frequency-doubled Nd:YAG laser used during first clinical human studies in 1970.

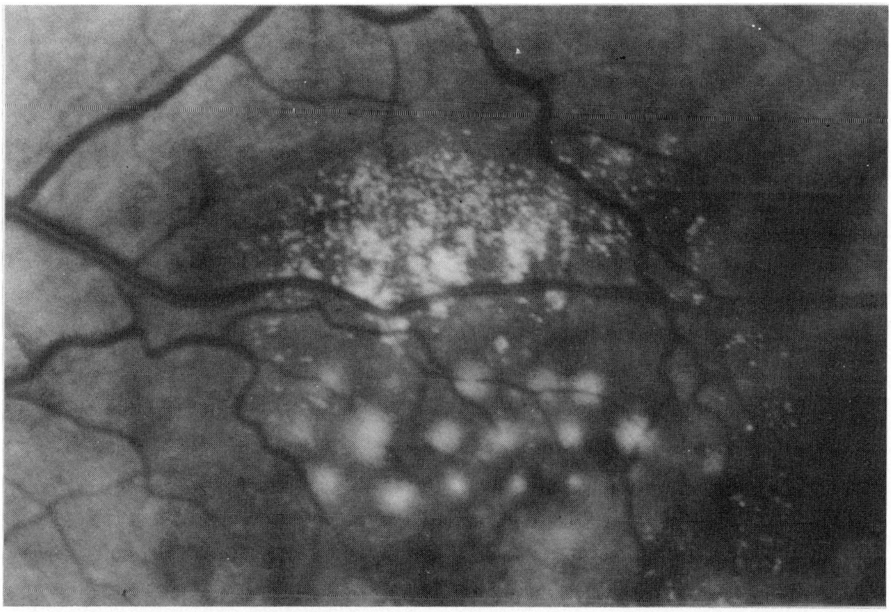

Fig. 15-2. First patient to be treated by frequency-doubled Nd:YAG laser (532.0 nm), using 100 to 150 μ coagulations at 0.2-second exposures and power levels ranging from 200 to 350 mW. This patient was treated in 1970 for localized paramacular retinal leakage caused by moderate nonproliferative diabetic retinopathy.

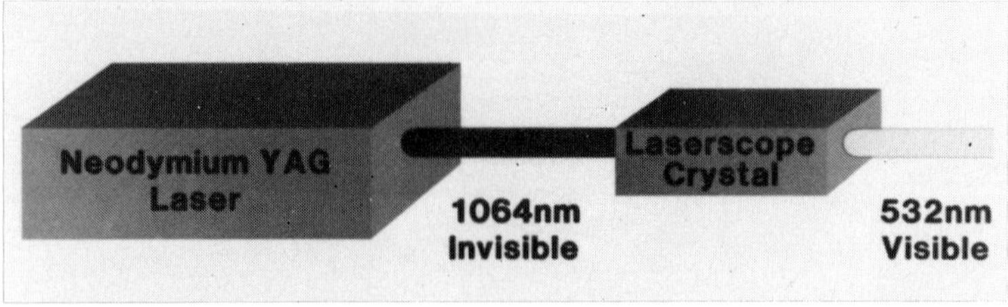

Fig. 15-3. Schematic drawing illustrating Nd:YAG laser producing invisible beam at 1064 nm that enters nonlinear KTP (potassium-titanium-phosphate) crystal and emerges with doubled-frequency and halved-wavelength of 532 nm in pea-green portion of spectrum. (Courtesy Laserscope, Inc.)

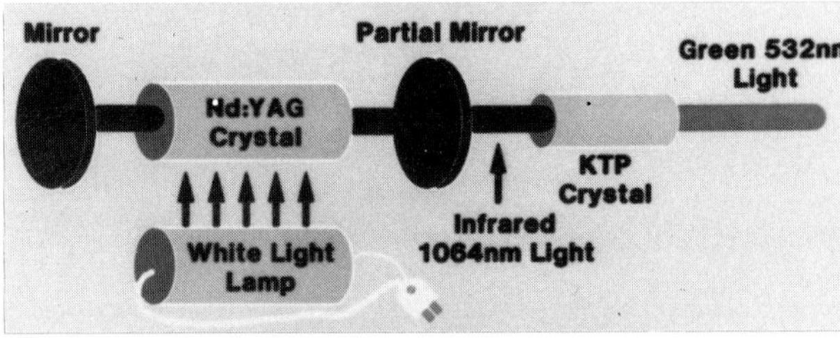

Fig. 15-4. Overall schematic drawing showing white-light pumping lamp that energizes Nd:YAG crystal to produce infrared beam, which is then converted by nonlinear KTP crystal to 532 nm laser beam. (Courtesy Laserscope, Inc.)

The pumping source that created the population inversion in the Nd:YAG crystal consisted of two tungsten filament lamps that operated directly from the AC line using a triac power supply. Electric power to the lamps, which were operated in parallel, was continuously variable from 120 V to full power.

The laser power was easily controlled within milliwatts because of the tungsten filament lamps and their inherently long reaction time, which also provided considerable electric output stability. At that time the power supply required an input of either 208 or 220 V with 50 to 60 Hz, single-phase electric requirements. The dimensions of this particular power supply were 5 × 5 × 9 inches.

During the past year a somewhat similar frequency-doubled Nd:YAG laser has been designed that eliminates many of the disadvantages and drawbacks of the original 1970 laser. The most significant changes with this new instrument are the following:

1. The doubling crystal is no longer a barium-sodium-niobate crystal, but rather a potassium-titanium-phosphate (KTP) crystal that has the capability of withstanding the potentially tremendous power generated by the solid-state Nd:YAG crystal and converting this wavelength from 1064 to 532 nm in the pea-green portion of the visible spectrum (Fig. 15-4). A potassium-deuterium-phosphate (KDP) crystal has been used with some success during the last several years, but even with this more sophisticated crystal, the potential power in the green portion of the spectrum was still limited. The KTP crystal allows the laser instrument to deliver full power in the frequency-doubled mode.

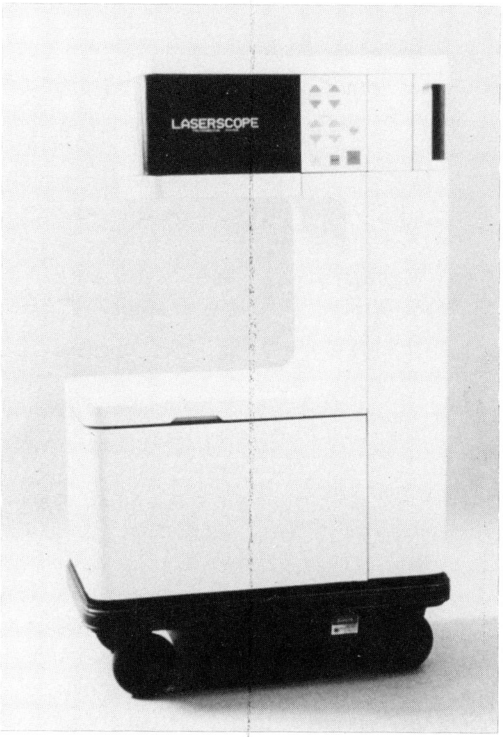

Fig. 15-5. Laserscope multispecialty frequency-doubled Nd:YAG laser console showing cathode ray tube readout area as well as controls for microprocessor unit. Unit has self-monitoring electronic surveillance and can produce output powers in the 20 W range at 532 nm wavelength.

2. The new frequency-doubled Nd:YAG laser designed by the Laserscope Corp. in conjunction with XMR Laser Co. utilizes a high-intensity flash source pulsing at 25,000 cycles per second (25 kHz) and producing powers in excess of 20 W emission from the laser port. This highly efficient system requires minimal cooling and can be self-contained and used in a portable fashion from the operating room to an outpatient surgical suite or other facility.
3. The entire laser was designed in a modern—if not futuristic—cabinet with the features of automatic self-diagnosis of any problems within the electronic circuitry of the system and with the appropriate method to solve these problems immediately (Fig. 15-5). The entire workings and intermanipulation of the laser and its energy output is under microprocessor control, and the output wattage, pulse duration, and potential mode of operation are displayed on a cathode ray tube. The system is therefore under complete electronic surveillance at all times, with minimal activation or interchange with the surgeon during the actual photocoagulation or photovaporization procedure.
4. The Laserscope frequency-doubled Nd:YAG laser system has the capability of producing extremely high powers and has been designed for ophthalmic use as a photocoagulator comparable to the argon green laser. It also has the potential of being used with 21 other peripheral devices. These fiberoptic-linked therapeutic

devices range from all types of endoscopic cauterization probes to dermatologic tattoo and port-wine stain eradicators and photovaporizers (Figs. 15-6 to 15-8). This multipurpose laser should therefore have considerable medical and surgical advantages, as well as provide an economic medical service.

Beam characteristics

Regardless of the nature of the laser or incandescent source, the main concern of the ophthalmologist is the nature of the beam entering the eye and its effectiveness in photocoagulation. This section summarizes the various features of the frequency-doubled Nd:YAG laser beam in terms of photocoagulation ability.

Collimation

The beam of any laser is extremely collimated or parallel as it travels from its source, and the Nd:YAG laser is no exception. However, the average 3 to 5 milliradians divergence of the beam makes it considerably less parallel than the average argon laser emission and therefore less able to focus to the small retinal spot produced by the argon laser photocoagulation system. This relative lack of collimation is an inherent property of all crystal lasers, such as the Nd:YAG, nd:glass, ruby, and frequency-doubled Nd:YAG lasers. Gas lasers produce less divergent beams and therefore can be focused more precisely for paramacular or individual vascular coagulations. Optical devices can reduce this divergence disparity, but only at the expense of power output.

It should be emphasized that this small amount of divergence from a crystal laser appears to be insignificant, particularly since the delivery system from the Laserscope frequency-doubled Nd:YAG source is through fiberoptic cables. When a laser beam emanating directly from a laser source enters a fiberoptic system, much of its coherence is broken down, with a significant divergence at the emission end of the fiberoptic cable. This divergent cone of light must be captured in most instances and refocused for the

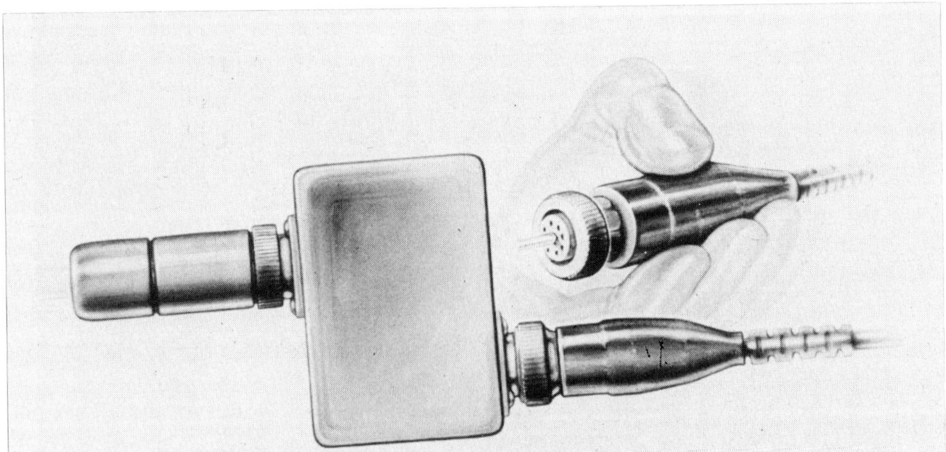

Fig. 15-6. Laserscope fiberoptic coupler for various medical uses of 532 nm beam. Interlock is designed to be recognized by main electronic console, so that each fiberoptic system has its own parameters for precise operation.

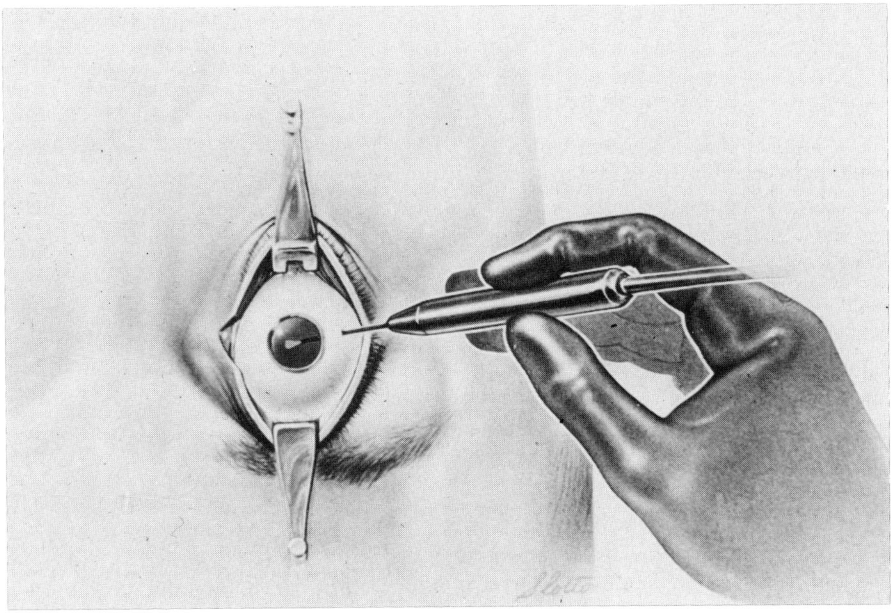

Fig. 15-7. Hand-held intraocular probe for endophotocoagulation of chorioretinal structures with 532 nm output. (Courtesy Laserscope, Inc.)

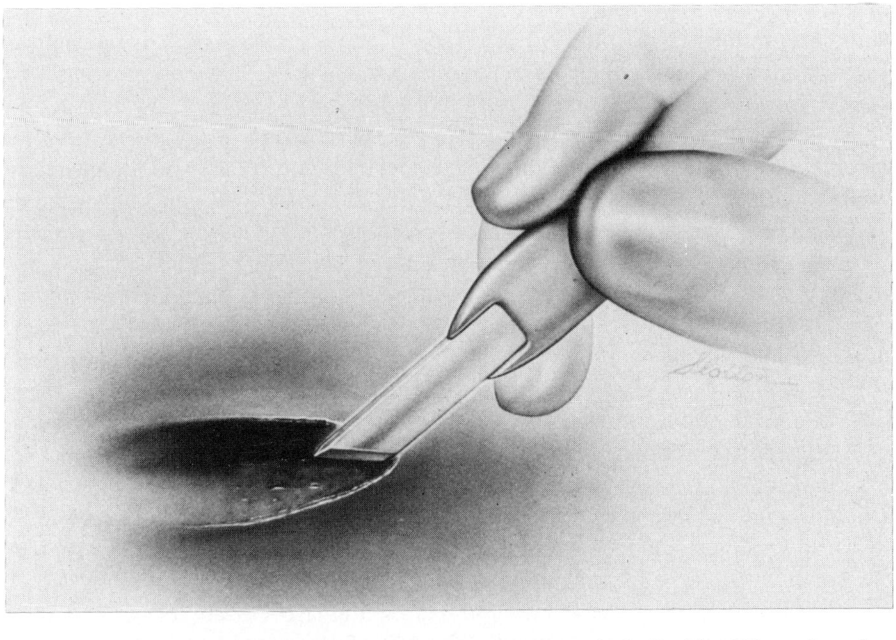

Fig. 15-8. Laserscope peripheral hemostatic quartz or diamond (Auth) knife. The 532 nm laser beam is channeled to cutting tip of knife to produce hemostasis during actual incisional process.

purpose of eventual photocoagulation. This has not posed a significant problem and may be advantageous in certain uses of the frequency-doubled Nd:YAG beam.

It must be noted, however, that this frequency-doubled Nd:YAG laser, produced in the pea-green region of the visible spectrum, will not be used directly after emission from the laser source. In all applications this laser beam will be interfaced with a fiber-optic cable in exactly the same manner as most photocoagulation systems, including the argon laser photocoagulation devices now in use. Because of the use of fiberoptic cable channeling devices from the laser to the photocoagulation instrument, the obvious advantageous property of minimal spot size is disregarded in favor of transmission of the laser beam over longer distances. With the use of fiberoptic coupling from the laser to the surgical instrument, the laser beam loses both its spatial and temporal coherence and becomes simply a monochromatic light source of high potential energy output. In essence, in ophthalmology it is the monochromaticity and the high power output that determine the effectiveness of a laser beam as a photocoagulation, photoradiation, or photovaporization device.

Monochromaticity

The Nd:YAG laser produces an output beam in the infrared portion of the electromagnetic spectrum at 1064 nm, which, when doubled in frequency (and therefore halved in wavelength) by the proper nonlinear crystal, is converted to a green beam at 532 nm. This single color can then be focused without chromatic aberration onto the retina or other ocular tissue. This factor has always been considered advantageous, and lasers have had the capability of producing retinal coagulations many times smaller than incandescent sources such as the xenon-arc instrument. It is also a law of laser physics that the potential size of the ocular photocoagulation varies directly with the wavelength, although much of this property is compromised by the use of fiberoptic channeling systems. The frequency-doubled Nd:YAG laser may actually gain some advantage because only one wavelength is being emitted, whereas the argon laser emits eight wavelengths, from 457.9 to 527.9 nm. Only two argon emissions are powerful—488 and 514.5 nm—and they are so closely approximated with regard to focus that they can be considered as one wavelength at 500 nm for calculation purposes. In addition, individual wavelengths can be selected from the argon laser emission spectrum so that the argon system can be considered as either a blue or green photocoagulation device, with focusing potential similar to the frequency-doubled Nd:YAG laser beam.

Focusing potential

It is possible to calculate the minimal size of a retinal image of any laser beam by employing a series of formulas described elsewhere.[2] From these figures it can be established that the theoretic minimal retinal image size produced by a frequency-doubled Nd:YAG laser is approximately 10.2 μ in diameter, as compared with a minimal retinal image diameter of 8.4 μ for argon laser radiation and 13.2 μ for krypton red laser radiation. Therefore, by the factor of wavelength only, the frequency-doubled Nd:YAG laser can theoretically produce a smaller retinal coagulation than the krypton laser, but not as small as the argon laser. In addition, the inferior collimation of the Nd:YAG beam may further decrease the focusing ability of this laser for any direct system.

The theoretic minimal retinal image diameter refers to an open, direct system from the laser source to the ocular tissue using optics other than fiberoptic systems. When a

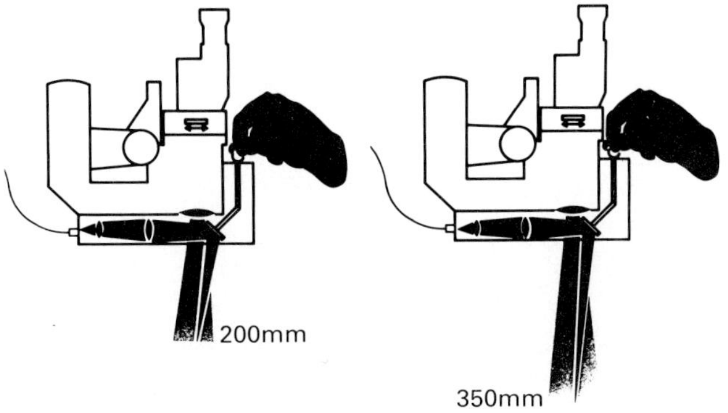

Fig. 15-9. Schematic drawing illustrating fiberoptic input to operating microscope, with manipulation of beam by a joystick and potential of varying focus of 532 nm beam from 200 to 350 mm from exit port of operating microscope. (Courtesy Laserscope, Inc.)

fiberoptic system is used not only the collimation but also the coherence of the laser beam is sacrificed, as previously mentioned, and new optical systems must be introduced to create a minimal spot size (50 μ) that is essentially the same for all of the visible laser photocoagulation instruments. Therefore, unless focusing becomes an extremely critical matter, all laser beams can be brought to a 50 μ coagulation size and perhaps smaller with fiberoptic channeling couplers. This has proved highly satisfactory with all photocoagulation, photodynamic, and photovaporization surgical procedures (Fig. 15-9).

Specific tissue response

Histopathology. The histopathologic response of monochromatic laser energy at 530.8 nm produced by a krypton laser has been described, and the chorioretinal tissue changes created by a frequency-doubled Nd:YAG laser beam at the closely related wavelength (532 nm) have been shown to be similar.[3] The most apparent histologic damage with the Nd:YAG laser was the coagulation and destruction of the outer nuclear area and the inner portion of the receptor layer in the impact zone. In sagittal sections of rabbit eyes, at 48 hours after irradiation with the green YAG laser emission at 532 nm, there was buckling of the inner retinal layers with some edema of the nerve fiber layer. Little histopathologic damage could be noted in the region of the ganglion cell to the outer plexiform layer. The locus of heat production appeared to be in the area of the outer nuclear rod/cone junction. A moderate pigment epithelial disruptive effect was observed, but there were only minimal choroidal changes. This histopathologic picture is similar to that produced by argon radiation, and both lasers have the potential to destroy the deep vascular plexus in the area of the coagulation (Fig. 15-10).

Hemoglobin absorption. The absorption potential of a 100 μ film of oxyhemoglobin has been documented spectrophotometrically, and 82% of incident monochromatic laser radiation at 532 nm is absorbed (Fig. 15-11). This figure represents an 8% increase over a comparable monochromatic argon laser beam at 488 nm. Both laser radiations are more highly absorbed by blood than the red krypton (647.1 nm) laser beam (11%) and similarly produce intense coagulation in vascular tissue by the conversion of the absorbed energy to heat.

A

B

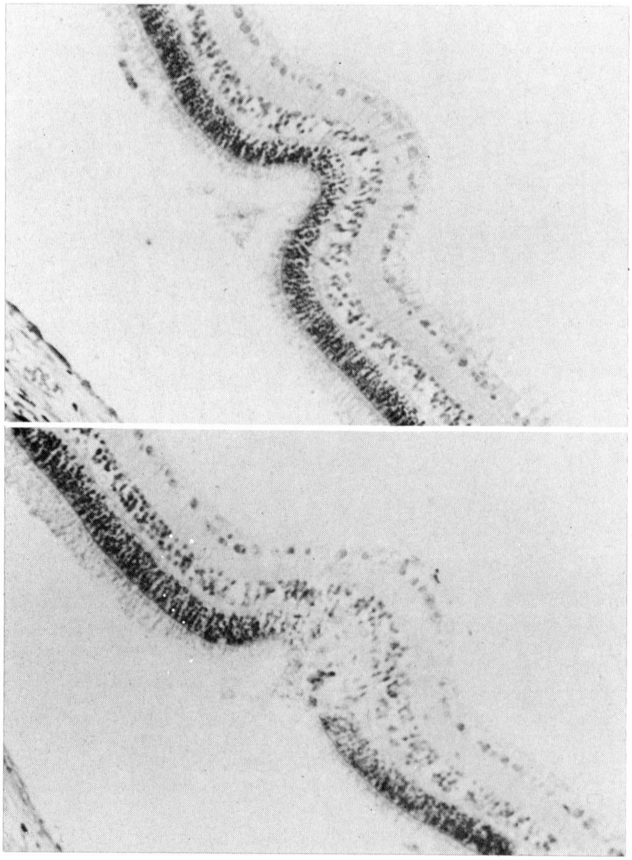

Fig. 15-10. A, Histopathologic microphotograph illustrating effect of 532 nm beam on rabbit retina 48 hours after treatment (see text). **B,** Histopathologic microphotograph showing effect of argon laser beam on rabbit retina after 48 hours. Effect is very similar to that seen with 532 nm wavelength. (Courtesy Laserscope, Inc.)

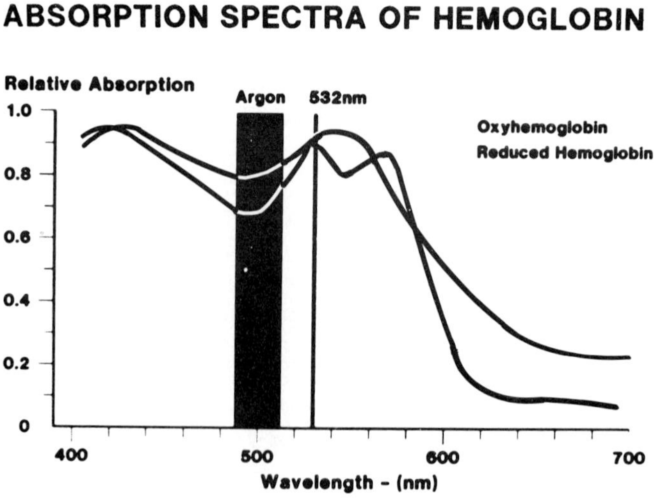

Fig. 15-11. Relative absorption for wavelengths emitted from argon laser and from frequency-doubled Nd:YAG laser at 532 nm by oxyhemoglobin and reduced hemoglobin. Note that a large differential exists between absorption potential of 532 nm and the basic wavelengths of argon laser system.

Melanin absorption. The peak of the absorption curve for melanin has been determined to exist at 550 nm,[6] whereas the pigment epithelium absorption peak has been plotted at 530 nm.[1] This would indicate that the frequency-doubled Nd:YAG output would be highly absorbed by pigmented particles in the retina and the pigment epithelium. Therefore, an exudative choroiditis could be produced with less transmitted Nd:YAG energy than with any existing laser source. The beam energy would be slightly dissipated at the nuclear retinal layers, where partial absorption takes place, but the existing transmitted energy would be sufficient to create a firm chorioretinal adhesion.

Xanthophyll absorption. The absorption peak for xanthophyll has been determined to exist at approximately 460 nm, with a rapid decrease in absorption with the longer wavelengths. The more powerful argon laser wavelengths at 488 and 514.5 nm absorb approximately 70% and 11%, respectively, of the energy that would be absorbed by a tissue pigment with maximal absorption at 460 nm (Fig. 15-12). Therefore, the argon blue and the argon green laser wavelengths can be sufficiently absorbed with high input powers to cause sufficient conversion of the light energy to heat energy at the inner and outer plexiform layers of the macula, where the xanthophyll pigment is found. It has been advised by numerous authorities that the argon blue not be used in the macular region because of the high possibility of coagulation of the nerve fiber, outer plexiform, and inner plexiform layers containing the xanthophyll pigment.[9] The argon green (514.5 nm) has been considered to be sufficiently safe—with minimal energy absorption by this pigment—in cauterization of subretinal neovascularization defects of the macular zone.

The frequency-doubled Nd:YAG laser at 532 nm produces a pea-green laser beam that is only absorbed 3% to 4% by the xanthophyll layers in the macular region. Therefore, it is apparent that this wavelength has a considerable inherent safety margin when used in the macular region with the minimal absorption by xanthophyll, while retaining the highest absorption of the commonly used laser emissions with oxyhemoglobin or

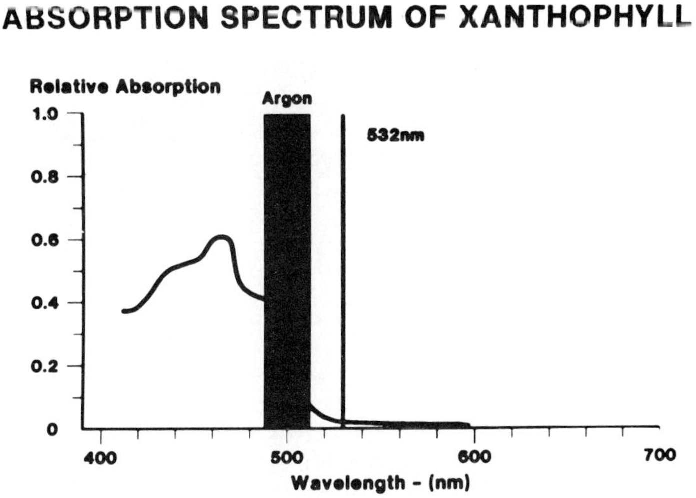

Fig. 15-12. Relative absorption of argon laser and frequency-doubled Nd:YAG laser (532 nm) beams by macular xanthophyll pigment. The 532 nm wavelength is highly transmitted by xanthophyll pigment, whereas argon green is slightly absorbed and argon blue beam highly absorbed.

reduced hemoglobin and other hemoglobin-filled vascular abnormalities. The 532 nm wavelength should be considered as the ideal wavelength for the treatment of subretinal neovascularization, macular macroaneurysms, microaneurysms, macular telangiectatic defects, and other pigment-related or structural defects in the macular region.

Discussion

The technologic advances in physics have allowed ophthalmologists to approach the ideal condition in which various portions of the eye can be selectively photocoagulated by the use of specific monochromatic laser beams. As lasers emitting different colored beams are developed, the production of a predictable specific target response in an ocular tissue becomes possible. This would mean that a certain chorioretinal layer could be coagulated without disruption of other zones by carefully matching the absorption potential of that layer to the proper laser emission.

The frequency-doubled Nd:YAG laser produces one of the most ideal wavelengths for vascular photocoagulation or production of an adhesive chorioretinitis. The Nd:YAG emission occurs at 1064 nm in the infrared spectral region and after passage through a nonlinear (KTP) crystal is converted to a green wavelength at 532 nm. The

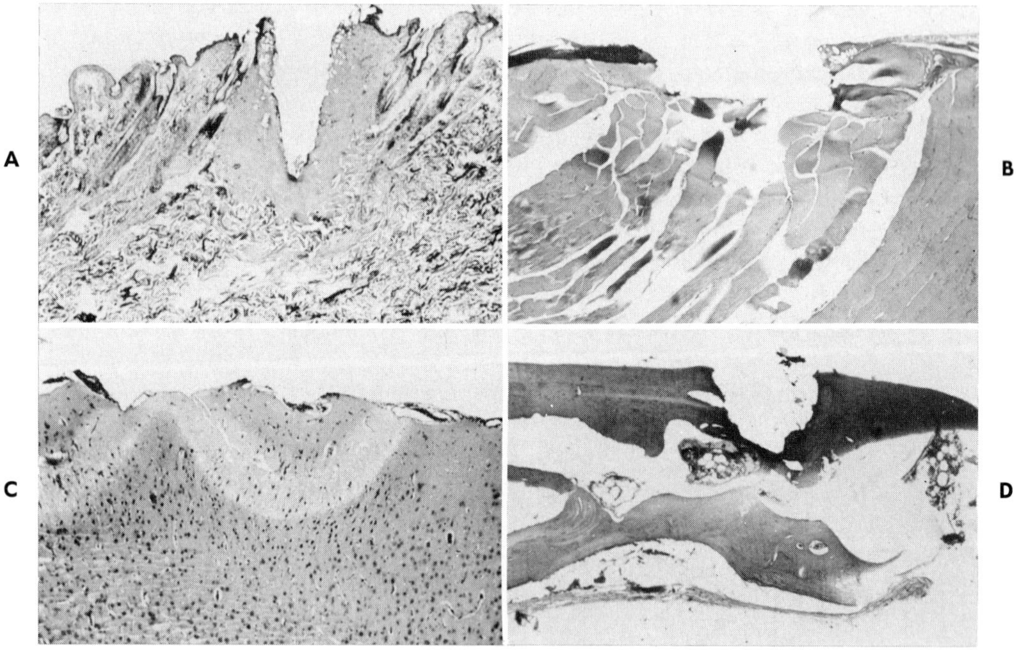

Fig. 15-13. A, Histopathologic appearance of skin impacted with sufficient power density to create incision. Note thermal destruction of sides of incision as well as cauterization of nearby vessels. **B,** Histopathologic appearance of section of muscle tissue incised with 532 nm—focused beam showing slight charring and slight thermal damage to sides of incision. **C,** Histopathologic appearance of brain tissue after minimal incision by 532 nm–focused beam. Note slight charring at incisional site, with area of coagulation extending deeper into brain tissue. **D,** Histopathologic appearance of bone tissue incised with higher power densities at 532 nm wavelengths. Power density of frequency-doubled Nd:YAG laser is sufficient to cut through bone, cartilage, or other biologic structures, with optimal hemostasis and minimal thermal effects to nearby tissue. (Courtesy Laserscope, Inc.)

green beam exists at a location in the visible spectrum very near one of the peak absorption regions of oxyhemoglobin (542 and 576 nm) and also near the maximum absorption of reduced hemoglobin (552 nm). Therefore, less energy is necessary for spasm, occlusion, and obliteration of ocular blood vessels, since the Nd:YAG photocoagulation beam is more highly absorbed, with greater conversion to heat energy. Under ideal conditions in vitro studies indicate that the frequency-doubled Nd:YAG laser emission would be 8% more highly absorbed by a 100 μ film of oxyhemoglobin than the argon laser, 71% more highly absorbed than the red krypton (647.1 nm), and similarly absorbed as the green krypton laser emission (530.8 nm), although 2% less well absorbed than the yellow krypton laser beam (568.2 nm).

The frequency-doubled Nd:YAG laser should thus offer distinct advantages in photocoagulation therapy of vascular disease over other lasers, such as the ruby (694.3 nm) or longer wavelengths of the krypton (647.1 nm). The Nd:YAG laser should be comparable to certain krypton (568.2 and 530.8 nm) laser emissions and slightly advantageous when compared to the argon (488 and 514.5 nm) laser emissions in efficiency and effectiveness for therapy of vascular diseases such as diabetic retinopathy, angiomas, Coats' disease, sickle cell retinopathy, Eales' disease, and retrolental fibroplasia.

The Nd:YAG green laser may also prove more effective than any laser for the creation of a chorioretinal adhesion or for the therapy of diseases related to the pigment epithelium. Minton[6] showed that the peak absorption of melanin from a choroidal melanoma occurred at 550 nm, with decreased absorption at shorter and longer wavelengths. This would indicate that less energy would be required for the coagulation or thermal irritation of the pigment epithelium because of the close approximation of the green Nd:YAG emission wavelength and the melanin absorption maximum.

Less photocoagulation energy passing through the ocular media or retina is always an advantage, especially when corneal, lenticular, or vitreal haze or opacities are present. The use of the green Nd:YAG laser in the treatment of retinal tears, peripheral retinal degeneration, retinoschisis, and postretinal detachment surgery can be anticipated to be highly effective because of the superior absorption characteristics.

Undoubtedly the potential uses of the frequency-doubled Nd:YAG laser operated at 25 kHz pulsing frequency at powers in excess of 20 W will provide a role for this particular laser emission beyond retinal or ocular photocoagulation. A laser source capable of producing powers of this magnitude and at this frequency (532 nm) can be used via fiberoptic transmission to multiple other peripheral devices. This particular laser beam should prove extremely valuable in the destruction of tumors of the bronchi and gastrointestinal tract; miniscusectomies; dermatologic procedures, including the eradication of port-wine stains and other skin defects; endoscopy; and bronchoscopy (Fig. 15-13). The use of this laser should have enormous potential in all areas of medicine and surgery, as well as in photocoagulation, photodynamic, and photovaporization therapy in ophthalmology.

EXCIMER LASERS

Excimer lasers are pulsed gas lasers that use a mixture of a rare gas and a halogen as the active medium (Fig. 15-14, *A*). Excimers are molecules that exist only in the electronically excited state. As these molecules return to the ground state, they emit short wavelength radiation and dissociate into single atoms because the ground state is nonbonding (Fig. 15-14, *B*). Thus excimers are an ideal laser medium, since the lower laser level is automatically depleted as a result of dissociation.

A

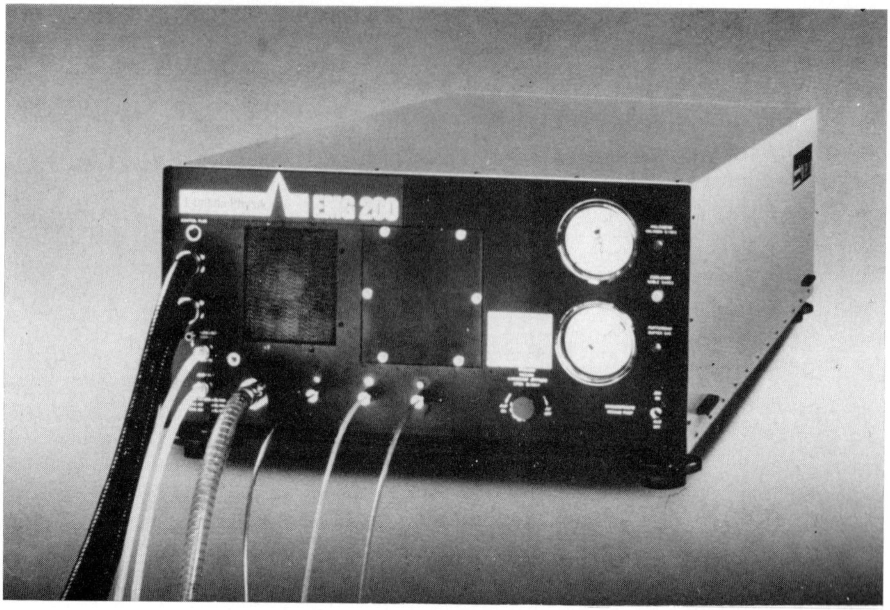

B

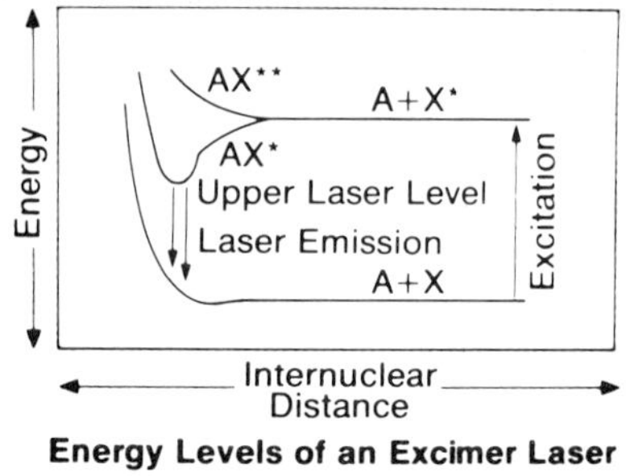

Fig. 15-14. A, Typical appearance of excimer ultraviolet laser showing various input tubes and laser exit port. (Courtesy Lambda Physik.) **B,** Schematic interpretation of method of population inversion present with excimer laser. Because of unstable ground state, most molecules are in excited or upper laser level and are subject to stimulated emission and laser action.

Table 15-1. Ultraviolet laser wavelengths (including excimer lasers*)

Laser media	*Principal wavelength (nm)*
Fluorine (F_2)	157
Argon fluoride (ArF)*	193
Krypton chloride (KrCl)*	222
Krypton fluoride (KrF)*	248
Xenon chloride (XeCl)*	308
Nitrogen (N_2)	337
Xenon fluoride (XeF)*	351

The high output power and good efficiency agree with theoretic calculations when losses caused by fluorescence or quenching processes are minimized by using a fast excitation. In some excimer lasers a fast electric discharge is used, with its energy first transmitted into a buffer gas such as helium or argon. The output from the excimer molecules can have an efficiency as high as 2%.

The fast discharge circuit allows the laser to be operated with other gases as well, such as fluorine (F_2), operating at 157 nm; or even carbon dioxide (CO_2), operating at 10.6 μ.

The choice of gas mixture determines the output wavelength. Typical line width of an excimer emission is about 0.3 nm but tuning the output over a region of about 3.0 nm is possible at lower output energy.

Certain excimer lasers (Lambda Physik) incorporate a gas processor into the laser to increase the gas-fill lifetime, in some cases approaching as many as 20 million electric discharges. Because the gas processor removes impurities from the gas as the laser operates, power output from the laser deteriorates much more slowly than in conventional excimer lasers. The Lambda Physik technique of cleaning the laser gases is more efficient and reliable than the brute-force technique used in some excimer lasers of automatically increasing discharge power as the laser gas becomes contaminated. Most excimer lasers are multigas lasers in that operation is permitted at a number of wavelengths simply by selecting the appropriate gas mixture. All the common ultraviolet excimer wavelengths shown in Table 15-1 are available. No modification of the laser hardware is required when changing excimer gases, and only the mirrors need be replaced when changing from the ultraviolet to infrared output emissions.

A typical example of an excimer laser (Lambda Physik EMG 103 E) produces 40 W at 249 nm (KrF), 20 W at 193 nm (ArF), or 20 W at 308 nm (XeCl). The standard repetition frequency of the EMG 103 E is 200 Hz, but a slight factory modification allows higher repetition frequencies. Another special configuration, the S-version of the EMG 103 E, allows pulse energy up to 500 mJ at either 249 or 308 nm at a reduced repetition frequency. For the maximum output in the vacuum-ultraviolet mode, an optimized F_2 version of the EMG 103 E produces 1.5 W average power at 157 nm. These reliable, economically priced lasers can be an attractive alternative to the Nd:YAG lasers in such applications as optical pumping of dye lasers.

The heart of an excimer laser is the gas reservoir, with its integrated laser channel and low-inductance discharge circuit. The gas reservoir is fabricated from a single piece of thick-walled aluminum extrusion in some excimer lasers. It serves not only as a 30/L gas reservoir, complete with gas circulation and cooling mechanisms, but also as a stable optical bench to which the resonator mirrors are attached. A fast transverse flow of laser gas through the electrodes ensures high pulse energy independent of repetition frequency. As noted, with the EMG 103 E frequencies up to 500 Hz are possible.

There are three factors that contribute to the high efficiency of an excimer laser: (1) properly designed electrode shape, (2) efficient preionization of the laser gas and an ultrafast mode, and (3) a low-inductance electric discharge circuit. In effect these factors are combined into a single, unique design for the new preionization scheme of the EMG-series lasers as an integral part of the discharge circuit. It is a simple and reliable design that produces a uniform field of ions, and the discharge is completely free of arcs. In some other excimer lasers the peaking capacitors have to be placed very close to the electrodes inside the gas chamber to avoid arcing. The Lambda Physik approach of optimizing the energy transfer from one capacitor to another before the onset of the laser discharge results in a much higher efficiency.

It is extremely important for excimer lasers to be engineered to allow a maximum life of the laser gases. For the user this means reduced operating cost as well as more reliable laser operation at steady power levels.

Only fluorocarbon insulators and metals such as aluminum and nickel, which passivate quickly in a fluorine or hydrogen-chloride environment, are used in Lambda Physik lasers. All electric circuit components, except the electrodes themselves, are outside the gas system, where they do not need to be passivated.

Significant improvements, both in reduced power deterioration and in-fill lifetime, have been observed when a gas processor is added to a laser. For example, 20 million shots can usually be obtained from a XeCl laser before the power decreases to 50% of its original value. Without the processor, the same laser might only produce 4 million pulses before requiring a gas change. Similar improvements in gas-fill lifetime have been observed for other standard gases, including KrF, XeF, and ArF.

Extended lifetime means reduced operating costs for the excimer lasers, particularly in comparison to Nd:YAG lasers, which might alternatively be used as dye laser pumps. The flashlamps of Nd:YAG lasers must be replaced about as frequently as the gas of a XeCl laser must be changed, or about every 20 million shots, but a gas change is much less expensive. Based on current prices for research-grade xenon, the gas costs of a XeCl laser are 40 cents per hour less if the laser is operated at a 100 Hz repetition frequency. The corresponding operating costs for a Nd:YAG laser are significantly greater.

Excimer laser surgery

Laser applications in ophthalmology include the processes of photocoagulation, photovaporization, photoradiation, photodisruption,[5] and more recently photodecomposition. Photocoagulation and photovaporization are tissue interactions that involve the thermal effects of laser radiation; photoradiation occurs through a photon interacting with a sensitized chemical bonded to malignant tissue. Photodisruption uses laser-induced optical breakdown to section tissues by forming a plasma and associated shock waves. The excimer laser has provided a fifth form of laser interaction with tissues called *photodecomposition*. The use of this far-ultraviolet laser radiation (150 to 200 nm) creates a specific photochemical reaction and results in the ablation of corneal or other ocular tissues without thermal damage to the remaining adjacent structures (Fig. 15-15). Therefore, incisions of controlled depth and shape can be made in defined areas of the cornea or other ocular tissue, and any amount of tissue can be removed by ablating that tissue to a predetermined depth.

Srinivasan[7,8] reported that the far-ultraviolet radiation acts on organic polymers by a process described as ''ablative photodecomposition.'' The irradiated molecules are broken into smaller volatile fragments by direct photochemical interaction without heating the remaining adjacent tissues (Fig. 15-16). Ultraviolet light at this frequency is highly energetic, with each photon having 6.4 electron volts. This provides the photochemical energy that directly breaks intramolecular bonds.

It is known that the longer-wavelength lasers vaporize tissues but also produce changes in remaining adjacent structures. Histologic studies have demonstrated irregular edges in various tissues such as bone and muscle are caused by the heat of the cutting

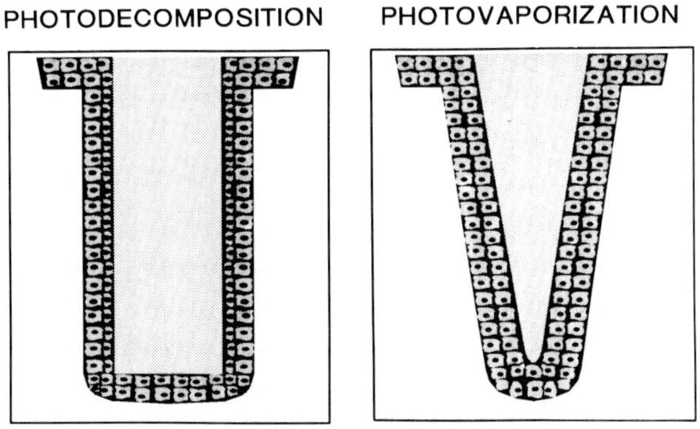

Fig. 15-15. Comparison of photodecomposition and photovaporization illustrating precise cleavage of cells in rectangular fashion without charring with photodecomposition, and minimal charring along the incision site with photovaporization. Photodecomposition is accomplished with far-ultraviolet lasers, and photovaporization can be created with high photon flux from any visible laser, most commonly with far-infrared CO_2 laser.

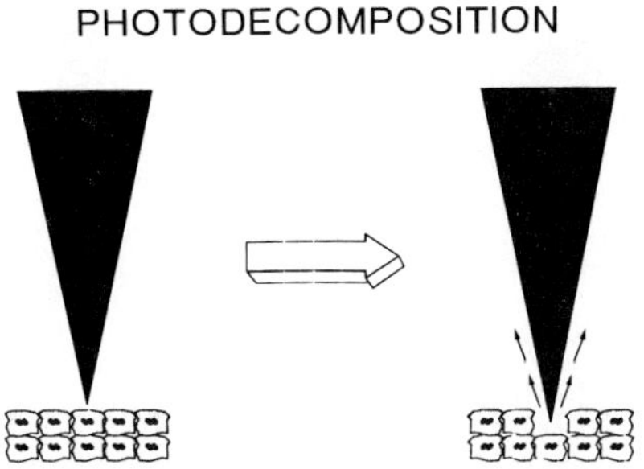

Fig. 15-16. Photodecomposition process showing impact of far-ultraviolet laser beam on individual cell or small area of cells, causing breakage of intramolecular bonds and disruption and disappearance of cellular matter from impact site.

thermal laser (Fig. 15-17). Far-ultraviolet laser irradiation, however, produces a trench with sharp and cleanly defined boundaries, as seen with light microscopy. There are no changes in adjacent tissues, nor are there observable thermal effects (Fig. 15-18).

Trokel, Srinivasan, and Branen[10] have found that the excimer laser produces an optimal biologic effect in the far-ultraviolet wavelength at 193 nm. At shorter wavelengths optical delivery systems are difficult to construct because of the limited availability of refracting materials. At available wavelengths longer than 200 nm thermal effects become more dominant, and the percentage of true ablative photodecomposition lessens. By using various types of masks over the corneas of cows' eyes, Trokel and co-workers were able to restrict the laser energy to narrowly defined areas (Fig. 15-19). Among those masks tested were configurations with a row of four slits measuring 150 to 800 μ in width and one drilled with a series of seven holes measuring 100 to 750 μ in diameter (Fig. 15-20). The laser output was delivered in a series of pulses, and it was found that 1 joule per square centimeter (1 J/cm^2) ablates corneal tissue to a depth of 1 μ. Thus a groove 200 μ deep requires the application of 200 J/cm^2 (Fig. 15-21).

Energy such as this was delivered in a series of pulses, ranging in intensity from 100 to 200 mJ/cm^2, depending on the area of the final laser focus (Figs. 15-22 and 15-23). The pulse rate used during these experiments ranged between 1 and 20 Hz. Similar mechanisms have allowed large areas of corneal tissue to be removed in a precise manner to form an effective laser lamellar keratectomy. Because of the high tissue absorption of ultraviolet light, defects of the laser appear to be localized to the site of the ablation.

The implications for the use of the excimer laser with operations such as keratomileusis or corneal transplantation appear to be a logical additional experimental avenue. The applications for refractive keratoplasty would seem to be of great interest, since the cornea can be reshaped in such a manner as to correct most moderate degrees of hyperopia, myopia, and astigmatic defects. This type of laser surgery is highly experimental at this time, but considerable research will be forthcoming.

Text continued on p. 203.

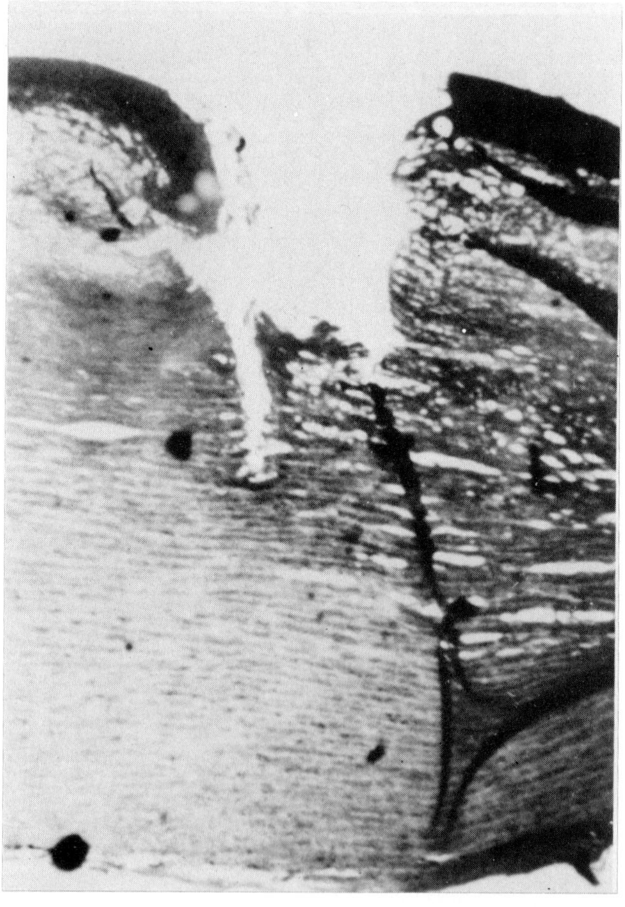

Fig. 15-17. A, 0.4 mm crater produced with 532 nm laser beam showing charring and irregular cauterization of edges of incision; original magnification ×40. (Courtesy Ralph Linsker, M.D., Ph.D.; R. Srinivasan, Ph.D.; James J. Wynne, Ph.D.; Daniel R. Alonso, M.D.; IBM T.J. Watson Research Center; and Cornell University Medical College.)

A 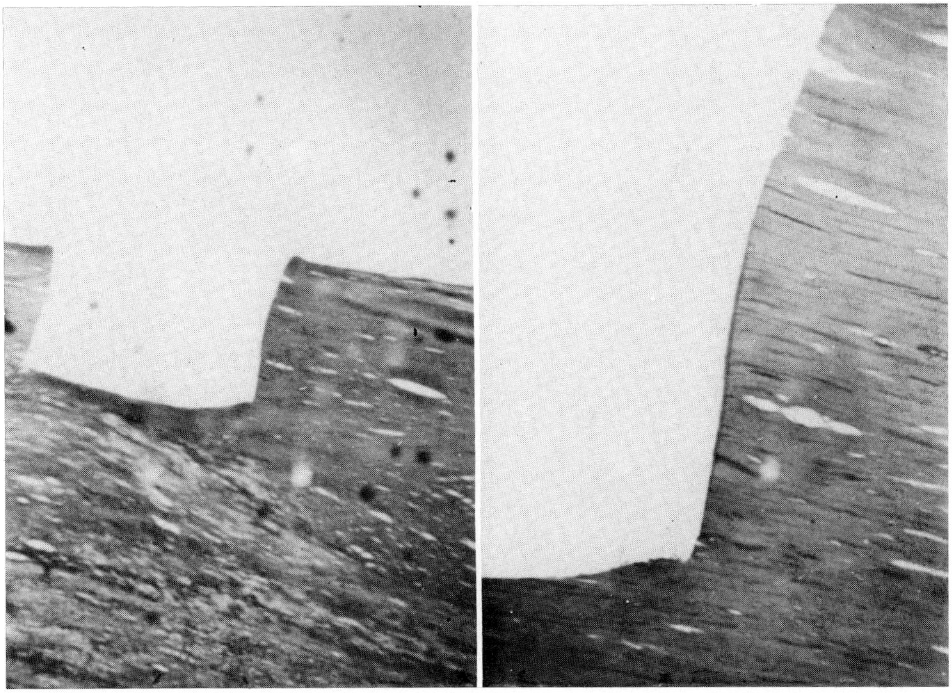 B

Fig. 15-18. A, Trench measuring 0.35 mm produced by excimer laser (193 nm) irradiation of luminal side of aortic wall showing exquisite precision and absence of damage to nearby cellular material; original magnification ×40. **B,** An enlarged view (×160) of same incision emphasizing lack of thermal or other damage and precise sculpting of aortic incision. (Courtesy Ralph Linsker, M.D., Ph.D.; R. Srinivasan, Ph.D.; James J. Wynne, Ph.D.; Daniel R. Alonso, M.D.; IBM T.J. Watson Research Center; and Cornell University Medical College.)

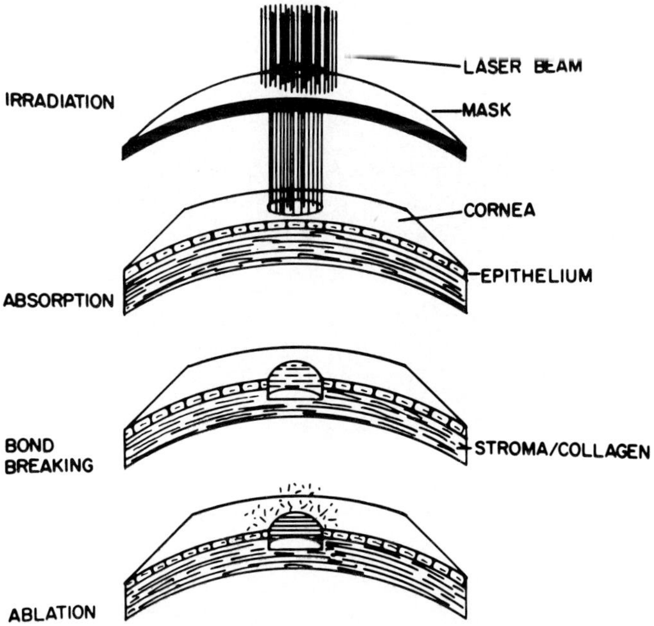

Fig. 15-19. Scheme of delivery of excimer laser to cornea. Series of masks are used to deliver various amounts of energy to preselected corneal areas. (Courtesy Stephen L. Trokel, M.D.)

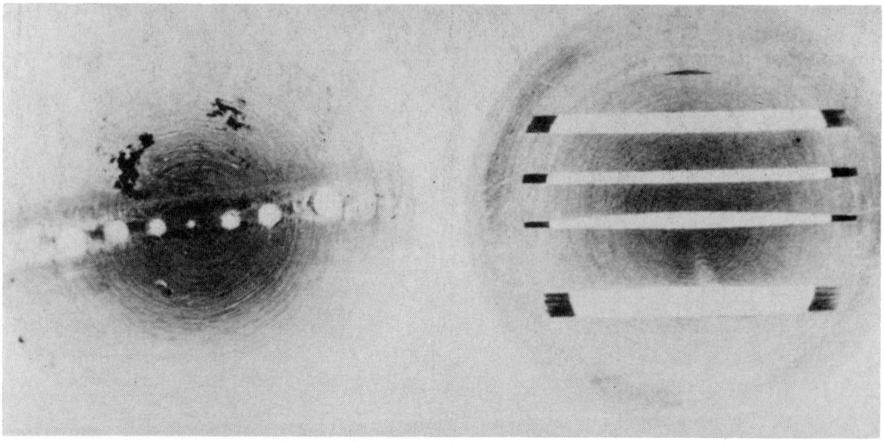

Fig. 15-20. Metal masks used to allow only small portions of excimer laser energy to impact on corneal epithelium and stroma to create incisions into those tissues. (Courtesy Stephen L. Trokel, M.D.)

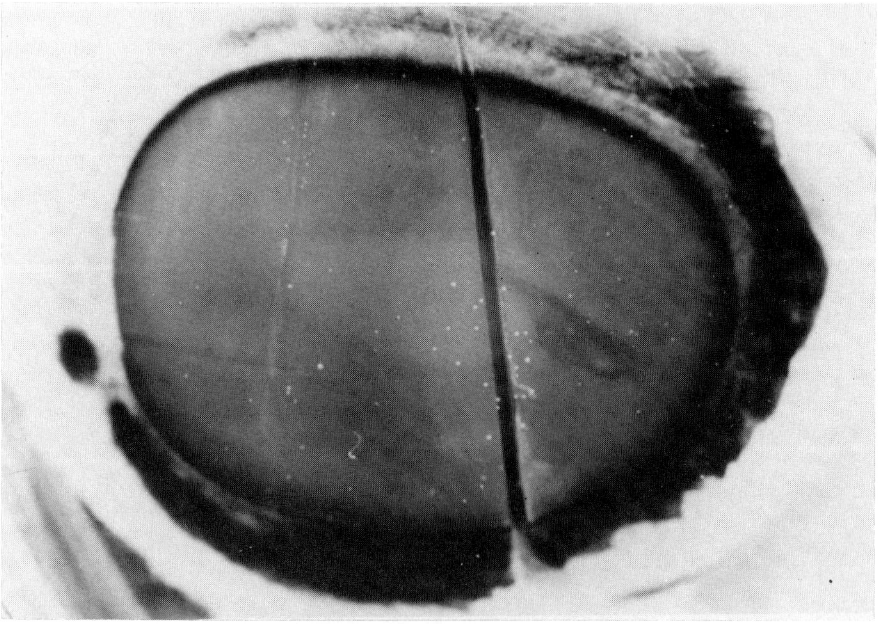

Fig. 15-21. First rabbit incised by excimer laser action, showing precise incision through outer layers of cornea without penetration into anterior chamber. (Courtesy Stephen L. Trokel, M.D.)

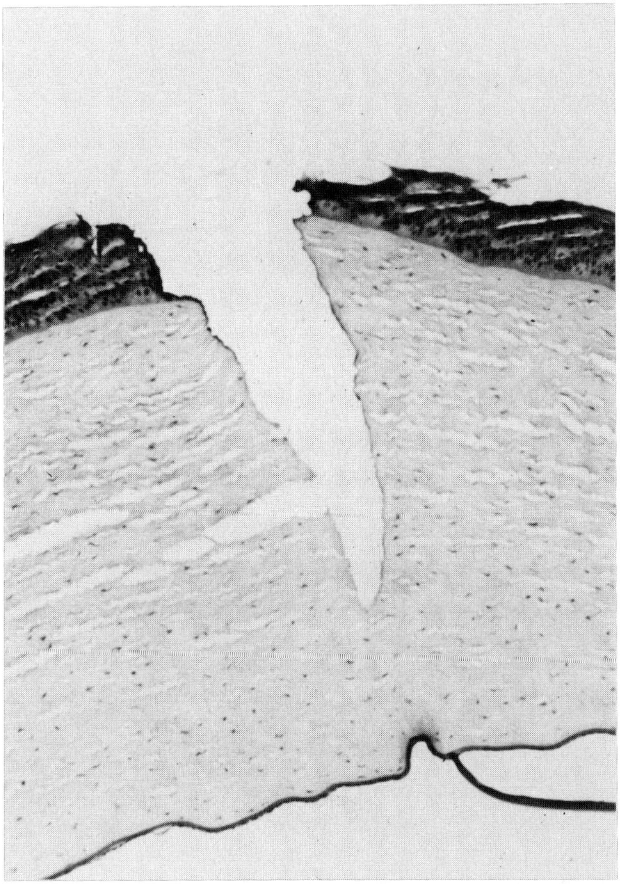

Fig. 15-22. V-shaped incision of cornea showing minimal damage to sides of incision with complete removal of impacted corneal tissue. (Courtesy Stephen L. Trokel, M.D.)

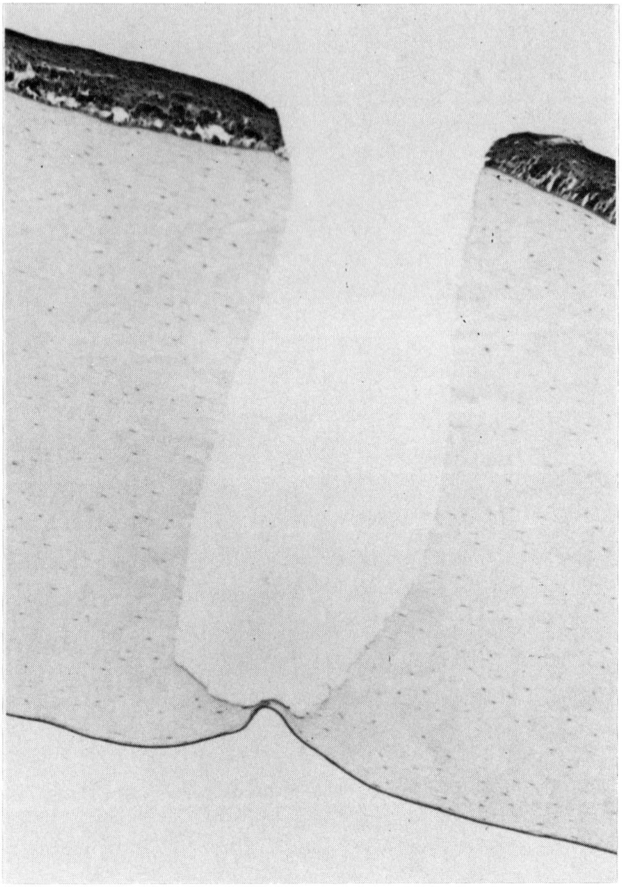

Fig. 15-23. Square-shaped corneal incision using 193 nm excimer laser beam. Note absence of tissue reaction on sides of incision and precision with which depth of incision and precision with which depth of incision can be determined. (Courtesy Stephen L. Trokel, M.D.)

Table 15-2. CW neutral atom gas laser wavelengths

Laser media	*Principal wavelength (nm)*
Helium neon	593.9
	632.8
	1152.3
	3391.3
Oxygen	844.6
Xenon	2026.2
	2651.1

CONTINUOUS AND QUASICONTINUOUS WAVE LASERS

Continuous-wave (CW) laser action will be achieved in almost all laser medias if the material will permit a permanent population inversion to be sustained. Although there are, in general, many competitive processes that may limit CW laser operation, such as heating of the media and "self-quenching" effects, it is often possible to achieve continuous or high-repetition-rate operation even with many materials previously considered as only "pulsed" laser media. The limiting factors are (1) the low efficiency of converting pump energy into laser emission, (2) retention of heat by the laser media, and (3) degradation of the components used for continuous pumping. This does not mean, however, that the same levels of instantaneous power, as achieved in the pulsed operation, will be achieved in CW operation. The rapid emission and subsequent high power levels achieved with a small ruby laser will be in the multikilowatt range, whereas the quasi-CW (60 Hz) operation of a ruby crystal will only reach a few watts, even in the most ideal system.

The most successful medias for pure CW operation have been gases (or gaseous mixtures) and the many diode lasers. Quasi-CW operation is possible in most of the solid medias common in pulsed operation, in addition to many gases.

CW neutral atom gas lasers

CW neutral atom gas lasers operate namely in the near-infrared range, from about 600 to 3400 nm. Representative lines of such gas media are shown in Table 15-2.

The first CW system was the helium-neon (HeNe) gas mixture. Although the first successful operation was at an infrared wavelength of 1152 nm, an HeNe laser is most well known operating at the red 632.8 nm transition. The more recent HeNe gas laser designs use direct current excitation, and the power output available from the low-efficiency HeNe laser ranges from a fraction of a milliwatt to about 100 mWs in the largest available systems. Because the HeNe laser may be easily operated with high-frequency stability and a single-mode operation, many applications have been found in precision measurement holography, but it has not been used in ophthalmology because of the low power output. The HeNe laser has found indirect use as a target beam for the pulsed Nd:YAG systems, as well as for invisible lasers such as the CO_2 photovaporization instruments.

CW ion gas lasers

CW ion gas lasers operate principally in the ultraviolet and visible range, from 235 to 800 nm. Representative lines of such gas media are shown in Table 15-3.

The gases mercury, argon, krypton, xenon, chlorine, iodine, oxygen, nitrogen, and neon have been successfully operated on the ion laser principle. The combination of gases has generated more than 50 spectral lines in the ultraviolet invisible spectral range. In general the mechanism of CW ion lasers is one in which an electronic collision—in either single or multiple successive steps—takes place for a double-ionization process to occur, with the power output proportional to the fourth power of the current through the laser tube. This successful series of lasers have made an enormous impact on the field of ophthalmology, particularly using the beneficial wavelengths of the argon and krypton lasers. Because of the precision, monochromaticity, and selective absorption by the ocular pigments, the argon laser is still used as the workhorse in ocular photocoagulation. Recently the krypton red laser (647.1 nm) has added immensely to our under-

Table 15-3. CW ion gas laser wavelengths

Laser media	*Principal wavelengths (nm)*
Neon (IV)	235.8
Argon (IV)	262.5
Helium-cadmium	325.0
	441.6
Helium-selenium	460.0
	480.0
	520.0
Neon (II)	332.4
Krypton (II)	467.2
	530.8
	568.2
	647.1
Argon (II)	476.5
	488.0
	514.5
Xenon (II)	526.2
	597.1

Table 15-4. CW molecular gas laser wavelengths

Laser media	*Principal wavelengths (cm)*
CO	5,600
CO_2	10,600
H_2O	27,974
	47,693
	118,650
	220,340
HCN	310,887
	336,558
ICN	773,500

Table 15-5. Quasi-CW gas and solid-state laser wavelengths

Laser media	*Principal wavelengths (nm)*
Nitrogen (molecular)	337.1
	540.1
Copper vapor	510.0
	578.0
Frequency-doubled Nd:YAG	532.0
Mercury (ion)	614.9
Gold vapor	628.0
Chromium (ruby)	694.3
Chromium (alexandrite)	701.0-818.0
Chromium (emerald)	750.0-759.0
Neodymium (YAG)	1064.0
(glass)	1060.0

standing and therapy of macular diseases and other conditions complicated by retinal or vitreal hemorrhagic problems.

CW molecular gas lasers

CW molecular gas lasers operate in the infrared region in a range extending from 5500 to more than 750,000 nm. Representative lines of such gas media are shown in Table 15-4.

There are several molecular gas mixtures that can generate laser emissions. Of these, the CO_2 laser has been found to be the most efficient and consequently the most powerful of all CW laser devices. Continuous powers have been reported above 5000 W in the infrared spectral region at the 10,600 nm wavelength. Unlike the other molecular lasers, the CO_2 laser is chemically stable enough to function with an electric discharge occurring within the gas itself. This function contributes to its high efficiency and its usefulness in many areas other than medicine. This laser has proved to be one of the most useful lasers in all fields of medicine for photovaporization of tumors, as well as an incisional device in areas of potential hemorrhage or with patients with various bleeding disorders. The water vapor laser and the hydrogen cyanide laser have had little practical application in any branch of medicine.

Quasi-CW gas and solid-state laser

The quasi-CW gas and solid-state laser classification includes both molecular and ion gas lasers and solid-state systems that cannot be operated except in rapid pulse (quasi-CW) mode (Fig. 15-24). Representative lines are shown in Table 15-5.

One of the most promising sources at present uses the nd-doped crystal made of YAG. This sytem is pumped by special tungsten lamps and is capable of an average CW output approaching 100 W at the 1064 nm wavelength. Pulse repetition rates are normally the 60 Hz of the alternating line current. The recent emergence to popularity of the YAG laser has been stimulated by better growth techniques of longer YAG crystals. YAG systems are also ideal for high-repetition-rate, Q-switched operation. Opera-

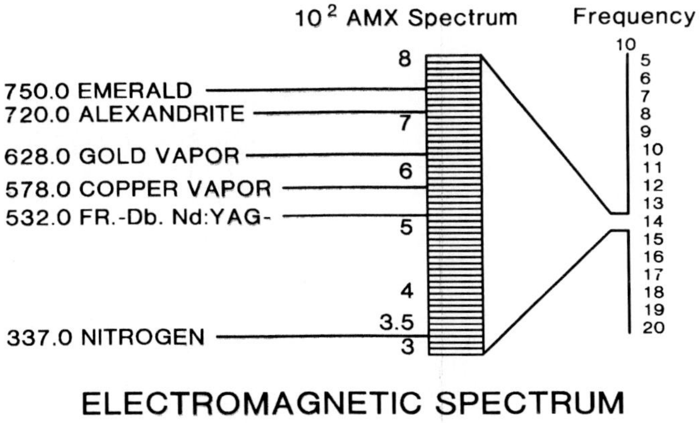

Fig. 15-24. Positions in visible portion of the electromagnetic spectrum of the emerald (750.0 to 759.0 nm), alexandrite (701.0 to 818.0 nm), gold vapor (628.0 nm), copper vapor (578.0 nm), frequency-doubled Nd:YAG (532.0 nm), and nitrogen (337.0 nm) lasers. These new lasers should have significant impact on the therapy of various diseases in medicine, especially in the field of ophthalmology.

tion at repetition rates of over 20,000 Hz are now commonly reported with and without frequency-doubling of the basic laser wavelength.

The increasingly common use of the pulsed Nd:YAG laser at its fundamental frequency (1064 nm) in the Q-switched or the mode-locked type of operation produces extremely short pulses of energy at either 10 to 12 nanoseconds (ns) or 20 to 30 picoseconds (ps) duration, respectively. The formation of an optical breakdown at the focal point of the laser, as well as an acoustic and hydrodynamic shock wave, have been instrumental in lysing membranes within the eye, such as the posterior capsule, vitreous stands, and anterior synechiae, and for performing peripheral iridotomies. The expansion of the intravitreal uses of the pulsed Nd:YAG laser, as well as its application in other anterior segment conditions, will undoubtedly be occurring within the near future.

High repetition rates for ruby lasers have been created with pulse rates of up to 100 Hz. To achieve this high repetition rate, special mercury-vapor flash tubes are operated in an ellipsoidial cavity in which the flash tube and ruby rod are coaxial. Powers greater

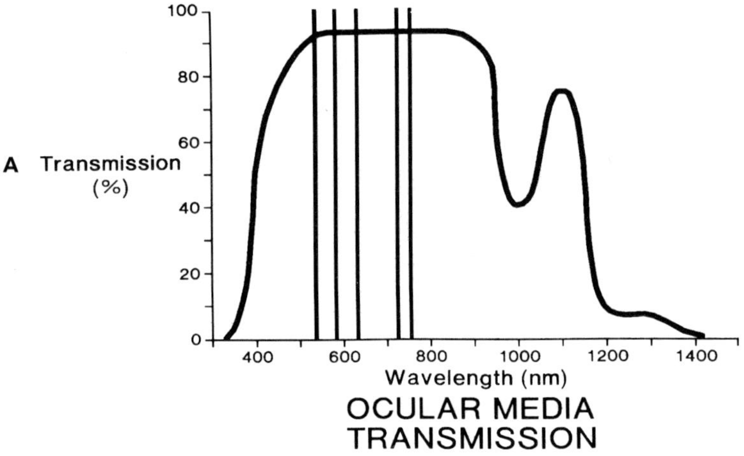

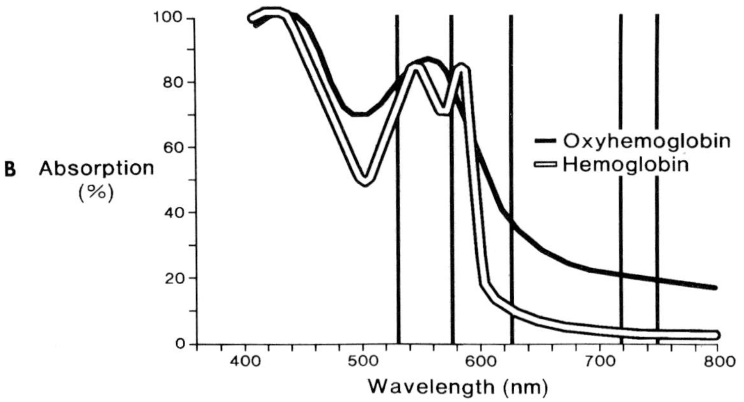

Fig. 15-25. A, Ocular media transmission *(right* to *left)* for emerald (750.0 nm), alexandrite (720.0 nm), gold vapor (628.0 nm), copper vapor (578.0 nm), and frequency-doubled Nd:YAG (532.0 nm) laser emissions. **B,** Percent absorption of oxyhemoglobin and reduced hemoglobin for wavelengths *(right* to *left)* represented by emerald, alexandrite, gold vapor, copper vapor, and frequency-doubled Nd:YAG laser emissions (per wavelengths in **A**).

than 2 to 3 Watts in the quasi-CW configuration can be produced at the 694.3 nm wavelength. The red beam from this particular solid-state laser may have significant application in the future, when moderate amounts of blood in the vitreous or inner retina has prevented effective photocoagulation of the pigment epithelium or external chorioretinal structures.

A rapidly pulsed molecular nitrogen laser emits energy in a quasi-CW train of 10 ns pulses, each pulse at 100 kW peak power levels. A maximum average power of several hundred milliwatts is produced at the ultraviolet 337.1 nm wavelength, which may be advantageous for some photodecomposition applications. Other lasers may be more applicable in the field of ophthalmology because of greater stability and higher power output (Fig. 15-25).

C

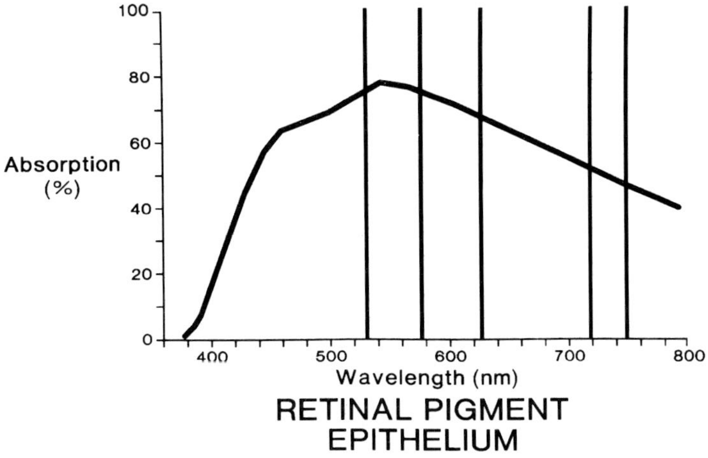

D

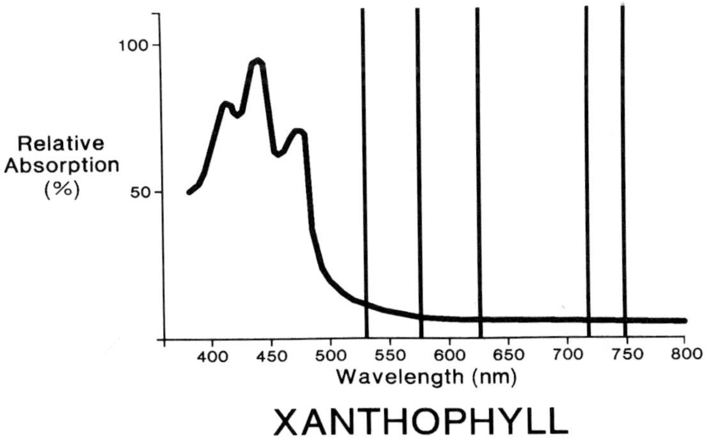

Fig. 15-25, cont'd. C, Percent absorption of retinal pigment epithelium for various wavelengths represented *(right* to *left)* by emerald, alexandrite, gold vapor, copper vapor, and frequency-doubled Nd:YAG laser emissions (per wavelengths in **A**). **D,** Relative absorption of xanthophyll macular pigment for various wavelengths *(right* to *left)* represented by emerald, alexandrite, gold vapor, copper vapor, and frequency-doubled Nd:YAG laser emissions (per wavelengths in **A**). *Continued.*

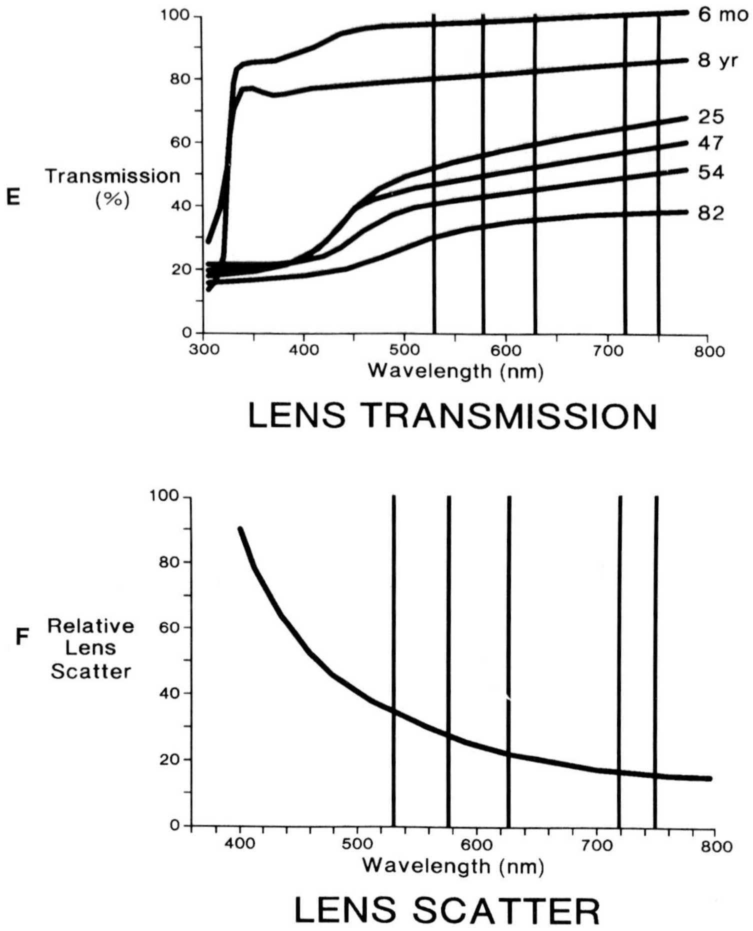

Fig. 15-25, cont'd. E, Percent transmission of lens for various wavelengths *(right* to *left)* represented by emerald, alexandrite, gold vapor, copper vapor, and frequency-doubled Nd:YAG laser emissions (per wavelengths in **A**). **F,** Relative lens scatter for various wavelengths *(right* to *left)* represented by emerald, alexandrite, gold vapor, copper vapor, and frequency-doubled Nd:YAG laser emissions (per wavelengths in **A**).

Table 15-6. CW diode laser wavelengths

Laser media	*Principal wavelengths (nm)*
Zinc sulfide	330
Cadmium sulfide	490
Zinc telluride	540
Gallium arsenide	850
Indium arsenide	3100
Indium antimonide	5400

CW diode lasers

The CW diode laser classification includes both electron-beam and *p-n* junction diode devices. Wavelengths range from the ultraviolet through the infrared spectral region. Representative wavelengths are shown in Table 15-6.

The semiconductive diode lasers have the advantages of being extremely small, being able to convert electric power directly into coherent light, and being capable of changing their output by simply modulating the diode current. However, despite these apparent advantages, semiconductive lasers have not been used in any of the fields of medicine, except in a minor diagnostic capacity.

SUMMARY

Many interesting lasers are rapidly appearing on the medical scene, such as the liquid dye lasers discussed in Chapter 5, the copper and gold metal vapor lasers, the free-electron laser, and a multitude of other configurations. The most powerful of all lasers, at present, is the free-electron laser, which is pumped by a linear accelerator or its equivalent. This laser will provide hundreds of watts of power in any portion of the electromagnetic spectrum, from the x-ray to the far infrared region. Copper and gold metal vapor lasers, as well as several of the other metal vapor lasers, provide specific wavelengths, some of which are useful in photodynamic therapy or in specific ophthalmic use. In general the adage first coined with the invention of the laser, that "the laser represented a solution looking for a problem," is especially true in the field of ophthalmology, where therapeutic solutions by laser intervention have shone brilliantly.

ACKNOWLEDGMENT

I would like to acknowledge the invaluable assistance of Beth Ann Hughes, Ruth J. Helmich, and Paul Saivetz.

REFERENCES

1. Geeraets, W.J.: The relative absorption of thermal energy in retina and choroid, Invest. Ophthalmol., **1:**340, 1962.
2. L'Esperance, F.A., Jr.: An ophthalmic argon laser photocoagulation system: design, construction, and laboratory investigations, Trans. Am. Ophthalmol. Soc. **66:**827, 1968.
3. L'Esperance, F.A., Jr.: The ocular histopathologic effect of krypton and argon laser radiation, Am. J. Ophthalmol. **68:**362,1969.
4. L'Esperance, F.A., Jr.: Clinical photocoagulation with the frequency-doubled neodymium yttrium-aluminum-garnet laser, Am. J. Ophthalmol., **71:**631, 1971.
5. L'Esperance, F.A., Jr.: Ophthalmic lasers: photocoagulation, photoradiation, and surgery, St. Louis, 1983, The C.V. Mosby Co.
6. Minton, J.P.: A method to determine laser wavelength absorption capabilities of experimental malignant tumors, Life Sci. **3:**1007, 1964.
7. Srinivasan, R.: Action of far-ultraviolet light on organic polymer films: applications to semiconductor technology, J. Radiation Curing. (In press.)
8. Srinivasan, R.: Kinetics of the ablative photodecomposition of organic polymers in the far-ultraviolet (199 nm), J. Vacuum Sci. Technol. (In Press.)
9. Trempe, C.L.: Macular photocoagulation—optimal wavelength selection, Ophthalmology, **89:**7, 1982.
10. Trokel, S.L., Srinivasan, R., and Branen, B.: Excimer laser surgery of the cornea, Am. J. Ophthalmol., **96:**710, 1983.

16

Technical considerations in laser trabeculoplasty

James B. Wise

Laser trabeculoplasty (LTP) is capable of producing marked reduction in intraocular pressure (IOP) with long-term control of open-angle glaucoma.[1,2,4,8,10,11,13] Although the procedure is simple in concept—placing approximately 100 laser burns of 50 μ each evenly spaced around the trabecular ring—several technical points can greatly influence the result of the procedure. This chapter discusses some pitfalls that can alter the results of LTP.

Before performing LTP, the ophthalmologist must focus and test the laser to ensure that it is producing a precise 50 μ spot with adequate power. An external power meter should be used to check the accuracy of the built-in meter of the laser, since losses in the optical system can cause a marked disparity between indicated and delivered power. At least 1500 mW should be available at the cornea. The slitlamp biomicroscope must then be focused at the same aerial focal point as the laser beam. The laser should be set on 50 μ spot size and 0.02 second exposure. A piece of orange paper should be taped in position to represent the patient's eye. The eyepieces should be set at every diopter setting from +8 to −8; at each setting a burn should be made by focusing on the paper fibers and using enough power to burn halfway through the paper. The burn should appear the same size as the aiming spot. The eyepiece setting giving the smallest burns and the smallest aiming spot should be used for treatment, regardless of its numeric value. The smallest burns should be measured with a microscope to determine precise spot size. In a study of 27 lasers by this method,[12] 44% would not burn a spot size smaller than 70 μ which is double the area of a 50 μ spot.

The Ritch trabeculoplasty lens (Ocular Instruments, Inc., Bellevue, Wash.) is the trabecular analog of the Abraham iridectomy lens. The magnifying buttons over the mirrors reduce the spot diameter by 30%, doubling the power density and halving the spot area. This lens should be used for pale trabecular meshworks and should always be used if the laser gives oversized spots.

Topical anesthesia is usually adequate for LTP. In sensitive patients it can be supplemented with subconjunctival lidocaine, without epinephrine. For severe blepharospasm a facial nerve block injected in front of the ear can be used. Retrobulbar anesthesia is never necessary for LTP.

The patient's head should be stabilized by an assistant standing behind him; straps and bands do not work as well. A three-mirror-type lens is preferred because of easier gripping and greater range of tilting. Leftover sodium hyaluronate (Healon) makes an excellent gonioscopy medium for filling the lens. A large sponge block extending beneath the full length of the surgeon's arm gives a much steadier and more comfortable support than a box or block.

The original description of LTP[11,13] recommended a spot size of 50 microns, exposure time of 0.1 second, power level to give a small bubble or depigmented spot, and 100 burns spaced 360 degrees. Subsequent clinical experience has supported the validity of these parameters. The 0.1 second exposure is the longest time available before eye movement can occur. With longer exposure times the burns can be linear or smeared and are not reproducible. Shorter burns of 0.05 second or less do not adequately shrink the meshwork. This is best visualized on the iris, where the shorter burns are useful for excavating iridectomies without pupil distortion. The shorter burns also give less burn depth and may not shrink the deep trabecular layers, which are the site of most of the

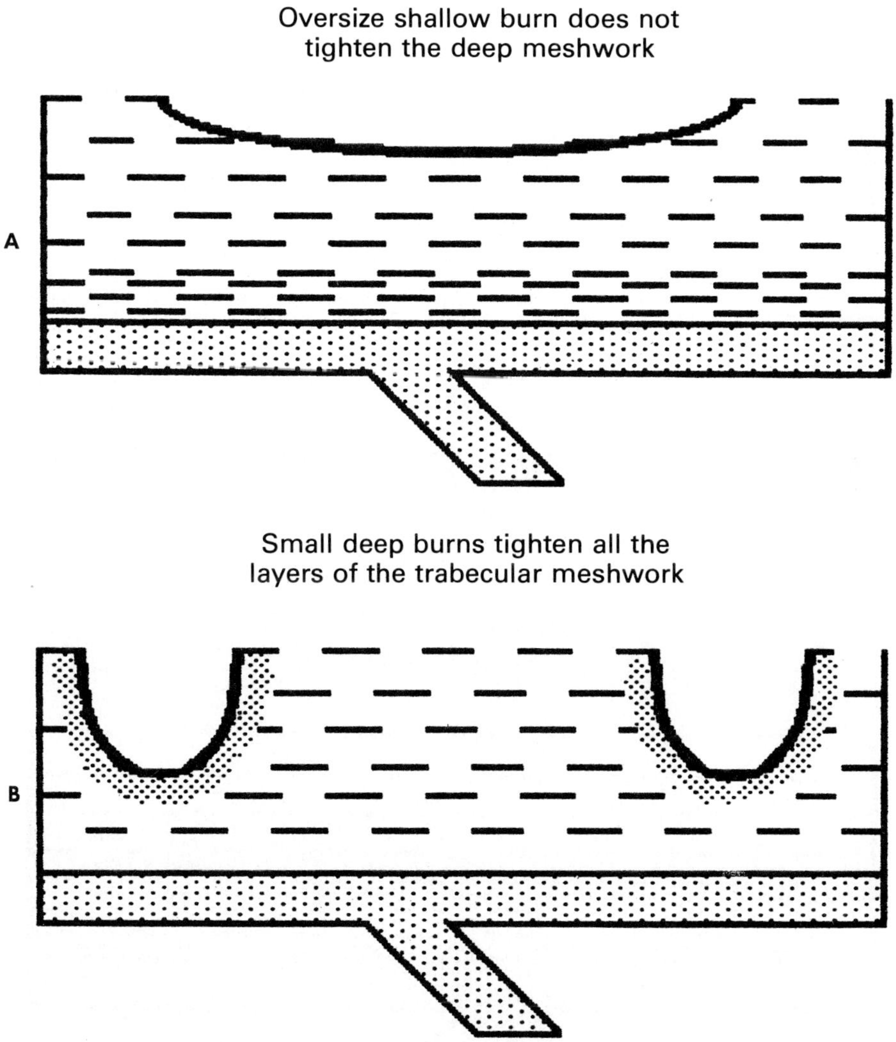

Fig. 16-1. A, Oversized shallow burn does not tighten deep trabecular meshwork. **B,** Small, deep burns tighten all layers of meshwork.

Table 16-1. Results of phakic eyes treated with various numbers of burn—prelaser IOP 26-30 mm Hg (retreatment 1-13 weeks later excluded)

Burns	*Eyes*	*Retreatment (%)*	*Surgery (%)*	*Total (%)*
50	14	36	0	36
60	30	33	6.7	41
70	11	37	0	37
80	13	14	0	14
90	14	7	21	28
100	34	12	3	15
110	33	0	9	9
120	21	14	5	19
130	8	0	12	12
140	6	0	0	0

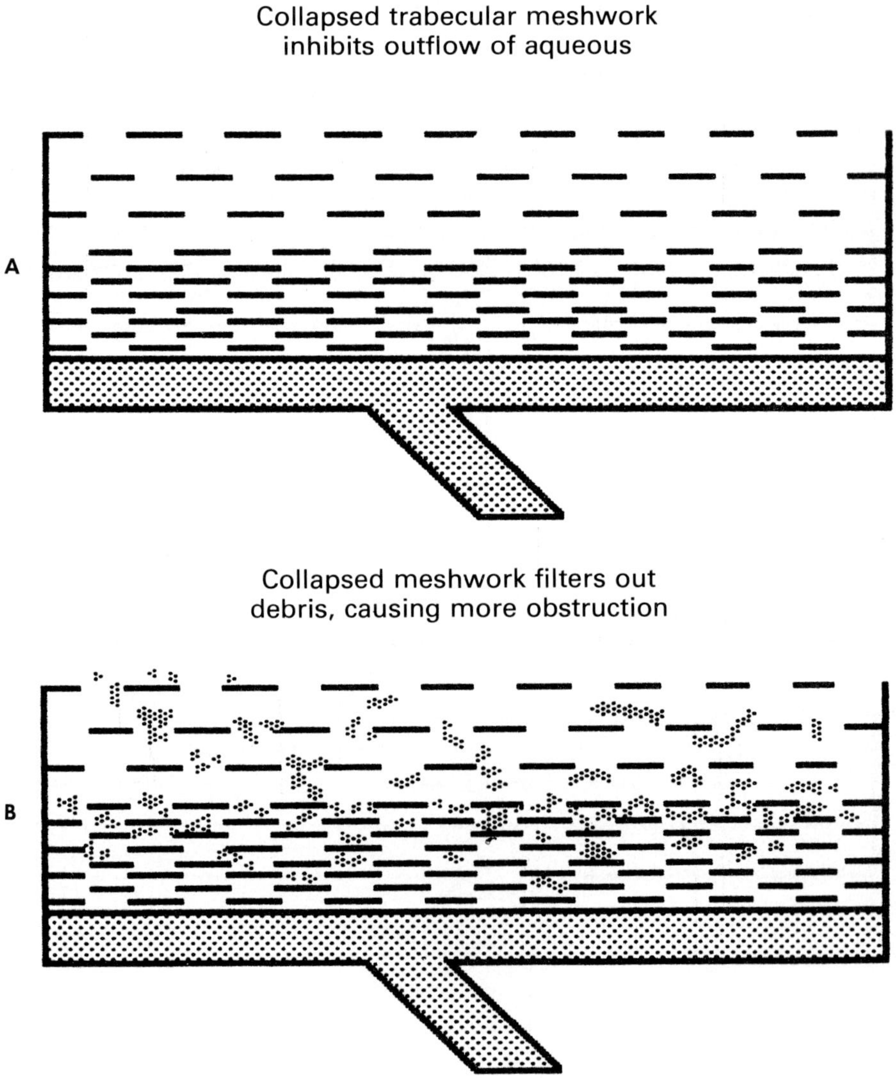

Fig. 16-2. A, Collapsed trabecular meshwork inhibits outflow of aqueous. **B,** Collapsed meshwork filters out debris, causing more obstruction.

outflow impairment. From the standpoint of iritis and synechiae, the anterior half of the pigmented band appears to be the best location for the placement of the burns.[3] However, the original patients were treated in the middle of the pigmented band, and they are maintaining good control 6, 7, and even 8 years later. The optimum power level still appears to be that producing a small bubble, which is a good indicator of adequate tissue temperature rise. Histologically such burns penetrate about halfway through the meshwork, leaving open intertrabecular spaces and an open Schlemm's canal beneath them.[10] If the beam is defocused or the power too low, no bubble will be seen. The defocused spot gives a large but shallow burn (Fig. 16-1, *A*), which sears the surface but does not tighten the important deep trabecular layers (Fig. 16-1, *B*).

The principal controversy in LTP concerns the number of burns to be used. Thomas, Simmons, and Belcher[4,5] modified the original 100-burn, single-session protocol by giving 50 burns in 180 degrees and then delivering the other 50 burns in the remaining 180 degrees 1 month later. Schwartz and co-workers[3] found that 25 burns in one quadrant gave little effect, but 50 burns in 180 degrees produced almost as much effect as 100 burns in 360 degrees. Wilensky and others[6,7,9] advocate only 50 burns and no additional treatment unless the first was not effective.

The present study covers 1450 eyes that I treated, with a total of 2004 trabeculoplasty sessions. Data were stored on a 5 megabyte hard disk and analyzed with an Apple III computer using the PFS File and PFS Report programs. The computer was used to retrieve data on eyes that were phakic, patients over age 39, patients with no previous surgery, cases with a minimum 2 years of follow-up, and patients with IOP prelaser of 26 to 30 mm Hg. All eyes were treated in a single session. I found that the maximum pressure drop at 6 months and at 2 years occurred with 110 laser burns of precise 50 μ size. A second study meeting these criteria was done with 184 eyes, with the additional requirement that any laser retreatment had to be done more than 13 weeks after the first, eliminating planned two-stage LTPs. A much higher retreatment or surgery rate (failure rate) was found in eyes that had received fewer than 100 burns (Table 16-1). The lowest failure rate was found at 110 burns and at 140 burns. It appears half-angle treatment with 50 or 60 burns will indeed give temporary control, but the control obtained will fail in 6 to 18 months. Larger numbers of burns, approximately 110 burns of true 50 μ diameter, are required to give the 7 and 8 years of control now observed in the original eyes treated.

Case report. A 72-year-old male patient had an IOP of 28 mm Hg in his left eye while taking medication. Laser trabeculoplasty was done using 124 burns in 360 degrees in a single session. The IOP fell to the middle teens, without medication, and has remained stable for more than 3 years.

The patient's right eye had an IOP of 27 mm Hg while he was taking medication. The right eye was treated with laser trabeculoplasty, with 64 burns in 360 degrees. The IOP fell to 21 mm Hg without medication, but 6 months later rose to 27 mm Hg. Additional laser trabeculoplasty of 54 burns in 360 degrees was done. The IOP fell to the upper teens without medication and has remained stable for 3 years.

There does appear to be the hazard that, when the first low-dose trabeculoplasty fails, recurrent trabecular collapse and plugging by debris has occurred (Fig. 16-2). A second treatment will not therefore be additive with the first and will also subsequently fail, so that the eye ultimately goes blind or requires glaucoma surgery. The object of trabeculoplasty should be to pull the meshwork wide open, separating the layers so that the cells and debris found in the aqueous of every eye can pass through the meshwork and be eliminated. If this is achieved, the meshwork becomes self-cleaning and will remain open for years—an important consideration in a lifetime disease such as glaucoma.

It is my present practice to treat all eyes in two sessions, with 55 to 60 burns per session. Since many eyes have been controlled for 7 and 8 years by the 100-burn protocol, the advocates of smaller numbers of burns must demonstrate equally good long-term control rates before recommending general adoption of their methods.

REFERENCES

1. Schwartz, A.L., and Kopelman, J.: Four year experience with argon laser trabecular surgery in uncontrolled open-angle glaucoma, Ophthalmology **90:**771, 1983.
2. Schwartz, A.L., and others: Argon laser trabecular surgery in uncontrolled phakic open-angle glaucoma, Ophthalmology **88:**203, 1981.
3. Schwartz, L.W., and others: Variation of techniques on the results of argon laser trabeculoplasty, Ophthalmology **90:**781, 1983.
4. Thomas, J.V., Simmons, R.J., and Belcher, C.D., III: Argon laser trabeculoplasty in the presurgical glaucoma patient, Ophthalmology **89:**187, 1982.
5. Thomas, J.V., Simmons, R.J., and Belcher, C.D., III: Complications of argon laser trabeculoplasty, Glaucoma **4:**50, 1982.
6. Weinreb, R.N., and others: Influence of the number of laser burns on the early results of argon laser trabeculoplasty. Am. J. Ophthalmol. **95:**287, 1983.
7. Weinreb, R.N., and others: Immediate intraocular pressure response to argon laser trabeculoplasty, Am. J. Ophthalmol. **95:**279, 1983.
8. Wilensky, J.T., and Jampol, L.M.: Laser therapy for open angle glaucoma, Ophthalmology **88:**213, 1981.
9. Wilensky, J.T., and Weinreb, R.N.: Low-dose trabeculoplasty, Am. J. Ophthalmol. **94:**423, 1983.
10. Wise, J.B.: Long-term control of adult open angle glucoma by argon laser treatment, Ophthalmology **88:**197, 1981.
11. Wise, J.B.: Glaucoma treatment by trabecular tightening with the argon laser, Int. Ophthalmol. Clin. **21**(1):69, 1981.
12. Wise, J.B.: Errors in laser spot size in laser trabeculoplasty. Ophthalmology **91:**186, 1984.
13. Wise, J.B., and Witter, S.L.: Argon laser therapy for open-angle glaucoma; a pilot study, Arch. Ophthalmol.**97:**319, 1979.

17

Laser treatment of macular disease: procedure and follow-up

Robert C. Watzke

After detecting subretinal membranes and selecting the appropriate laser, the physician is ready to treat the patient for macular disease. An angiogram should be used to guide treatment and should be taken no later than 72 hours before surgery. A frame of the angiogram should be available for reference at the photocoagulator.

The physician should obtain an informed consent and should be sure that the patient understands that vision will be worse immediately after treatment because of the retrobulbar injection and the retinal edema surrounding the burn. I give patients and their families a leaflet describing macular degeneration, laser treatment, and possible complications. I think that it is good practice to ask patients, "What do you expect from this treatment?" It is illuminating to listen to their answers, and the ensuing dialogue is helpful in avoiding unrealistic expectations.

A retrobulbar injection of a short-acting local anesthetic without epinephrine is necessary. Retrobulbar injection is required because of the intensity of photocoagulation and its juxtafoveal location.

SUBRETINAL NEOVASCULAR MEMBRANES MORE THAN 200 μ FROM CENTER OF FOVEAL AVASCULAR ZONE

The argon blue-green laser should be selected. The membrane should be outlined and surrounded with several 100 μ burns placed at the margin of the surrounding pigment ring (or blocked fluorescence in the angiogram) in normal appearing retina (Fig. 17-1, *A*). Intensity should be sufficient to produce visible burns of the pigment epithelium. These "surround" burns are placed as a guide for more intense treatment to the membrane itself. The burns should not be deep or placed on the edge of a membrane within the zone of blocked fluorescence, since such small burns to neovascular tissue might cause hemorrhage. Placing these surrounding burns also enables the physician to judge the effectiveness of the retrobulbar anesthetic and the patient's stolidity. It is best to always start photocoagulation on the nonfoveal edge of the membrane.

Following this, the membrane, surrounding pigment, and blood are treated with 200 to 500 μ, overlapping burns of 0.2- to 0.5-second duration (Fig. 17-1, *B*). The pilot burn should be placed at the nonfoveal edge of the subretinal membrane. The physician should increase intensity rapidly and aggressively to produce intense whitening of the

A 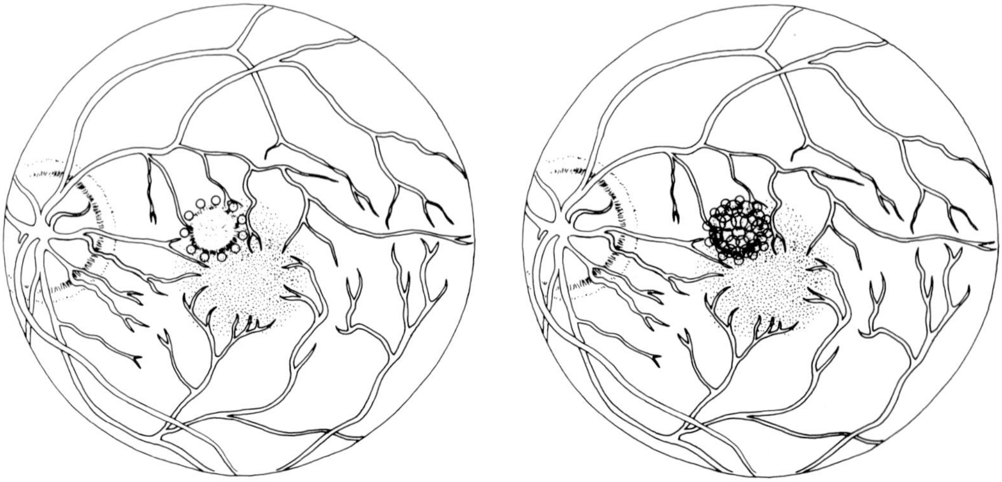 B

Fig. 17-1. A, Treatment of membrane more than 200 μ from foveal center with argon blue-green laser. Membrane is surrounded by 100 μ, 0.1- or 0.2-second burns of light intensity. **B,** Membrane is treated directly and heavily with 200 or 500 μ, 0.2- to 0.5-second, overlapping heavy burns to produce intensely white end point. Foveal edge should be treated with 200 μ spots.

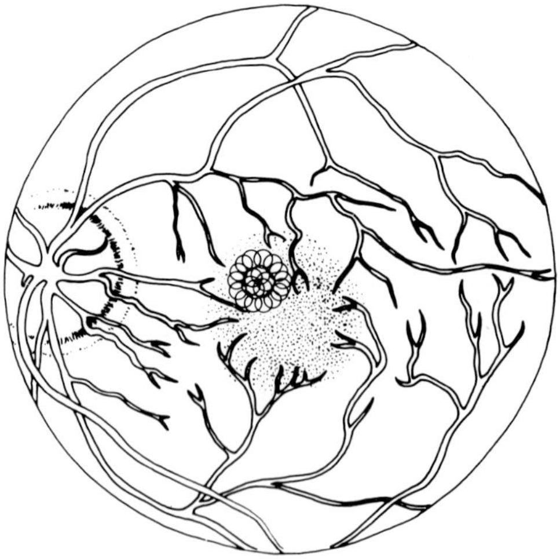

Fig. 17-2. Treatment of membrane less than 200 μ from foveal center with krypton red laser. Entire membrane and zone of blocked fluorescence is connected with overlapping 0.2- to 0.5-second, 200 or 500 μ burns sufficient to produce white burn.

membranes[1]; some hypopigmented membranes, however, can never be turned white. Retreatment over less intense burns is less effective. Although 500 μ, 0.5-second burns will produce contraction of the internal limiting membrane, there is less tendency for hemorrhage or perforation of Bruch's membrane with larger burns. If hemorrhage occurs, it is usually small and self-limited, but it may be stopped by direct treatment.

SUBRETINAL NEOVASCULAR MEMBRANES LESS THAN 200 μ FROM CENTER OF FOVEAL AVASCULAR ZONE

Neovascular membranes whose foveal edge is at or within the margin of the foveal avascular zone cannot be delimited with outlining burns in that area. Such membranes should be treated with either overlapping argon green or krypton red laser photocoagulation burns of 200 or 500 μ spot size and 0.2- or 0.5-second duration (Fig. 17-2). When using krypton red, I advise 500 μ spots for 0.5 second, which allows the burn to expand to its full extent to cover the entire membrane and zone of blocked fluorescence. Krypton red intensity should be at least great enough to produce white burns. Another technique is to treat the extrafoveal part of the membrane with argon blue-green and the foveal part with argon green.

After concluding laser therapy, the physician should check the extent of treatment against the angiogram to be absolutely sure that the entire membrane and zone of blocked fluorescence has been intensely burned with heavy photocoagulation.

FOLLOW-UP AND RETREATMENT

Because laser photocoagulation is new, guidelines for follow-up and retreatment are not standardized. There is disagreement, particularly with krypton red photocoagulation, on the frequency of follow-up visits and posttreatment angiograms.

Argon blue-green or green

It is worthwhile but not essential to see patients 2 weeks following argon blue-green or green photocoagulation. Vision can be checked, and questions about blurred vision or paracentral scotomas can be answered. If the lesion is becoming pigmented and there is less serous retinal detachment, prognosis is good. If there is still a serous detachment and the edge of the lesion appears gray and swollen, the physician can order an angiogram. However, I usually defer angiography for another 2 weeks; this assumes that photocoagulation has been meticulous and intense and has definitely covered the entire membrane.

At 4 weeks following argon blue-green or green treatment a fluorescein angiogram is done. The macula is then examined by contact lens biomicroscopy. The fluorescein angiogram should be used to delineate the extent and location of remaining or recurrent neovascular tissue. If a serous detachment is still present, with continued gray, subretinal pigmentation beyond the treatment scar, retreatment will be necessary.

Krypton red

Since the average krypton red burn produces less inner retinal destruction and retinal vasculitis than argon blue or green wavelengths, the physician can do a fluorescein angiogram earlier after treatment and find hypofluorescence of the treated area caused by vessel closure and necrosis of the pigment epithelium. An angiogram done within 24 hours after krypton red treatment can show complete hypofluorescence of the treated membrane. An early posttreatment angiogram could be obtained as a guide to completeness of treatment, but I believe that an angiogram at 2 weeks is sufficient if treatment is meticulous and effectively covers the lesion.

Long-term follow-up

Argon

After the first post treatment examination and angiogram the patient should be seen at 1-month intervals for two additional follow-up visits and then, if stable, at 6 months. Patients should be urged to check their vision daily and their paracentral scotoma with an Amsler grid. If there is no subjective change and no serous detachment surrounding the scar on contact lens examination, a fluorescein angiogram is probably not necessary at 2 and 3 months. However, this scheme assumes an alert and reliable patient and a meticulous and experienced examiner. If in doubt, an angiogram should be obtained.

Krypton red

Since krypton red photocoagulation is a new modality and recurrences may occur more often, follow-up visits should be more frequent.[2]

After the first postoperative visit and angiogram at 2 weeks the patient should be examined at least twice more at 2-week intervals. A favorable evolution of the scar is indicated by an absent or regressing serous detachment, resolving hemorrhage, and increased pigmentation and flattening of the scar. Most physicians obtain angiograms at each visit. By the third postoperative visit a good impression of prognosis should be possible, and postoperative visits should be planned every 1 to 3 months.

REFERENCES

1. Macular Photocoagulation Study Group: Argon laser photocoagulation for senile macular degeneration: results of a randomized clinical trial, Arch. Ophthalmol. **100:**912, 1982.
2. Yannuzzi, L., and others: Recurrence of subretinal neovascular membranes following krypton red laser photocoagulation. Delivered at the annual meeting of The Macula Society, Jan. 26-28, 1984, San Diego.

18

Unilateral shallow anterior chambers and glaucoma

Robert N. Shaffer

The relative rarity of shallow anterior chambers in the normal population is not generally appreciated. In the 2185 refraction patients in our offices graded by slitlamp and checked by gonioscopy, 4% had shallow anterior chambers, and less than 2% had anterior chamber angles capable of closing.[10]

The clinician who fails to note a shallow chamber has missed a sign of great prognostic significance for the patient. This applies to untouched eyes and those that have had surgery or trauma. The most common cause for bilaterally shallow anterior chambers is genetic, predisposing the person to the risk of angle-closure glaucoma (see Chapter 3). Unilateral shallowing of the chamber, which suggests a secondary process, is the subject of this chapter.

The tonometer is often the most important instrument in investigating the cause of a flat anterior chamber. An extremely low intraocular pressure (IOP) usually means a wound leak or a cyclodialysis. an increased pressure indicates either a block to anterior flow of aqueous humor or a sudden increase in posterior chamber volume, such as in a choroidal hemorrhage.

SHALLOW ANTERIOR CHAMBERS WITH LOW PRESSURE

Anterior chambers can be moderately shallow without causing angle closure. Until there is iridotrabecular block, the pressure is not elevated. The condition should be recognized and an episode of angle closure avoided if possible.

Excessive aqueous outflow: leaking wounds

All the filtration operations for glaucoma create larger openings than are necessary. Even a 1 mm trephine makes a 1000 μ hole. Only 12 μ are needed to provide sufficient aqueous humor outflow. The added resistance produced by the trabeculectomy flap has decreased postoperative flat chambers, although surprisingly few became problems even with trephines and sclerectomies. The healing power of nature increases the resistance to outflow, and the anterior chamber usually forms within hours or days, even with large openings.

Thin-walled blebs that are obviously leaking aqueous humor are often seen, yet the anterior chamber usually remains full. I do not favor attempts to thicken such blebs, despite the risk of infection, since plastic repair frequently results in a recurrence of increased pressure. Such repair is needed if there is a gross fistula or if the hypotony has caused macular edema with marked visual reduction.

Any penetrating wound of the cornea can result in a flat anterior chamber. After glaucoma surgery the physician usually should defer repair 3 to 4 days, depending on the presence of a bleb and a quiet, soft eye. If the lens is against the cornea, we customarily fill the anterior chamber with air through a small paracentesis opening. This acts as a cork and gives time for the fibroblasts to decrease the outflow. If hypotony and flat chamber persist, two or more posterior sclerotomies are performed to drain choroidal edema, and the anterior chamber is again filled with air.

If the flat anterior chamber occurs in an aphakic eye, reformation of the chamber is more urgent, particularly if the vitreous is against the posterior cornea. Endothelial damage and corneal edema can result within 2 or 3 days. Injection of air into the anterior chamber is the simplest method to gain time while a leaking area is healing. If the wound continues to leak and the site can be visualized, the best procedure is prompt resuturing. Seidel's fluorescein test can be useless in such eyes. There is no aqueous in the anterior chamber to be pushed out, and the hypotonous eye produces little aqueous. When in doubt, the best method is to fill the anterior chamber through a paracentesis with fluorescein-stained, balanced salt solution under pressure. The site of the leak is then easily determined.

Posterior space-occupying lesions

Choroidal edema is invariably present in the hypotonous eye. It is not the cause of the flat anterior chamber, but rather the result of the hypotony. Draining of the choroidal fluid and reformation of the anterior chamber usually resolve the problem. Choroidal edema with increased IOP is only produced by increased choroidal venous pressure, such as found after closure of vortex veins by an encircling band in retinal detachment surgery.

The other cause of a shallow to flat anterior chamber with hypotony is cyclodialysis, either surgical or traumatic. If sufficient aqueous flows back through a cyclodialysis cleft, it produces a space-occupying posterior collection that moves the iris forward. At the same time there is a profound decrease in aqueous production, which prolongs the problem. Closure of the cleft can result in an abrupt, high rise in IOP, which can sometimes be relieved by intensive miotics to reopen the cleft. Often a filtering procedure becomes necessary.

When the anterior chamber is very shallow, it is difficult or impossible to identify the exact site and extent of a cyclodialysis cleft. Indentation gonioscopy should be tried but may also be ineffective. When repair of a cleft is contemplated, balanced saline should be used to reform the anterior chamber. In a full anterior chamber clefts are easily seen by Koeppe gonioscopy at the time of surgery. If IOP can be raised above 12 mm Hg, the choroidal edema will be resorbed.

Profound hypotony leads to choroidal edema, which often includes the posterior pole. Macular edema causes a central scotoma, with a vision of 20/200. It is this reduction in vision that forces the ophthalmologist to take steps to relieve the hypotony, even though it risks a return of the glaucoma. No entirely reliable method for closure of the cyclodialysis cleft has been found. Procedures have included laser treatment to the cleft, diathermy or cryotherapy over the cleft, a scleral buckle over the cleft, or suturing of the ciliary body to the sclera to close the cleft. It was correctly pointed out by Maumenee[5] that the ciliary body must be brought in contact with the sclera to effect a cure. He used laser application through the cleft to produce the irritation, then injected air into the posterior chamber to hold the ciliary body in contact with the sclera.

It is important to remember that this edema is very different from cystoid macular edema, which can permanently destroy useful vision. A delay in repair for at least several weeks is justifiable. Even after many years of hypotony restoration of useful vision is possible. A patient of mine had hypotony of 4 to 6 mm Hg and 20/400 vision for nearly 10 years after a cyclodialysis with macular edema. Nine penetrating scleral diathermies over 2 years, including penetrating Pischel pins, eventually raised the pressure to 8 to 15 mm Hg and a surprising 20/40 vision. Over a 15-year period a cataract formed and was removed. Thirty years after the cyclodialysis, the patient still has a corrected vision of 20/40.[8]

SHALLOW ANTERIOR CHAMBERS WITH INCREASED PRESSURE

Pupillary block

Bilateral shallow chamber

Bilateral shallow chambers are almost always genetic in origin. Pressures become elevated if enough of the angle is blocked by peripheral iris. However, a monocular shallow anterior chamber must always be considered to have a secondary etiology, such as a swollen lens. The etiology of this glaucoma is pupillary block, just as in the primary glaucoma, but the therapy is usually lens removal rather than iridectomy.

After a lens has been removed, a shallow chamber indicates either a wound leak, in which IOP will be low, or iridovitreal pupillary block, in which IOP will be increased. Immediate use of mydriatics and cycloplegics can break the block, but surgery is often needed. When a flat anterior chamber is caused by wound leak, a delay of a day or two is justifiable. When the pressure is elevated, intervention is mandatory.

To perform a laser iridectomy, the anterior chamber must be formed to avoid burning the cornea. This can often be accomplished by hyperosmotic agents and a reformation of the chamber through a small corneal paracentesis. If an iridectomy is performed at a point of iridovitreal adhesion, nothing is accomplished. This is a particular problem with the small openings produced by the laser. We have seen several eyes with pupillary block following the use of an anterior chamber intraocular lens. Multiple openings in the iris peripheral to the lens were ineffective because vitreous was attached to the posterior iris. An anterior vitrectomy can clear the vitreous from behind the iris, and the Ocutome can be used to perform a new iridectomy; sometimes the lens must be removed. I have not seen an iris bombe with an intraocular posterior chamber lens, but pupillary block is certainly a possibility. For this reason I question the current tendency to avoid performing any peripheral iridectomy at the time of cataract extraction.

Posterior space-occupying lesions

A space-occupying lesion that is increasing slowly in size will not cause a shallow anterior chamber unless it becomes very large. The most common cause of an increase in posterior volume is hemorrhage, which can occur into a tumor, into the vitreous, or most commonly into the choroid following intraocular surgery. This is usually accompanied by moderate pain and increased IOP. If a patent iridectomy is present, the signs are exactly the same as in ciliary block (malignant) glaucoma, except the pressure is not usually as high, depending on the blood vessel involved. An arterial hemorrhage can rapidly destroy all sight. This ''expulsive hemorrhage'' usually occurs at the time of an intraocular surgery or within a day or two.

Typically during a cataract extraction the incision will suddenly begin to bulge, followed by the vitreous and retina, unless the surgeon is prepared immediately to perform posterior sclerotomies so that blood can drain outward. If the dark mound of blood-filled choroid and retina can be seen, the sclerotomy should be done over that quadrant, but speed rather than accuracy is the goal. The sclerotomies should be V shaped and should be placed in at least two quadrants. Cautery to the tip of the V will hold it open to continue drainage for a few days; the opening should not be sutured. A spatula in the suprachoroidal space can be used to search for other pockets of blood if the bleeding has stopped. Saline continuously injected into the anterior chamber will force more and more blood out. This choroidal blood remains unclotted for a surprising length of time and must be evacuated. If the hemorrhage occurs after the patient has left the operating room, the eye is usually lost. Occasionally patient and physician are lucky, as in the following example.

Case 1. A 79-year-old man with arteriosclerosis and vascular hypertension had advanced glaucoma under medical control and moderate cataracts. When seen 2 years later, his vision was reduced to finger-counting in one eye. The other eye had undergone a cataract operation and had no light perception. The patient stated that there had been a hemorrhage at the time of surgery. He was told to defer cataract extraction in the remaining eye until he could no longer get around his home.

Two years later, when the patient was 83, the cataract was removed intracapsularly. Temporary glasses were given after 3 days, and the patient was delighted with his 20/50 vision. On the 13th postoperative day the patient had sudden, severe pain and loss of vision. When seen 1 hour later, vitreous was hanging out of the wound, and the pupil was occupied by the retina!

He was taken to surgery, where 2 V-shaped sclerotomies were performed in the inferior quadrants. After the wound dehiscence had been sutured, blood poured out of the sclerotomies as saline was injected into the anterior chamber. The retina was pushed back halfway before stopping the operation. Three days later, there had been no change; only light perception was present. The patient returned to surgery. Both sclerotomies were reopened, and two more sclerotomies were placed in the superior quadrants. Unclotted blood again poured out of all four as saline was forced into the anterior chamber; suddenly black choroid appeared at the four sites. Ophthalmoscopically a pink reflex could be seen everywhere. The patient died 1 year later, still with 20/200 vision.[7]

This patient and his physician were lucky, but the case does show that salvage is possible in difficult situations. Undoubtedly minor choroidal hemorrhages that we are not aware of do occur. Others are sufficient to cause a flat anterior chamber and increased pressure. Unless the hemorrhage is visible ophthalmoscopically or by ultrasonography, the clinician can only distinguish between this entity and ciliary block glaucoma by a posterior sclerotomy; in ciliary block no edema or blood will be found.

Nanophthalmos and choroidal edema

Nanophthalmos, or "dwarf eye," is a genetically determined bilateral condition with hyperopia, small corneas, shallow anterior chambers, and narrow angles. The sclera seems to be abnormally thick and interferes with the posterior drainage of venous blood through the vortex veins. If the eye is opened, the abrupt drop in IOP causes a marked choroidal effusion, angle closure, frequently choroidal hemorrhage, and retinal detachment. The eyes are usually lost. Surgery is to be avoided if at all possible. Laser iridectomy and iridoplasty to shrink the iris away from the trabeculum is the safest treatment after medical therapy has failed.

Choroidal edema with increased pressure can also be seen following panretinal photocoagulation and after an encircling scleral band for retinal detachment. It is often difficult to reform the anterior chamber after filtering surgery for glaucoma in Sturge-Weber syndrome caused by choroidal edema or dilation of a choroidal hemangioma. In these eyes the edema usually subsides and the chamber reforms in 2 to 4 days. A central retinal vein thrombosis can occasionally cause enough choroidal edema to flatten the chamber. Finally, there are occasional cases of ''idiopathic edema.''

Ciliary block (malignant) glaucoma

This relatively rare but devastating cause of flat anterior chamber and increased pressure usually follows filtering surgery in glaucomatous eyes with shallow anterior chambers. Before development of hyperosmotic agents and carbonic anhydrase inhibitors it was more common. The diagnosis is made by observing a flat anterior chamber and increased IOP in the presence of a patent iridectomy.

The glaucoma is caused by a block to anterior flow of aqueous humor at the interface between peripheral lens, anterior vitreous body, and anterior ciliary body. Frequently the physician can see that the ciliary processes extend anterior to the equator of the lens. Opening the anterior chamber allows the lens to drop forward into the scleral ring. The adherence of lens to vitreous to ciliary body prevents anterior aqueous flow, which is diverted posteriorly into the vitreous body. This lifts the iris-lens diaphragm forward, closing the angle. Pilocarpine loosens the pull on the zonules; the lens drops anteriorly, making the condition worse, as do all forms of conventional glaucoma operations. This is the reason that the condition has been known as *malignant glaucoma*. This term, with its cancerous connotation, should be discarded and supplanted by the term *ciliary block glaucoma*. This locates the site of obstruction and is a term comparable to pupillary block.

Rarely ciliary block can occur in an unoperated eye. The condition can be recognized when one eye has a shallow chamber and the other is of normal depth.[4,6] It is common to find the shallowness aggravated by pilocarpine. Cycloplegics, on the contrary, increase the ciliary body tension on the lens, pulling it posteriorly and permitting forward aqueous flow; the anterior chamber thus deepens. Both the medical and the surgical management of ciliary block glaucoma have been devised by Chandler, Simmons, and Grant[1] with a marked improvement in results.[3]

The advised medical regimen is prompt lowering of IOP by hyperosmotic and carbonic anhydrase–inhibiting agents and the intensive use of cycloplegics and sympathomimetics. Atropine, 1%, and Neo-synephrine (phenylephrine hydrochloride), 10%, are instilled at least four times a day. If successful, the anterior chamber should reform promptly or within 2 to 3 days. This intensive treatment can slowly be reduced, but cycloplegics should be continued indefinitely. One of our patients titrates her ciliary block by noting the slight increase in myopia when her lens begins to move forward. She then instills a drop of atropine, which controls the block for about 5 days, when another drop is needed. She has been successfully controlled for the past 6 years.

When medical regimen fails, the surgical approach is used, as described by Simmons.[9] First, a corneal paracentesis is prepared for future injections into the anterior chamber. Second, two posterior sclerotomies are placed in both lower quadrants to test for suprachoroidal hemorrhage. A cyclodialysis spatula should be passed in both directions to make sure there are no unsuspected pockets of blood. If none is found, the condition is proved to be ciliary block. Then, after placing a ring of scleral diathermy to guard against ciliary body hemorrhage, a Wheeler knife is passed through the sclera 3.5 mm from the limbus and halfway into the vitreous. An 18-gauge needle is then passed through that incision for a measured depth of 12 mm; 1.5 cc of vitreous is then aspirated. A large air bubble is injected into the anterior chamber through the previous paracentesis, pushing the lens back and forming an anterior chamber depth greater than that of the usual myopic eye. Cycloplegics should be continued. The procedure can be repeated, but if it fails more than twice, lens removal and anterior vitrectomy are usually needed.

If ciliary block glaucoma occurs in an aphakic eye, the medical regimen is unlikely to be of help. Laser applications to the ciliary body, when possible, have been shown to break the block.[2,11] An anterior vitrectomy may be necessary.

• • •

In summary, two cases are instructive. The first summarizes the shallow chambers that are caused first by pupillary block, then by ciliary block, and finally by a wound leak.

Case 2. A 65-year-old patient with chronic angle closure had bilateral peripheral iridectomies. Angles opened to grade 2, but pressure remained elevated, necessitating the use of pilocarpine. Shortly after starting miotic therapy, the patient returned with a flat anterior chamber, a patent iridectomy, and a pressure of 65 mm Hg in one eye. Since this occurred before modern therapy was available, lens extraction was performed to break the ciliary block; the anterior chamber reformed; and the tension was reduced to 14 mm Hg.

Ten days later the patient returned with another flat anterior chamber, this time with an extremely soft eye. Fluorescein-stained salt solution injected into the anterior chamber showed the position of the wound dehiscence, which was repaired. The future course was uneventful.

Case 3. A 62-year-old patient with severe open-angle glaucoma had a trabeculectomy performed. The following day the anterior chamber was flat, and the IOP was 21 mm Hg. Atropine was instilled and temporarily restored the chamber, suggesting the mechanism was ciliary block. Ophthalmoscopy was negative. The next day the chamber was flat, and the pressure was 20 mm Hg. The intensive medical regimen did not improve the situation. On the third day the patient was taken to surgery, with plans to perform a vitreous aspiration and air injection. When the posterior sclerotomy was made, there was an immediate flow of xanthochromic fluid followed by bright red blood. Saline, then air, restored the anterior chamber. The cause of the flat chamber was subchoroidal hemorrhage. Evacuating the hemorrhage permitted the anterior chamber to reform, and the postoperative vision was 20/30.

These examples indicate the care the ophthalmologist must take to ascertain the exact cause of shallow anterior chamber in any patient. Only with accurate diagnosis of the cause can appropriate therapy be instituted.

REFERENCES

1. Chandler, P.A., Simmons, R.J., and Grant, W.M.: Malignant glaucoma: medical and surgical treatment, Am. J. Ophthalmol. **66:**495, 1968.
2. Herschler, J.H.: Laser shrinkage of the ciliary processes: a treatment for malignant (ciliary block) glaucoma, Ophthalmology **87:**1155, 1980.
3. Kolker, A.E., and Hetherington, Jr., editors: Becker-Shaffer's diagnosis and therapy of the glaucomas, St. Louis, 1983, The C.V. Mosby Co.
4. Levene, R.: A new concept of malignant glaucoma, Arch. Ophthalmol. **87:**497, 1972.
5. Maumenee, A.E.: Discussion. In New Orleans Academy of Ophthalmology: Symposium on glaucoma, St. Louis, 1981, The C.V. Mosby Co., p. 438.
6. Rieser, J.C., and Schwartz, B.: Miotic induced malignant glaucoma, Arch. Ophthalmol. **87:**706, 1972.
7. Shaffer, R.N.: Posterior sclerotomy with scleral cautery in the treatment of expulsive hemorrhage. Am. J. Ophthalmol. **61:**5, 1307 (part II), 1966.
8. Shaffer, R.N., and Weiss, D.I.: Concerning cyclodialysis and hypotony, Arch. Ophthalmol. **68:**25, 1962.
9. Simmons, R.J.: Malignant glaucoma. In Chandler, P.A., and Grant, W.M., editors: Glaucoma, Philadelphia, 1979, Lea & Febiger.
10. van Herick, W., Shaffer, R., and Schwartz, A.: Estimation of width of angle of anterior chamber, Am. J. Ophthalmol. **68:**626, 1969.
11. Weber, P.A., and others: Argon laser treatment of the ciliary processes in aphakic glaucoma with flat anterior chamber, Am. J. Ophthalmol. **97:**82, 1984.

19

CO_2 laser

Hugh Beckman

The unique optical properties of the eye, in which the transparent media serve to transmit visible laser wavelengths to the pigmented structures, caught the imagination of ophthalmic investigators early in the development of lasers. Absorption by the pigment epithelium, as in retinal photocoagulation or vaporization in laser iridectomy, created interest in procedures developed in the 1960s and have subsequently given way to techniques that are standard treatments.

All ocular media are opaque to the 10.6 μ (infrared) energy of the carbon dioxide (CO_2) laser. This laser has found great acceptance in many medical fields, such as gynecology and otolaryngology, where its ability to destroy such tissues as cervical carcinoma in situ and vocal cord nodules has established it as a valuable addition to the surgical armamentarium. In general the applications in these specialties have been directed to the ablation of relatively large amounts of tissue.

Interest in high-powered (20 to 50 W), continuous-wave (CW) CO_2 lasers with 2 to 3 mm spot sizes have focused the laser industry's attention toward the production of these larger lasers, leaving the ophthalmic field as yet relatively unexplored and undeveloped.

We first reported in 1971[2] a laser designed especially for use in ophthalmology (Fig. 19-1). This laser functions in both the CW and the rapid-superpulsed (RSP) modes. In CW mode it has a maximum output of 20 W; in RSP mode it has a peak output of 10,000 W, with average output of 20 W. The average power is a function of the pulse rate, which is continuously variable from 75 to 200 per second; the pulse width in RSP mode is 5200 microseconds. The higher peak powers yield a high power density, which develops less tissue heat. This energy cuts better, with less charring and shrinking of tissue—both desirable with ocular tissue—and slightly less hemostasis than with CW CO_2. The RSP laser operates optimally in the TEM^{00} mode and can be focused to a 0.75 mm spot through a 200 mm focal length lens. A helium-neon (HeNe) marking laser is directed coaxially with the CO_2 beam through a Zeiss OPMI 6. Through this microscope the surgeon can direct the beam by means of a "joystick." Until recently no commercial model of this type of laser was available, but we have just recently succeeded in modifying a Sharplan 743 laser for emission of the RSP energy and can deliver it both through the operating microscope or by means of an articulated arm into a handpiece, which can deliver a 0.5 mm spot size.

With the original laser we[2] described the formation of penetrating sclerostomies into the anterior chamber to cause external filtration of aqueous humor in rabbits. Ticho and

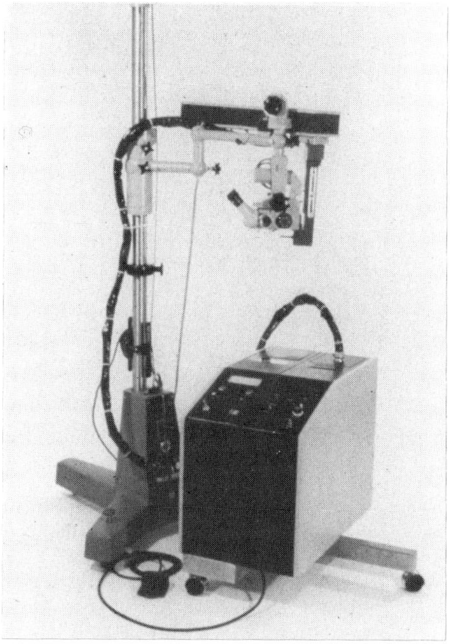

Fig. 19-1. Rapid-super pulsed CO_2 laser.

co-workers[5] and Fuller and I[1] described using the CO_2 laser to perform filtering procedures in the treatment of human glaucoma. Ticho and others used 3.8 W of CW CO_2 laser energy to form full-thickness sclerostomies at the limbus. In their eight cases of patients with neovascular glaucoma, four were successful and maintained filtering blebs and intraocular pressures (IOPs) below 20 mm Hg. No iridectomies were performed, and in the four cases that failed, twigs of peripheral iris adhered to the inner surface of the opening, giving the impression that, had iridectomies been created, the success rate might have been better.

With the RSP laser Fuller and I created a two-layer filtering procedure that might best be described as a subscleral CO_2 laser sclerostomy, similar to that described by Schimek and Williamson[4] with the electrocautery. A 5 × 5 mm, one-third thickness scleral flap is outlined with the laser and then dissected surgically down to the limbus. At first only a 1.5 mm laser sclerostomy was vaporized into the anterior chamber at the anterior border of the corneoscleral interface, but more recently we have etched furrows into the base of the flap in the hope that possibly this might (1) create more surface area within the flap, augmenting absorption of aqueous; (2) help direct fluid from the sclerostomy to the external filtering edges of the flap; or (3) inhibit scarring of flap surfaces rubbing together. Surgical iridectomies are performed in all instances. The scleral flap is closed with 9-0 supramid sutures. The original limbal-based conjunctival flap has recently been replaced by a fornix-based flap.

Using the original procedure, we obtained the following results in the 20 eyes treated. In the 11 eyes with primary open-angle glaucoma (POAG) there was successful lowering of pressure below 20 mm Hg, with only one of the eyes requiring topical medication for control. Of the nine secondary glaucomas, failure occurred in 50% of the four cases of neovascular glaucoma and in the one eye with traumatic glaucoma.

Two other cases were controlled below 20 mm Hg, and two below 25 mm Hg. To date we have performed 32 filtering procedures using some modification of this technique. The results are shown in Table 19-1.

In 1982 L'Esperance[3] reported on the use of a CW CO_2 laser to perform full-thickness and guarded filtering procedures for the treatment of neovascular glaucoma. His initial results with this were encouraging, yielding a success rate in the 70% range. Of interest were three cases in which a silicone sheet was implanted as a seton, with success in all cases. We attempted such a procedure in one case of a young male with desperately intractable congential glaucoma that had been unsuccessfully treated by two guarded filtering procedures and three ciliodestructive procedures. An attempt with the silicone seton failed, and a subsequent full-thickness filtration attempt using 5 FU also failed. With the patient now down to 20/400 in his only seeing eye because of a cataract and with his intraocular pressure out of control, a seton custom fashioned out of supramid mesh (Fig. 19-2) was inserted under a scleral flap after phacoemulsification of the cataract had been performed. Ends of the seton protruded through the flap underneath the conjunctiva. Six months after surgery a healthy bleb was still present, and IOP was controlled in the low 20s range with topical medication. We encountered an additional desperate case of neovascular glaucoma unresponsive to two prior filtering procedures and three ciliodestructive procedures. We performed a laser trabeculectomy with the same supramid stint, and there was control of IOP in the high teens 5 months after surgical intervention.

Why use the CO_2 laser?

1. *Safety*. Since no blade enters the anterior chamber, lens damage or vitreous penetration is impossible. Infection rates are kept to a minimum.

2. *Technical ease*. The dissection is performed under direct observation by the surgeon through the microscope. No blade hides the incision. Depth of the wound can be easily regulated, and dissection may take place in a curved fashion if this is thought to be desirable. Hemostasis is obtained by the laser beam, with the CW being slightly more hemostatic than the RSP mode. Better visualization of the wound from lack of blood in the field permits better technique.

3. *Adjunct to filtration*. Thermal injury may possibly inhibit healing of wound margins because of the coagulation of tissue. It is thought to be difficult for fibroblasts to ''crawl'' over carbon, and one can see in Fig. 19-3 the internal stoma of the wound demonstrating carbonization. Creating a groove 0.5 mm wide when dissecting the flap may facilitate external filtration. Increasing the posterior surface area of the bed with

Table 19-1. RSP CO_2 laser treatment—total with revisions (success criterion: IOP less than 23 mm Hg)

Type	*Eyes*	*Failure*	*Success*	*Success with medication*
POAG	22	2	19 (86%)	1 (5%)
POAG (aphakic)	1	—	1 (100%)	—
Neovascular	4	2	2 (50%)	—
Traumatic	1	1	0	—
Secondary	4	2	2 (50%)	—
TOTAL	32	7	24 (75%)	1 (5%)

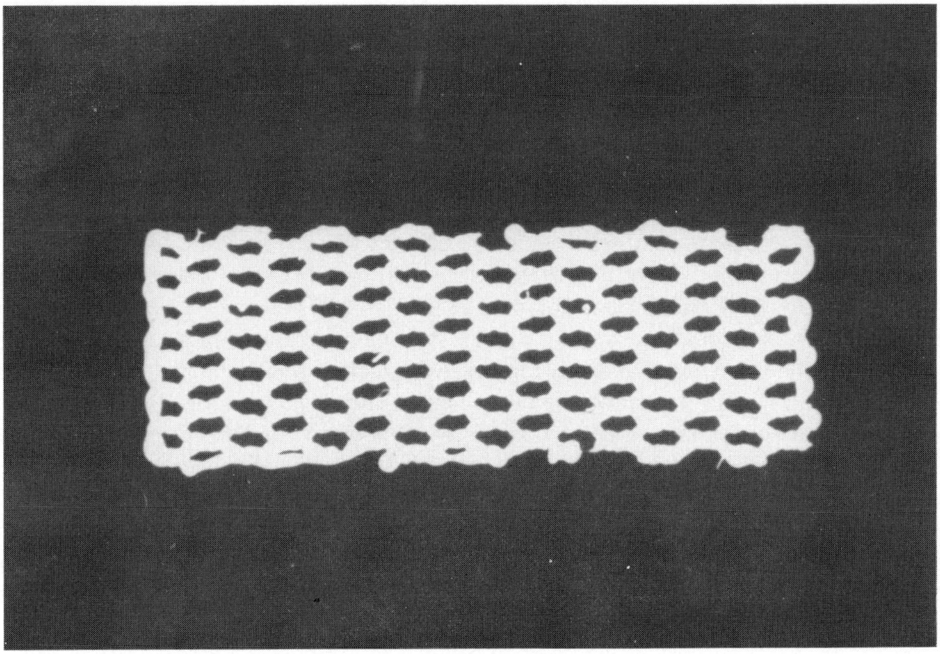

Fig. 19-2. Seton fashioned out of supramid mesh for insertion under scleral flap following phacoemulsification.

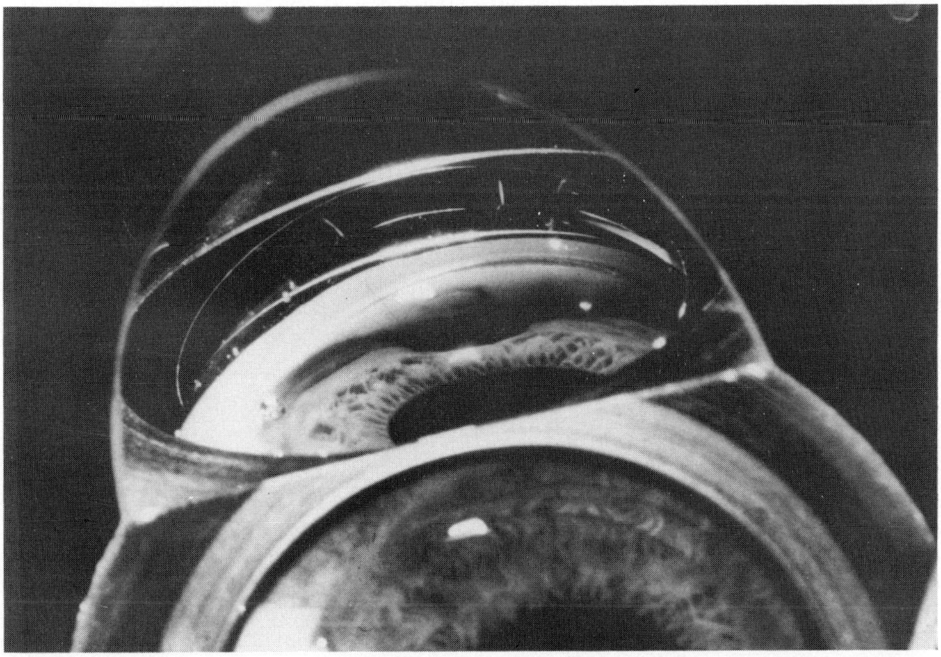

Fig. 19-3. Carbonization on internal stoma of wound.

furrows may result in an increased filtration bed or may cause delayed scarring of the flap down to the scleral bed.

4. *Transmission through fiberoptic material.* Because of the esoteric nature of the substances required to transmit 10.6 μ energy, the use of CO_2 lasers in endoscopic fiberoptic work has lagged behind those applications with lasers in the visible spectrum. Hollow infrared wave guides have been pioneered by Guarmire at the University of Southern California and by Marhic at Northeastern University. Unfortunately energy losses caused by bending the wave guides precludes these from being of practical use in endoscopic surgery. Pinnow in 1978 reported a new fiberoptic wave guide made of thalium bromide and thalium bromoiodide (KRS 5). When clad in a jacket, this fiber has fair transmission characteristics, although its bending characteristics are rather poor. The fiber is toxic, however, and this together with technical difficulties have limited its implementation. Fuller at Sinai Hospital of Detroit has developed the IRFLEX 3 fiber, which is currently capable of delivering 15 W of power with a bend radius of 13 cm (5.2 inches); the fiber system has a diameter of 0.875 cm (0.35 inches). Another fiber, the IRFLEX 4, has been manufactured as small as 20 μ and can be focused to small enough spot sizes to deliver the beam within the eye or onto the surface of the eye beneath the conjunctiva. In rabbits we have performed subconjunctival full-thickness laser sclerostomies using a 45-degree mirror at the end of the fiber wave guide. It is hoped in the near future that commercially available fiber will be wedded to RSP CO_2 lasers. Then, by making a needle incision beneath the conjunctiva and Tenon's capsule and placing the mirrored fiber at the limbus, a full-thickness CO_2 laser thermal sclerostomy cn be bored into the anterior chamber, the wound sealed with a single suture, and the patient sent home having had a filtering procedure.

The use of CO_2 lasers in ophthalmology has slowly gained momentum over the last 10 years. Research in the field has been hindered by industry concentrating its efforts on developing large-spot-size, ablative CO_2 laser systems. As the market turns its attention to more delicate application, such as in ophthalmology and plastic surgery, we believe that carbon dioxide will gradually take its place as a wavelength used in the armamentarium of every ophthalmologist.

REFERENCES

1. Beckman, H., and Fuller, T.A.: Carbon dioxide laser scleral dissection and filtering procedure for glaucoma, Am. J. Ophthalmol. **88:**73, 1979.
2. Beckman, H., and others: Limbectomies, keratectomies, and keratostomies performed with a rapid pulse carbon dioxide laser, Am. J. Ophthalmol. **71:**1277, 1971.
3. L'Esperance, F.A., Jr., Little, R.N., and James, W.A.: Carbon dioxide laser trabeculostomy for the treatment of neovascular glaucoma, Ophthalmology **90:**7, 821-829, 1983.
4. Schimek, R.A., and Williamson, W.R.: Trabeculectomy with cautery, Ophthalmic Surg. **8:**35, 1977.
5. Ticho, U., and others: Carbon dioxide laser filtering surgery in hemorrhagic glaucoma, Glaucoma **1:**114, 1979.

20

Current status of ophthalmic photovaporization therapy*

Francis A. L'Esperance, Jr.

A system for the photovaporization of intraocular malignant tumors of the choroid and retina, portions of the anterior segment, and extraocular lesions by carbon dioxide (CO_2) laser radiation has recently been developed. CO_2 laser radiation is highly absorbed by ocular tissue, with almost complete absorption and conversion to heat within a tissue depth of 100 to 200 μ. Therefore, malignant intraocular and extraocular tumors can be totally vaporized in an extremely precise manner by repeated surface burns with the CO_2 laser (Figs. 20-1 and 20-2).

The CO_2 laser is a continuous-wave (CW) laser of great power, with an emission located in the far-infrared part of the spectrum. This laser has characteristics that differ significantly from those of the pulsed ruby laser or other CW lasers, such as the argon laser or krypton laser, more familiar to clinical ophthalmologists. The very long wavelength of its emission (10.6 μ) means that its radiation is outside the visible region and that its absorption and transmission characteristics are significantly different from those generally encountered at shorter wavelengths, particularly in the visible portion of the spectrum.

This far-infrared radiation has interesting and potentially beneficial absorption characteristics, biologically as well as structurally. Most common nonmetallic materials absorb infrared energy, which is essentially heat, and most metals are fairly good reflectors. Substances such as plastics, glass, bone, and muscle tissue show that a high absorption of the radiation from the CO_2 laser is absorbed by water-containing tissues at a rate comparable to the absorption of visible light by the retinal pigment epithelium. Applications of the CO_2 laser in otolaryngology[10,20] and gynecology[5,13] are based on the finding that relatively inaccessible structures that can be visualized through a column of air, such as through a laryngoscope or a colposcope, can be photocoagulated or incised with excellent hemostasis and little damage to surrounding tissues. The recent interest in CO_2 lasers in ophthalmology focuses on these advantages and on the ability to directly vaporize extremely small particles of ocular tissue from the solid or semisolid state to smoke and vapor.

*This chapter contains slightly modified sections from L'Esperance, F.A., Jr.: Ophthalmic lasers: photocoagulation, photoradiation, and surgery, St. Louis, 1983, The C.V. Mosby Co.

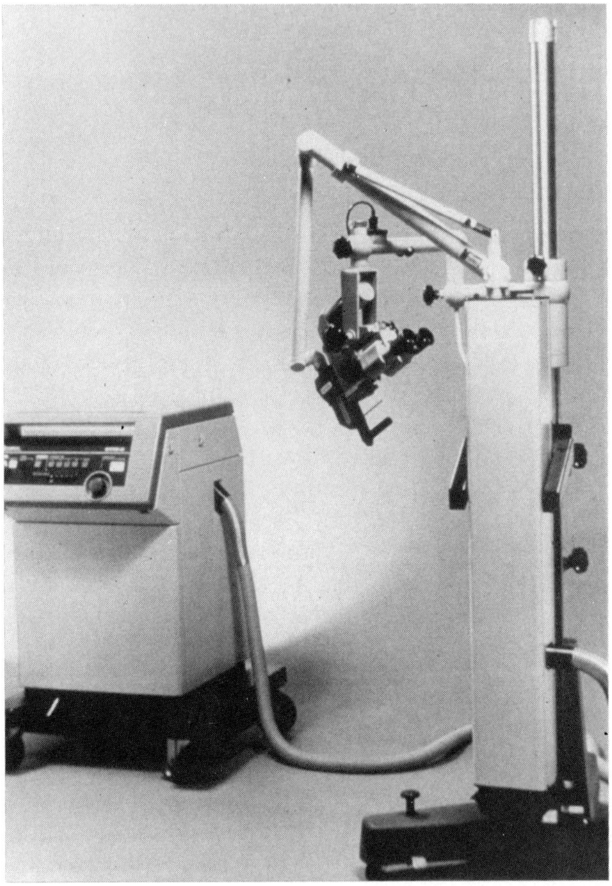

Fig. 20-1. Coherent Medical Group, Inc., CO_2 Laser Model 451 illustrating console *(left)*, laser tube *(right)*, attached articulated arm, and micromanipulator.

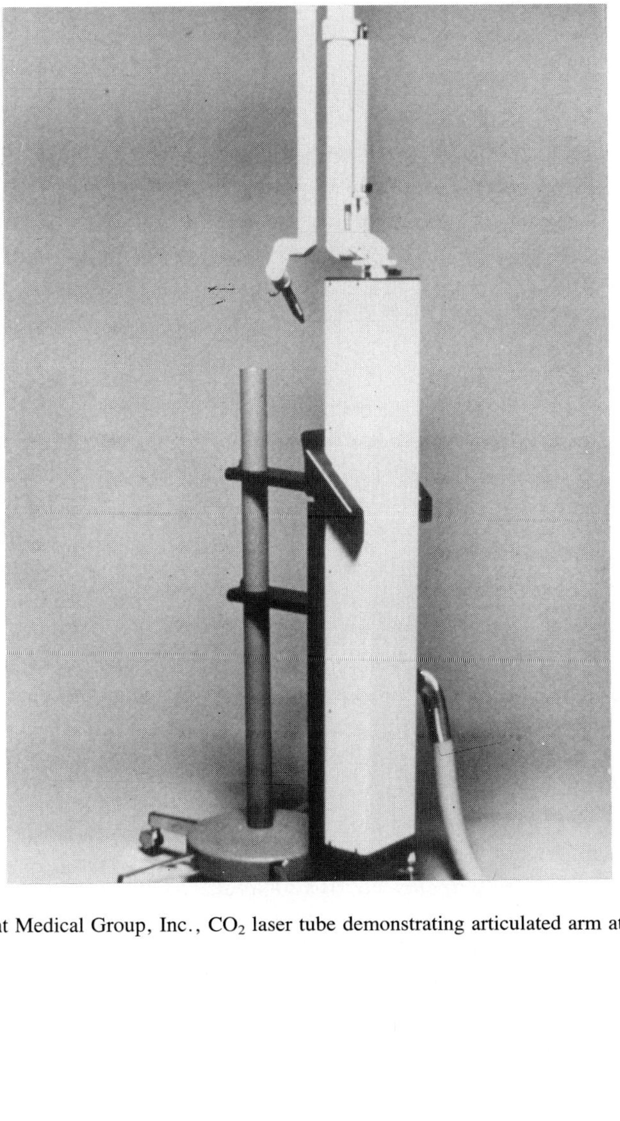

Fig. 20-2. Coherent Medical Group, Inc., CO_2 laser tube demonstrating articulated arm attached to hand-held external probe.

HISTORIC ASPECTS

The initial ophthalmic publications by Fine, Fine, and Peacock[8] followed the discovery of the CO_2 laser by Patel[17] in 1964. They demonstrated that energy at the wavelength of the CO_2 laser (10.6 μ, or 10,600 nm) is absorbed principally by the cornea. In these studies the corneas of rabbits were irradiated for 1 second over an area measuring 5 mm in diameter. The power ranged from 3 to 20 W. The corneal injury was characterized by opacification, ulceration with high energies, and finally perforation. The edges of the induced ulcer were charred, and it was the impression of the authors that the depth of penetration into the cornea was roughly proportional to the power density of the irradiation. There was no evidence of damage to the internal structures when nonpenetration of the eye occurred.

In 1968 Campbell and others[7] determined that the energy density for threshold lesions on the cornea was approximately 38.5 mW/mm^2. Besides summarizing the histopathologic effects on the cornea, these authors noted that ocular protection from this laser could be achieved at most ophthalmic power ranges by using ordinary spectacles without increased optical density. Regular eyeglasses were considered an effective shield from CO_2 laser radiation, since this particular wavelength is absorbed to an extremely high degree by glass.

In 1971 Beckman and others[4] introduced a new type of a rapidly pulsed CO_2 laser to perform limbectomies and keratectomies. This laser was able to pulse at a rate of 60 to 300 cycles per second. Although its rate was so rapid as to seem continuous, each laser burst was a discrete pulse, with each lasting a microsecond and reaching a very high energy level. Since each burst occurred so quickly, less total energy was required than with CW CO_2 emission, and less time was available for heat conduction to adjacent areas. Thus less tissue destruction occurred surrounding the vaporized area, and little charring was observed. This particular pulsed CO_2 laser provided energy emitted in the form of spikes at peak powers of 10,000 W or greater, providing power densities in excess of 10 mW/cm^2 when the incident laser beam was focused on the tissue. In this manner the high power density emission caused vaporization of the tissue in a short time. The limbectomies and keratectomies were relatively successful, and the authors pointed to the possible advantage of pulsed CO_2 laser trephination over mechanical trephination. They noted the following advantages:

1. The laser action is safe. As the CO_2 beam enters the anterior chamber, the aqueous fluid, which is opaque to this wavelength emission, bubbles. Under manual control it is simple to stop laser action when the bubbling is observed, without harm to underlying tissues.
2. The size of the hole into the anterior chamber could be well controlled by the focal length of the lens used.
3. Button-holing of the flap could be avoided, since the aiming light of the invisible CO_2 laser (helium-neon) beam gave a true representation of the beam's path and could be positioned accurately.
4. Less bleeding occurred from the sclera, as slight cauterization of the edges took place from the thermal component of the laser energy.

In 1972 Fleischman and I[14] designed and constructed a delivery system to conduct the CO_2 laser beam from its energy source to the eye (Fig. 20-3). This particular system incorporated a relatively low-powered CO_2 laser with a beam reduction device; a mechanical attenuator; moderately sophisticated power-monitoring equipment; an articulated arm, reflecting delivery system; and an intraocular probe to channel the laser beam to the eye. With this initial investigative instrument we could vary the laser power up to 10 W in a continuous fashion. Vaporization of lid papillomata in two patients and eradication of a pterygium and corneal neovascularization in one patient represented the first clinical ocular application of this particular laser. Minimal scarring of the lid and conjunctival region occurred, although the corneal neovascularization regrew 3 to 6 weeks after the laser cauterization, discouraging further therapeutic attempts at that time.

During the mid-1970s the CO_2 laser drew the interest of the medical profession as a potential tool for a variety of surgical procedures. This laser was successfully used in dermatology, otolaryngology, gynecology, and burn surgery.[15] The applications in these particular fields of medicine were possible because the laser could vaporize tissue with selected penetration, was hemostatic and lymphostatic, and was thought to promote excellent wound healing after vaporization.[9] Its use in plastic surgery[12] led to the consensus that the CO_2 laser had definite advantages over conventional surgical techniques in certain instances.

In 1978 Miller and others[16a] used a 1.5 mm–diameter probe with an infrared output window of zinc selenide for transvitreal photocautery of vessels at the posterior pole of an albino rabbit's eye. This represented the first successful use of the CO_2 laser in a fluid medium through a fluid-tissue interface, introducing a new dimension for its use. The infrared window placed at the tip of a needlelike probe allowed the infrared energy to be channelled through the vitreous fluid. The vessels were coagulated when the tip of the probe was placed in juxtaposition to the rabbit retinal vessels through a pars plana incision under binocular microscopic control. Approximately 0.4 W of CW CO_2 laser

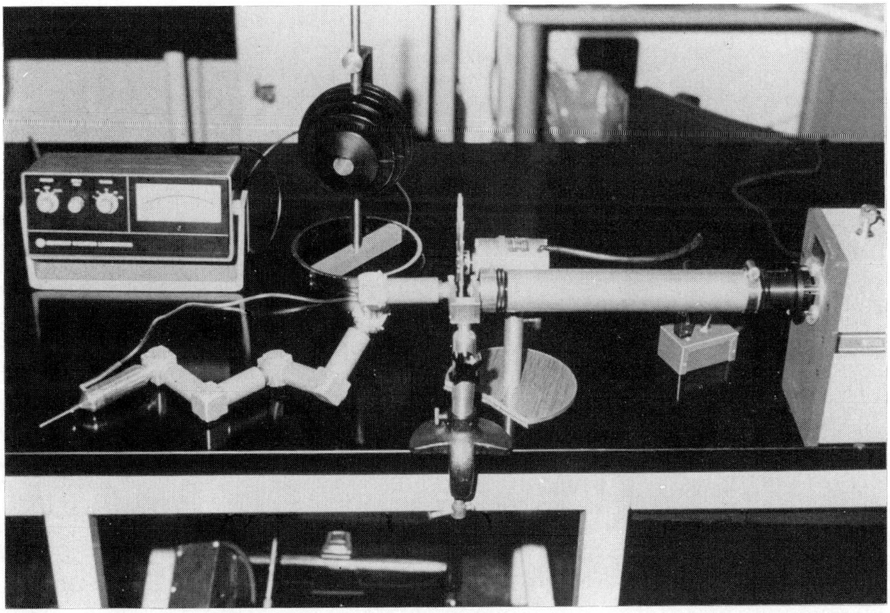

Fig. 20-3. Early model of CO_2 laser photovaporization system in our laboratory showing *(right* to *left)* beam reduction device, mechanical attenuator, power-monitoring equipment, articulated arm delivery system, and intraocular probe to channel laser beam to tumor or other abnormal tissue.

power for 4 seconds was used to coagulate the retinal vessels in this animal series. Miller and others also introduced a 3 mm vitrectomy probe with enclosed fluid irrigation, aspiration, and fiberoptic illumination. Their preliminary results demonstrated the ability to cut vitreal strands through a pars plana approach by using short bursts of peak CO_2 laser power.

In 1979 Miller, Smith, and Boyer[16] reported that CO_2 laser photocautery had been successfully used intraocularly in human patients to seal fibrovascular fronds and retinal tears at the time of vitrectomy. Closure of rubeotic vessels in the iris was demonstrated histologically. Six cases were described, although the authors recognized that much more experience was necessary and that caution should be exercised with such treatments.

Ticho and others[21] in 1979 reported moderate success in treating eight patients with severe neovascular glaucoma using the Co_2 laser beam. The focused CO_2 beam was used to penetrate the anterior chamber beneath the conjunctiva in the area of the limbus, thereby allowing the aqueous fluid to drain into the sub-Tenon's and subconjunctival space. Minimal bleeding at the laser incision site was reported, and the CO_2 laser was thought to be advantageous in treating this particular disease.

In 1979 Beckman and Fuller[3] reported their results with the CO_2 laser in creating filtering cicatrices in five glaucomatous eyes by using rapid-superpulsed Co_2 laser energy to perform the scleral dissection. The filtering procedures were performed on five patients with glaucoma resistant to medical therapy: one with chronic angle-closure glaucoma, two with neovascular glaucoma, one with chronic open-angle glaucoma, and

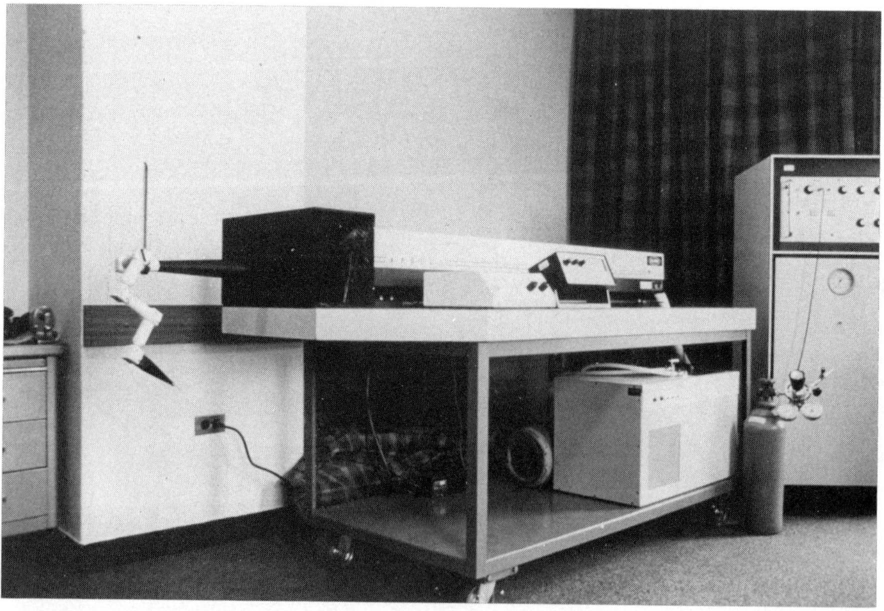

Fig. 20-4. Recent CO_2 system in our laboratory showing *(left* to *right)* articulated arm with shuttering mechanism, CO_2 laser, self-contained water cooling system, and power supply. This system was designed with SRI International and consisted of 50 W CO_2 laser system that could produce pulsed, superpulsed, and CW modes.

one with secondary glaucoma. This particular procedure revealed the possible technical advantages, which included: (1) the ease with which the microdissection is performed under direct microscopic observation, with absence of blood or instruments in the field; (2) the safety factor of penetration into the anterior chamber without the use of a sharp instrument, (3) the possible advantage of inhibition of healing at the wound edge by the laser beam, and (4) the bacteriocidal effect of thermal cutting. The results were encouraging and led to further interest in this particular laser instrument.

In 1977 work began in our laboratory on the construction of a high-powered CO_2 laser capable of producing 50 W of power in the continuous mode, although a variation of beam modes and configurations were available. Rapidly pulsed bursts at extremely short intervals (100 bursts per second at 1-millisecond duration), superpulses of high peak power, or any combination of pulse widths with varying numbers of pulsations per second can be produced by this unique machine. The delivery system from this laser was designed through the collaboration of our laboratory with Dr. Norman Peppers and SRI International, Inc. (Fig. 20-4). The laser beam is channeled through a series of devices that measure the power at various points along the delivery system and the articulated arm. A helium-neon (HeNe) red laser beam is channeled through the delivery

A

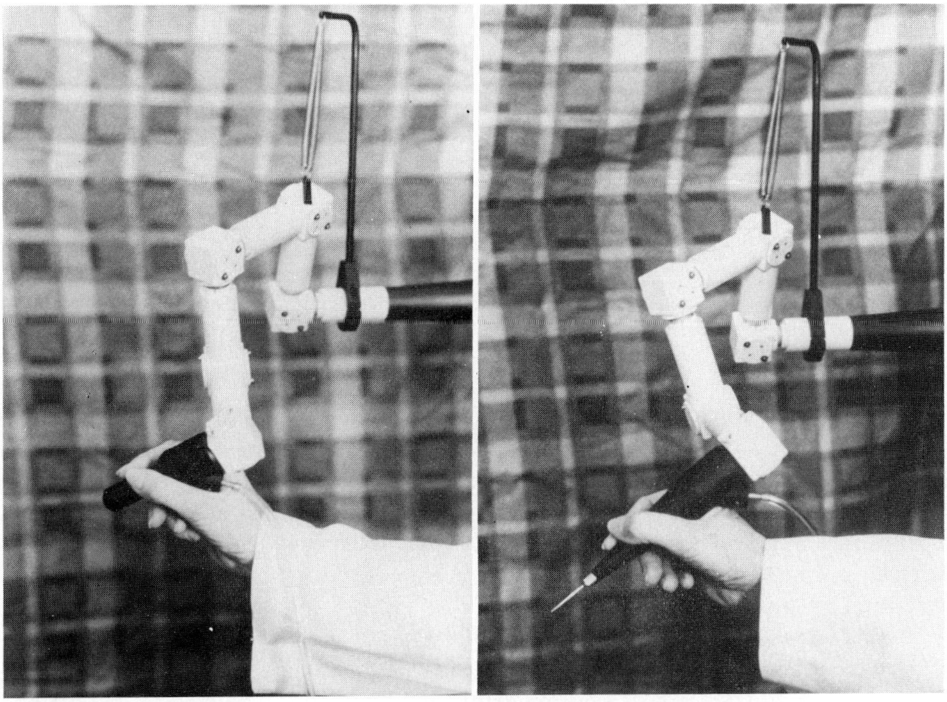

B

Fig. 20-5. A, CO_2 laser photovaporization articulated arm and handle for external vaporization of surface abnormalities and orbital tumors. Plastic tube delivers gentle flow of medical-grade nitrogen that removes smoke and vapor from operative field. Focus of CO_2 laser is determined by visualization of confocal red HeNe beam spot on surface of target tissue. **B,** Intraocular probe and articulated arm of our specially designed CO_2 laser photovaporization system. Laser and target HeNe beams are channeled through articulated arm and exit through small intraocular, needlelike probe that is kept clear by gentle flow of medical-grade nitrogen gas.

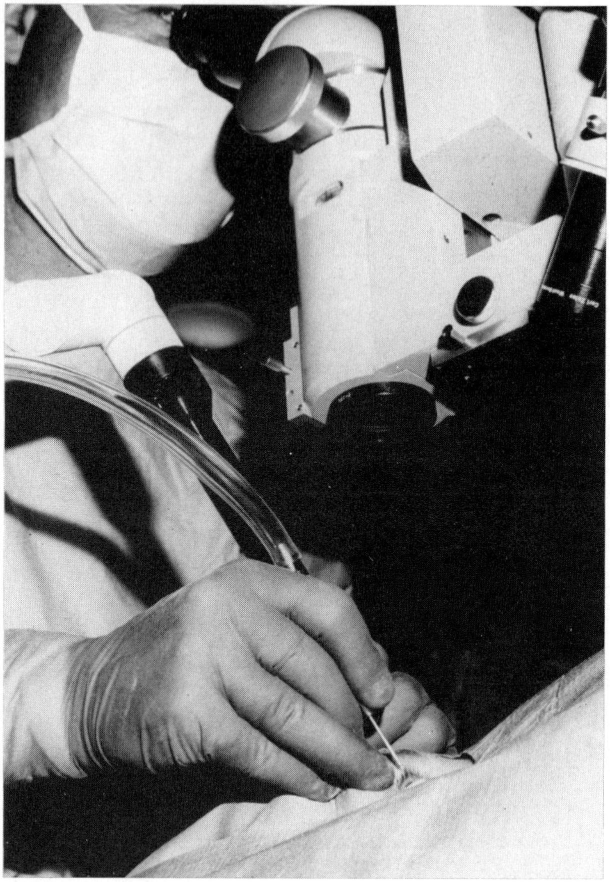

Fig. 20-6. Close-up view of intraocular probe and nitrogen gas flow system prior to intraocular CO_2 photovaporization.

system coaxially with the invisible Co_2 laser beam so that these laser beams travel together and focus to precisely the same spot with both the intraocular and extraocular delivery handpieces (Fig. 20-5). Thus the exact position of the invisible CO_2 laser beam is known at all times, and the surgeon can purposefully focus or defocus the beam. A sophisticated intraocular probe with a gold tip and a precise collimating system was designed in collaboration with Coherent Medical Group, Inc., to channel the beam into the central regions of the globe (Fig. 20-6).

Various types of animal and later clinical studies began in 1978 and, along with the work of other investigators, provide the basis for the following recommendations for the implementation of CO_2 laser surgery in ophthalmology.

ADVANTAGES OF CO_2 LASER SURGERY

Surgery with significant anticipated blood loss

In ophthalmology the use of the CO_2 laser for orbitotomies, removal of orbital tumors (Fig. 20-7), excision of lid and conjunctival tumors, and blepharoplasties[2] (Fig. 20-8) is apparent. Intraocular procedures, including penetration of the globe for tra-

A

B

C

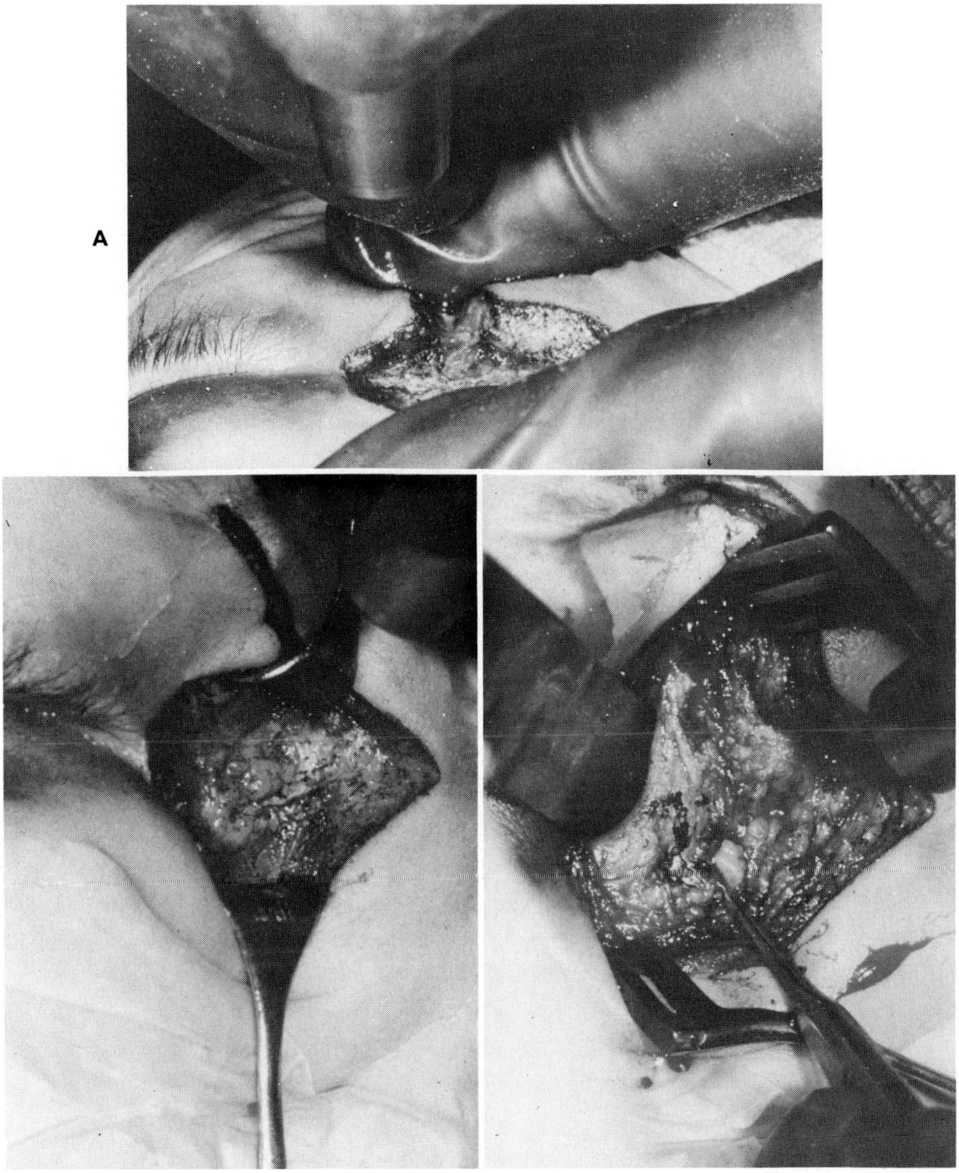

Fig. 20-7. A, Skin and subdermal incision extending posterior from lateral canthus during orbitotomy procedure for removal of lymphangioma in retrobulbar space of 2-year-old child. Entire incision and dissection was performed without loss of blood and with excellent cutting properties by CO_2 laser beam. **B,** Appearance of CO_2 laser through skin and superficial tissue down to zygomatic process. Note lack of bleeding and precision with which skin and subcutaneous tissue were dissected by laser beam. **C,** Deeper incision down to periosteum of zygomatic process with incision into bone. A moderately large piece of bony process was totally removed, according to Kronlein procedure, by the vaporization and cutting effect of CO_2 laser beam. Excellent hemostasis was maintained throughout procedure. (Courtesy Stephen L. Trokel, M.D.)

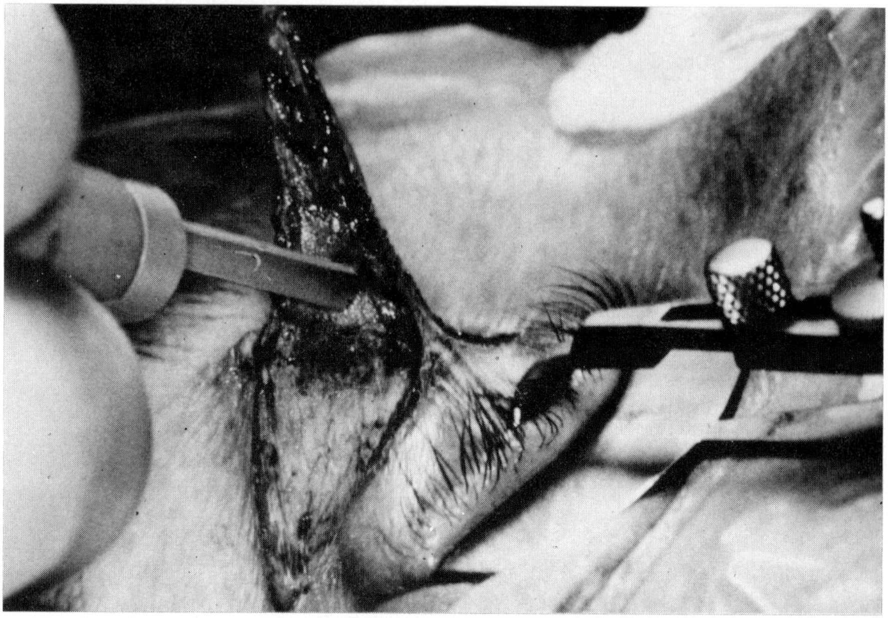

Fig. 20-8. CO_2 laser blepharoplasty showing removal of skin flap. All incisions are performed by hemostatic cutting action of focused CO_2 laser beam. (Courtesy Sterling Baker, M.D.)

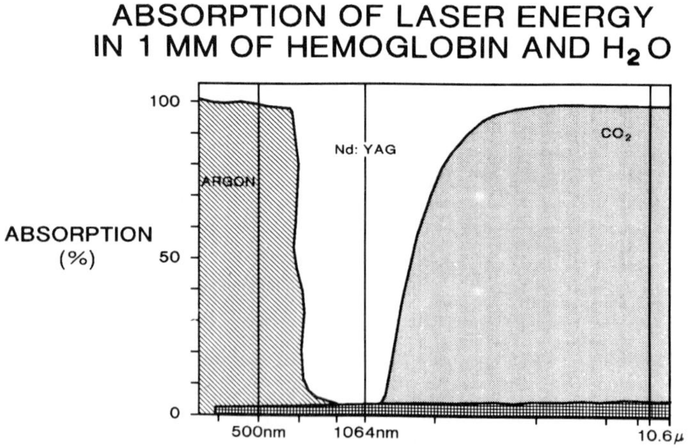

Fig. 20-9. Representative curve showing absorption characteristics of argon (500 nm), neodymium-YAG (1064 nm), and CO_2 (10.6 μ) lasers in hemoglobin and water.

beculostomies with neovascular glaucoma[14a] and full-thickness ocular wall resections for intraocular tumors,[18] are obvious uses for this highly hemostatic laser beam.

Surgery on patients with bleeding tendencies

Perhaps one of the most dramatic applications of the CO_2 laser lies in surgery performed on hemophiliac and thrombocytopenic patients. The reduction of blood loss and postoperative morbidity has been noted (Fig. 20-9), as well as the striking reduction in expenditure involved in the production of antihemophilic factors. In addition, patients who have been given heparin or dicoumarin can undergo incisions on most areas of the body without significant blood loss.

In the eye any surgery involving the lids, conjunctiva, or intraocular contents would yield to this highly advantageous form of therapy.

Surgery for malignant disease

It has been universally accepted by surgeons that surgery for cancer should be performed with minimal transsection of blood vessels, lymphatics, and manipulation of tissue, along with maximal visualization. Because the CO_2 laser seals blood vessels and lymphatics during surgery and concurrently permits an almost nontouching extirpation of the tumor while enabling the surgeon to distinguish between pathologic and normal tissue, its application in cancer surgery is obvious. Many surgeons are using the CO_2 laser for the incision of accessible malignant tissue because the laser beam exerts a cauterization and obstructive effect on the lymphatic and blood circulation. During ocular surgery the encirclement of the tumor by the laser beam interrupts the blood supply to and from the tumor, which could carry malignant cells into the surrounding circulation.

Surgery on highly infected tissue

Excisions of burns, synergistic gangrene, and decubitus ulcers are excellent examples of the application of the CO_2 laser in general surgery. Infected areas of the lids, as well as the extraocular structures, could be approached in a similar manner, with vaporization of the infected tissue and minimal underlying bleeding.

Vaporization surgery

The use of the CO_2 laser with its microscopic attachments and its other advantages over other modalities has been well established as a result of the pioneering work by otolaryngologists, in which tumors of the vocal cords, such as papillomata and nodules, have been vaporized directly.[11] Direct vaporization of tumors of the bronchi has also been performed and found to be highly advantageous in many instances. Perhaps the most highly successful surgery has been cauterization of the uterine cervix in cases of carcinoma in situ, in which the outer layers of the cervix have been vaporized down to the stromal layers.[6] Vaporization of cranial tumors in neurosurgery has also been accomplished, and this has become a highly practical and useful adjunct to regular neurologic procedures in many centers throughout the world.[19]

When one considers that extirpative surgery performed with a CO_2 laser on a clinical basis began within the last decade, it is apparent that its application in general surgery, as well as in ocular surgery, will become more and more universal as more surgeons introduce this modality into their armamentarium.

DISADVANTAGES OF CO_2 LASER SURGERY

Instrumentation

The CO_2 laser remains a difficult instrument compared to other lasers using a flexible fiber, since delivery of the infrared beam must be channeled through an articulated arm with special reflecting mirrors. The articulated arm is not as easily movable nor as flexible as a fiberoptic cable and can prove more awkward in the operating room. Experimental fiberoptic channeling systems for the CO_2 laser beam have been devised and may provide more adequate manipulation. Suction machines to keep the operating room free of steam, smoke, and odors must be vented with a special exhaust system. Eye protection and other safety features common with most laser instruments are required.

Surgical technique

The surgeon must learn new techniques to use the CO_2 laser. Instead of changing the mechanical pressure when using a scalpel to control the depth of cutting, the surgeon must learn to use an invisible beam and to change the power output, the spot size, the absorption coefficient, the tissue tension, and in some cases the blood supply to the operating field.

INCISIONAL AND VAPORIZATION CHARACTERISTICS OF CO_2 LASER

The CO_2 laser is the fastest-cutting laser and produces the least thermal damage to the sides of an incision. It achieves a greater irradiance or power density (watts per square centimeter) than other lasers for three reasons: (1) greater power output, (2) good absorption coefficient, and (3) nonspecific absorption for tissues involved in ocular surgery.

The greater power output results from the simplified nature of the laser device as compared with other lasers, such as the argon or krypton. The CO_2 laser is a molecular laser with an approximate efficiency of 15%, compared to the argon or krypton laser's efficiency of 1%. Therefore, extremely high powers can be produced using relatively low electric input energy for lasing action.

The good absorption coefficient (950 to 200 cm^{-1}) means that the beam is absorbed within 200 μ of tissue and quickly reaches the vaporization point of water (Fig. 20-10). The nonspecificity means the absorption coefficient remains high for all soft tissues of the body containing water. The 10,600 nm beam approaches an absorption coefficient of 950 cm^{-1} for water. Most tissues, with the exception of bone, contain about 40% to 60% of their weight in water and provide a range of absorption coefficients from 950 to 200 cm^{-1}. The tissue penetration of the CO_2 laser for 98% absorption can be calculated from the equation, $e^{\alpha X} = 0.02$, in which alpha (α) is equal to the absorption coefficient, and X is the tissue depth needed to absorb 98% of the incident energy *(e)*. The excellent absorption coefficient of tissues for the CO_2 laser decreases the volume of injured tissue, when compared to other lasers, and is comparable to the cutting mode of an electric knife, which causes less damage than the plasma scalpel.

The CO_2 laser, when used to cut through tissue, produces less conduction thermal damage to the sides of the incision than any other laser, with the possible exception of the new excimer lasers used in research. The amount of heat damage produced correlates directly with the cutting speed (or time the beam is held in one place) and the absorption coefficent (or amount of tissue needed to absorb the beam). Increased power permits faster movement of the laser beam for any given depth and therefore less heat damage.

The CO_2 laser has proved to be more advantageous than the argon and neodymium-YAG lasers for skin or tumor excison and vaporization, despite photocoagulation of blood vessels or the control of a bleeding surface being easier to achieve in pigmented surfaces with these lasers than with the CO_2 laser (Fig. 20-11). As noted by Goldmann and Rockwell,[9] the argon laser is hindered by three factors: (1) relatively poor power output, (2) a fair (37 cm^{-1}) absorption coefficient for pigmented tissue, and (3) marked specificity or absorption of the beam. A large part (35%) of the 488 nm argon beam is reflected from human skin or extraocular tissue, and although absorption increases with the amount of pigmentation, incision of lightly colored tissues is extremely difficult; this factor eliminates the argon laser for most excisional work. Similar arguments have been presented against the neodymium-YAG laser.[9] Its output is greater than that of the argon

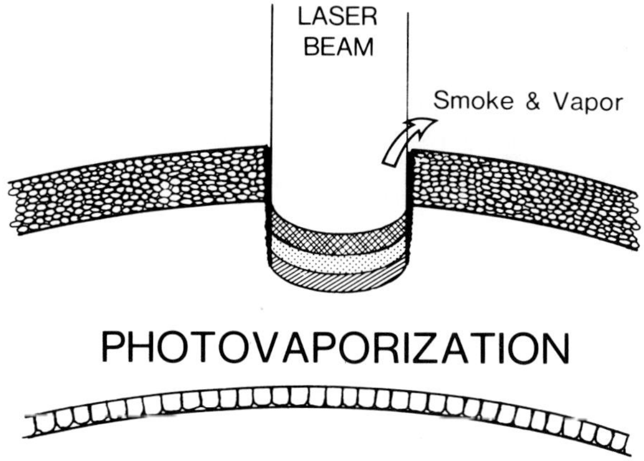

Fig. 20-10. Excellent absorption coefficient of biologic tissue allows CO_2 laser beam to be completely absorbed within 200 μ of tissue, causing that tissue to reach vaporization point of water and to be removed as smoke and vapor. Multiple burns with CO_2 laser beam result in "minishaving" and removal of multiple deeper layers at incision site.

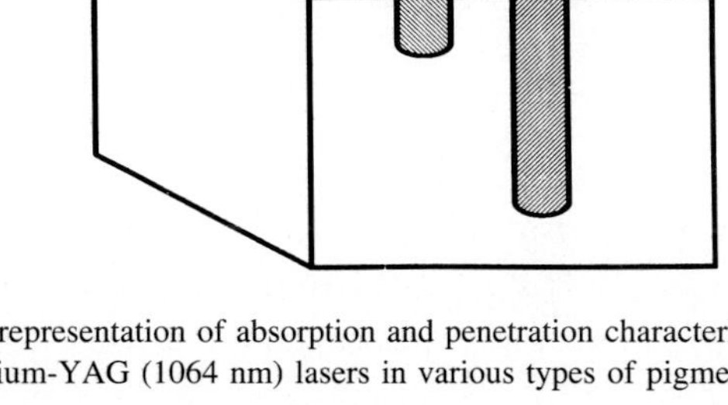

Fig. 20-11. Schematic representation of absorption and penetration characteristics of the CO_2 (10.6 μ), argon (500 nm), and neodymium-YAG (1064 nm) lasers in various types of pigmented tissues.

laser, but the absorption coefficient for excisional purposes is poor and makes this use equivocal. New machines now constructed have high-output energy in both the argon and the neodymium-YAG frequencies and make an incision with these instruments possible, but they result in greater depth of injury than does the CO_2 laser. An adaptation of the argon laser, in which the optical radiation is coupled with a transparent blade that mechanically cuts and photocoagulates, has been introduced by Auth.[1]

INSTRUMENTATION

Micromanipulator

Our laboratory has been working with a micromanipulator designed by Coherent Medical Group, Inc. (Fig. 20-12). The parallel laser beam, after leaving the plasma tube or the articulated arm, is focused by means of a concave mirror in the central portion of the micromanipulator. The main part of the micromanipulator is a gimbal-mounted concave mirror positioned at 45 degrees to the incident laser beam and deflecting it along the viewing axis of the microscope. Cutaway apertures on both sides of the mirror allow a visual path for the surgeon's eyes. A HeNe beam coincides with the impact point of the focused CO_2 laser beam.

The beam-reflecting, gimbal-mounted mirror can be moved by means of a control stick (''joystick''). The gimbaled mirror and control stick are arranged so that (1) the motion of the laser beam and the marker spot are directly proportional; and (2) the motion can be projected in any direction, much as the present joystick manipulators are used with the argon laser intraocular photocoagulator. The mechanical linkage of the control stick and gimbal makes it possible for the surgeon to move the focal spot with the speed considered appropriate for a particular situation. While a tumor or other ocular tissue is being vaporized, it is proper technique to adapt the speed of movement of the focal spot to the effect on the tissue, thus increasing the speed when vaporization penetrates too deeply and slowing down when deep tissue ablation is required. To achieve this, the direct mechanical transmission between the control stick and gimbal is a prerequisite.

Intraocular probe

The intraocular CO_2 laser probes have been designed in collaboration with Coherent Medical Group, Inc., to be used in two possible adaptations. First, the beam is focused by a zinc selenide lens as it exits from the articulated arm onto a cone-shaped, gold-plated tip leading to a 3 cm, needlelike probe with an inside diameter of 1mm. The CO_2 radiation, when focused at the proximal aperture of the probe, reflects from the gold-plated surface and spirals down the probe to the distal end for cauterization or vaporization of the intraocular tissue. The space between the zinc selenide lens and the tip of the probe is airtight, allowing the inflow of filtered, medical-grade nitrogen gas through the entire system and out the tip of the probe to keep the probe free of charred tissue and debris (Fig. 20-13). Thus, once a gas-fluid interchange of the vitreous body has been performed, an intraocular tumor can be approached directly, with vaporization occurring while the nitrogen gas is gently perfused down the intraocular probe into the central region of the eye and out through an exit port maintained near the pars plana. In this manner the intraocular probe is kept patent, and the smoke and vapor from the vaporization of the intraocular tumor are carried from the eye by the gentle passage of nitrogen gas through the system.

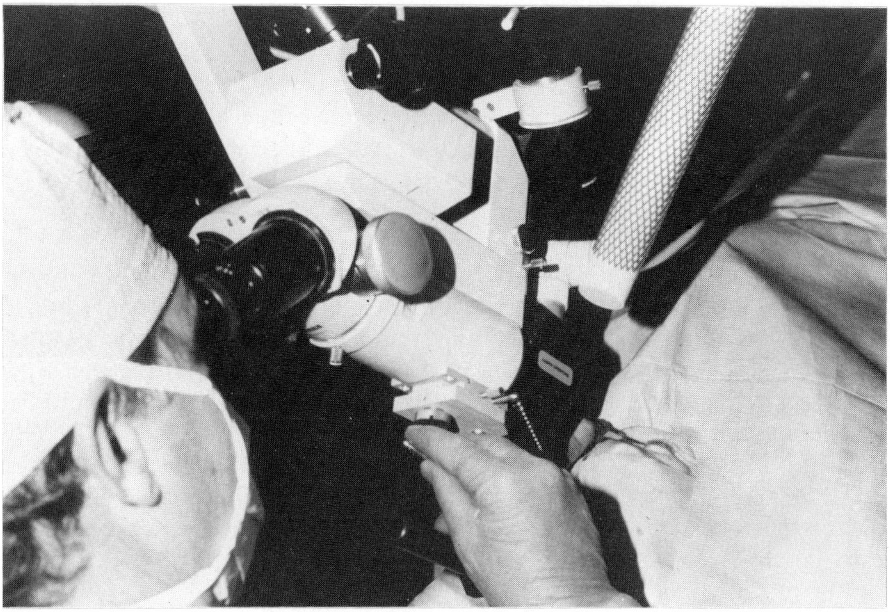

Fig. 20-12. Coherent Medical Group, Inc., CO_2 laser micromanipulator, with surgeon controlling beam by slight movement of joystick.

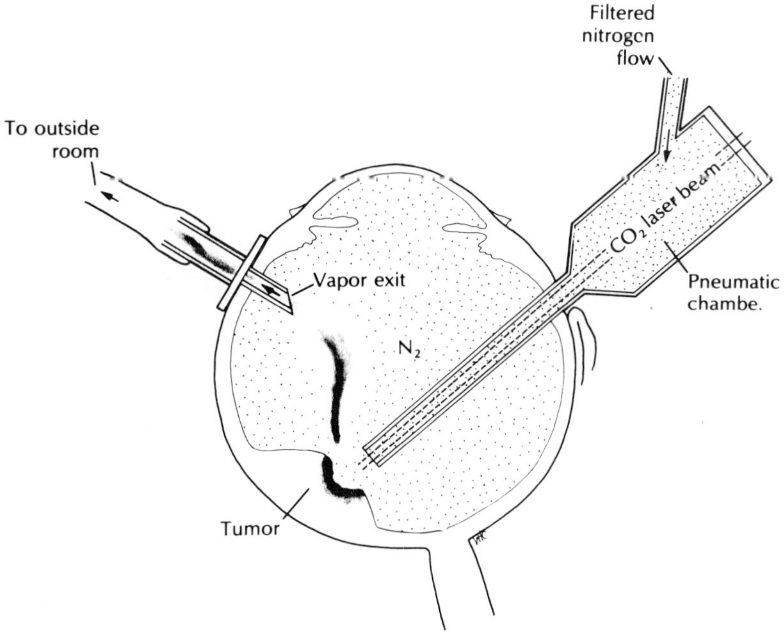

Fig. 20-13. CO_2 laser photovaporization of malignant choroidal or retinal tumors. Nitrogen gas is gently released through intraocular probe, after gas-vitreous exchange, to evacuate smoke and vapor from tumor through exit port.

A second similar system using a 3 cm intraocular probe has also been designed, in which a couplet of zinc selenide lenses is arranged to provide precise collimation and reduction of the beam diameter so that a greater portion of the beam energy is transported through the lumen of the intraocular probe. More critical adjustment of the lenses is required, but less heating of the intraocular probe tip is accomplished, with more uniform and efficient use of the laser energy.

External probe

An external CO_2 laser probe has been designed to attach to the end of the articulated arm; it contains a zinc selenide lens for focusing the target HeNe red spot and the CO_2 laser beam to a point approximately 30 mm from the lens. The protective cone at the distal end of the external probe is connected to a nitrogen gas system, which gently blows any smoke and vapor away from the vaporization site during use. This particular head has been used with great satisfaction for orbital surgery, and the red HeNe spot can be easily focused on all tissues in the orbital region, including bone and fascial planes. Orbital surgery, vaporization of lid tumors, eradication of pterygii and other growths on the conjunctiva, and corneal neovascularization have been performed with success.

A B C D

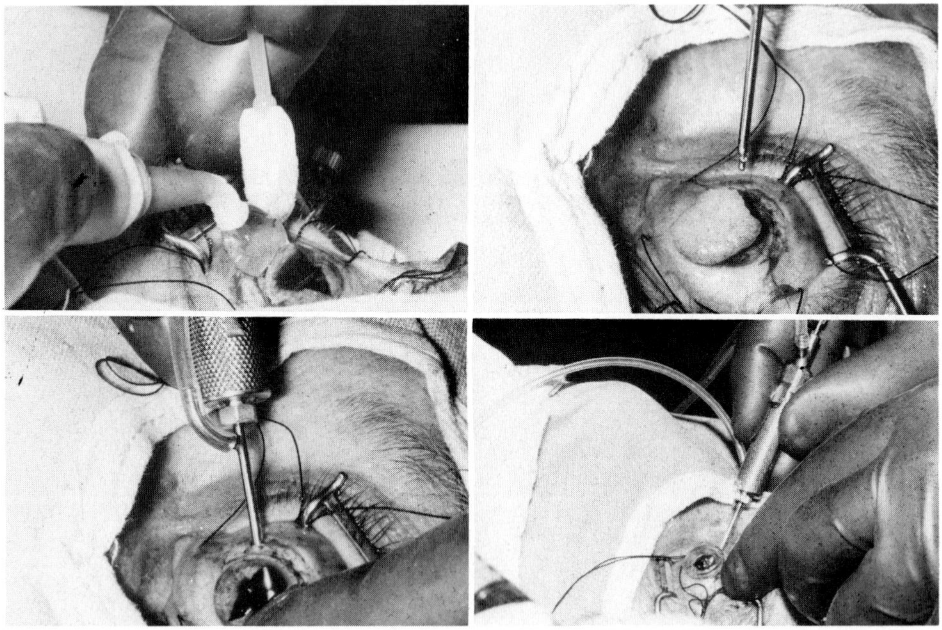

Fig. 20-14. A, Patient with 8 × 10 DD malignant melanoma of choroid extending 8 mm into vitreous body. Before CO_2 laser photovaporization, superior full iridectomy, inferior sphincterotomy, and intracapsular cataract extraction were performed for better visualization of posterior pole. **B,** Same eye after tight closure of cataract wound with 9-0 nylon sutures. Vitrectomy instrument is prepared *(above)* for insertion through pars plana incision into vitreous body. **C,** Cutting, infusion, and aspiration vitrectomy instrument removing vitreous from all parts of vitreous cavity. **D,** Removal of vitreous-saline mixture with replacement by medical-grade nitrogen during final stages of gas-fluid vitreous interchange.

REPRESENTATIVE PHOTOVAPORIZATION PATIENTS

Patient 1

A 76-year-old white female presented with an 8 × 10 disc diameter (DD) malignant melanoma of the choroid which extended approximately 6 to 8 mm. into the vitreous body. Photoradiation therapy had been attempted with some success, but because of the large size of the intraocular tumor, the red dye laser beam insufficiently penetrated the tumor for the creation of an adequate photochemical reaction. Therefore, it was decided to debulk the tumor by surgical means with CO_2 laser photovaporization.

During surgery the cataract was removed by the usual intracapsular cataract extraction technique, and a full superior iridectomy and inferior sphincterotomy were performed (Fig. 20-14). The cataract wound was sutured tightly, and pars plana vitrectomy was then accomplished. A gas-fluid interchange in the vitreous cavity was then performed by flowing medical-grade nitrogen through the vitrectomy probe, with the fluid removed through a side port. When the nitrogen had completely filled the eye, the intraocular CO_2 laser vaporization probe was placed into the vitreous cavity, with the nitrogen slowly flowing through the CO_2 laser intraocular probe and out through the vapor exit port. Direct visualization without a contact lens (or with a plano Lo-Vac lens) was accomplished in this aphakic patient.

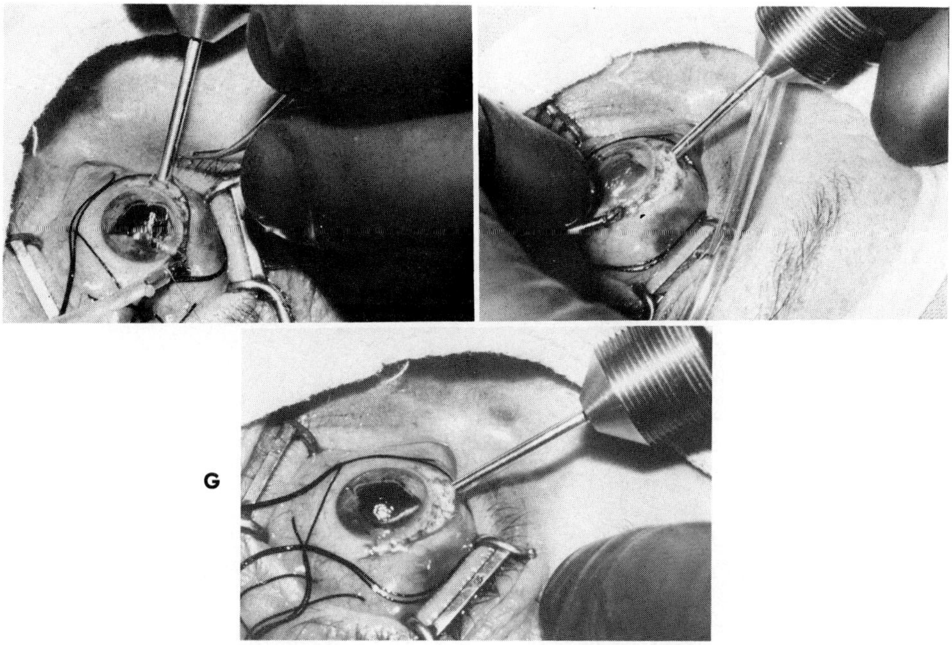

Fig. 20-14, cont'd. E, Gold-plated CO_2 laser intraocular probe during initial stages of photovaporization of choroidal malignant melanoma. **F,** Immediately following CO_2 laser photovaporization, with smoke filling anterior chamber and vitreous cavity for several seconds. Smoke and vapor were cleared through side port shown inserted at limbus. **G,** After multiple CO_2 laser photovaporization burns, tumor mass was reduced to approximately one quarter of its original size, and eye was refilled with balanced salt solution.

The photovaporization probe was kept constantly patent, and the intraocular pressure was stabilized by the gentle flow of nitrogen gas through the inside of the eye and out a previously placed 4 mm vitreous cannula to the room air. The intraocular probe was brought within 1 mm of the tumor surface, and the tumor was precisely vaporized to smoke and vapor, which was removed through the exit cannula port by the gentle flow of nitrogen gas through the laser probe within the vitreous cavity. Vaporization was continued until most of the tumor tissue had been removed. It was estimated that approximately 25% of the tumor remained after photovaporization (Fig. 20-15). The laser probe was then withdrawn, and the vitreous cavity was reconstituted with normal balanced salt solution as the residual nitrogen gas was removed. The various exit and entrance ports through the sclera were closed with sutures. Closure of the wound and

A

B

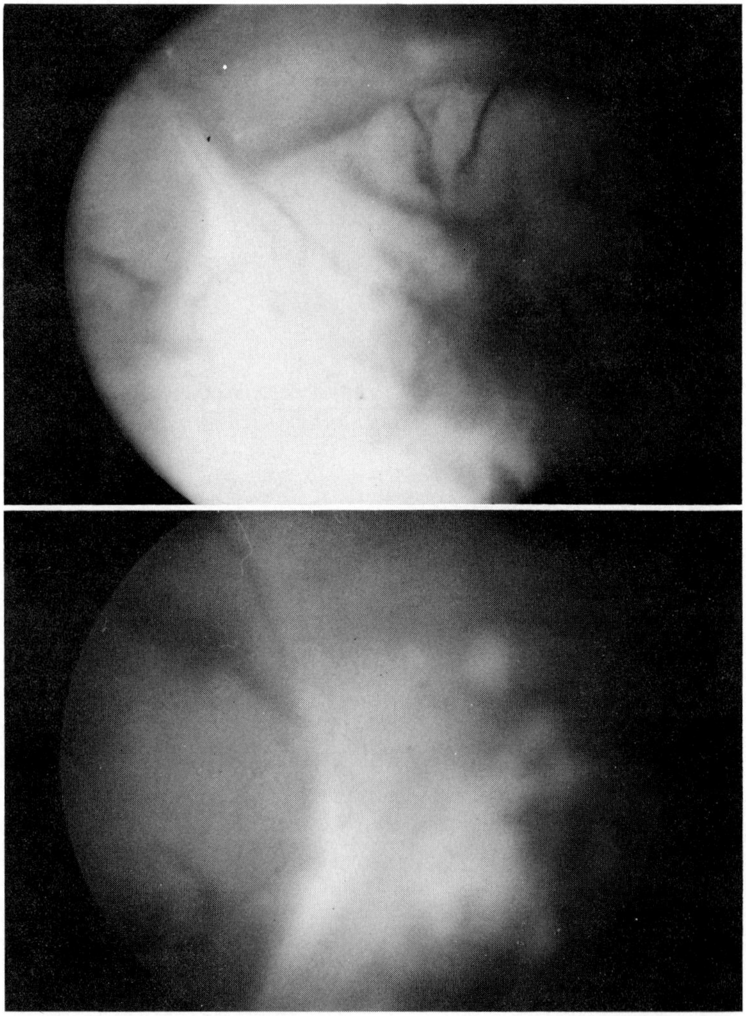

Fig. 20-15. A, Extremely large choroidal malignant melanoma extending 8 mm into the vitreous cavity before intraocular photovaporization of tumor. **B,** Same tumor 1 week after photovaporization of 75% of melanoma.

other aspects of the operative procedure were entirely similar to a routine pars plana vitrectomy with gas-fluid interchange. The only departure from this procedure was the actual vaporization of the tumor tissue by the CO_2 laser beam and the removal of the smoke and vapor by continuous flow of nitrogen through the vitreous cavity during photovaporization.

The patient healed well, and the tumor remained in its debulked state and was later subjected to additional photodynamic therapy using a hematoporphyrin derivative–dye laser therapeutic regimen. Since this procedure and the adjunct photodynamic (photoradiation) therapy, the tumor has remained in a regressed state and has been evaluated closely at monthly intervals.

Patient 2

A 42-year-old female was referred from France with an enormous infiltration of the conjunctiva of the left eye with a malignant melanoma (Fig. 20-16, *A*). Because there had been repeated attempts to excise this melanoma and great difficulty with manipulation of the tumor during surgery, the patient was prepared for CO_2 laser photovapori-

A

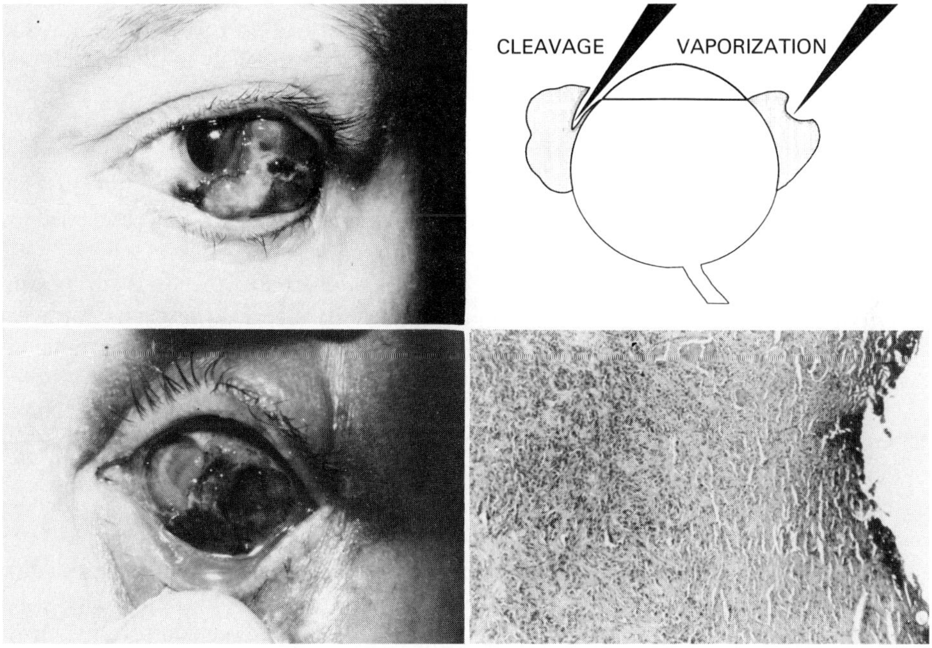

B

C

D

Fig. 20-16. A, Patient with malignant melanoma of conjunctiva that had undergone eight previous excisions. Regrowth required debulking procedure by CO_2 laser photovaporization followed by photodynamic therapy to remaining malignant cells. This original ocular appearance showed some areas of hemorrhage and extensive malignant melanoma growth in conjunctiva as well as along inner surface of upper lid of left eye. **B,** Methods of photovaporization of large, extraocular mass demonstrating knifelike incisional effect of cleavage technique and more expanded tissue vaporization process used with photovaporization therapy. **C,** Appearance of totally vaporized melanoma immediately after photovaporization with CO_2 laser beam. Both cleavage and vaporization techniques were employed to destroy the tumor down to healthy sclera and conjunctiva on globe and to tarsal plate on upper lid. **D,** Histopathologic appearance of conjunctival malignant melanoma removed by cleavage photovaporization technique. Note charring *(right)* of cells at cleavage site and some thermal damage to more centrally located cells.

zation debulking procedure. The extreme size of the tumor prevented the patient from closing her eyelid on most occasions, and a small portion of the upper lid showed a typical "kissing melanoma."

The patient was subjected to two distinct laser surgical techniques. After a small portion of the tumor had been surgically excised for histopathologic investigation, a large part of the tumor was excised by cleavage of the tumor from the sclera (Fig. 20-16, *B*). The CO_2 laser beam was directed along the surface of the sclera and tangent to it so as to incise portions of the tumor and excise them from the surface of the sclera. Another portion of the tumor overlying the cornea and a large part of the sclera was vaporized directly by the action of a slightly larger, defocused CO_2 laser beam. This portion of the tumor was completely destroyed and vaporized down to normal sclera (Fig. 20-16, *C*). The kissing melanoma on the upper lid was also completely vaporized by this method, so that the lesion was removed as well as a portion of the normal surrounding lid and conjunctival surface. At the end of the photovaporization procedure a superficial keratectomy had been performed by the laser, and all portions of the malignant melanoma had been either cleaved away or directly photovaporized so that none of the melanoma tissue remained visible on any portion of the eye or lid surface (Fig. 20-16, *D*). This patient was later subjected to photodynamic (photoradiation) therapy and appeared to do well for approximately 8 months but was lost to follow-up evaluation. When the patient did return, portions of the tumor had begun to regrow and enucleation was performed in Europe.

Other patients

Mittl, James, and I[14a] reported on a series of 23 patients who had severe neovascular glaucoma, markedly elevated intraocular pressure, complete angle closure by synechiae, moderate to severe pain, corneal disruption and disintegration and visual acuities in the range of 20/200 to hand movements. Because of the high risk of bleeding during filtration surgery, two procedures—CO_2 laser trabeculostomy and CO_2 laser sclerotrabeculostomy—were performed using the CO_2 laser to penetrate the anterior chamber and release the aqueous fluid beneath the conjunctiva or scleral flap (Fig. 20-17). A scleral flap was performed using routine trabeculectomy procedure, and the anterior chamber was entered with the CO_2 laser until a free flow of aqueous was demonstrated. With the sclerotrabeculostomy the full thickness of the sclera and the trabecular meshwork was incised with the CO_2 laser beam until the aqueous was free flowing into the subconjunctival–Tenon's fascial space. A 0.005 inch Chevron strip of medical-grade silicone rubber was inserted in the area of the trabeculostomy with both procedures to maintain the drainage system from the anterior chamber to the postequatorial region. Because of the acute inflammation in most of these eyes, it was found necessary to use the silicone seton to maintain drainage through the conjunctival and scleral scarring that usually occurred in the region of the filtration area.

Of the cases treated with CO_2 laser sclerotrabeculostomy or trabeculostomy, more than 70% have maintained a pressure of 18 mm Hg or less, with subsequent relief of corneal problems and discomfort (Fig. 20-18). More recently 90% of the cases in which a silicone seton was used have filtered well, with pressures also maintained below 18 mm Hg. The procedure appears to have considerable promise for the control of severe neovascular glaucoma, not only in eyes that are sustaining severe discomfort, but also in those that have some useful visual function remaining.

Senile keratotic lesions of the lid and conjunctiva (Fig. 20-19) and other tumors of

A

B

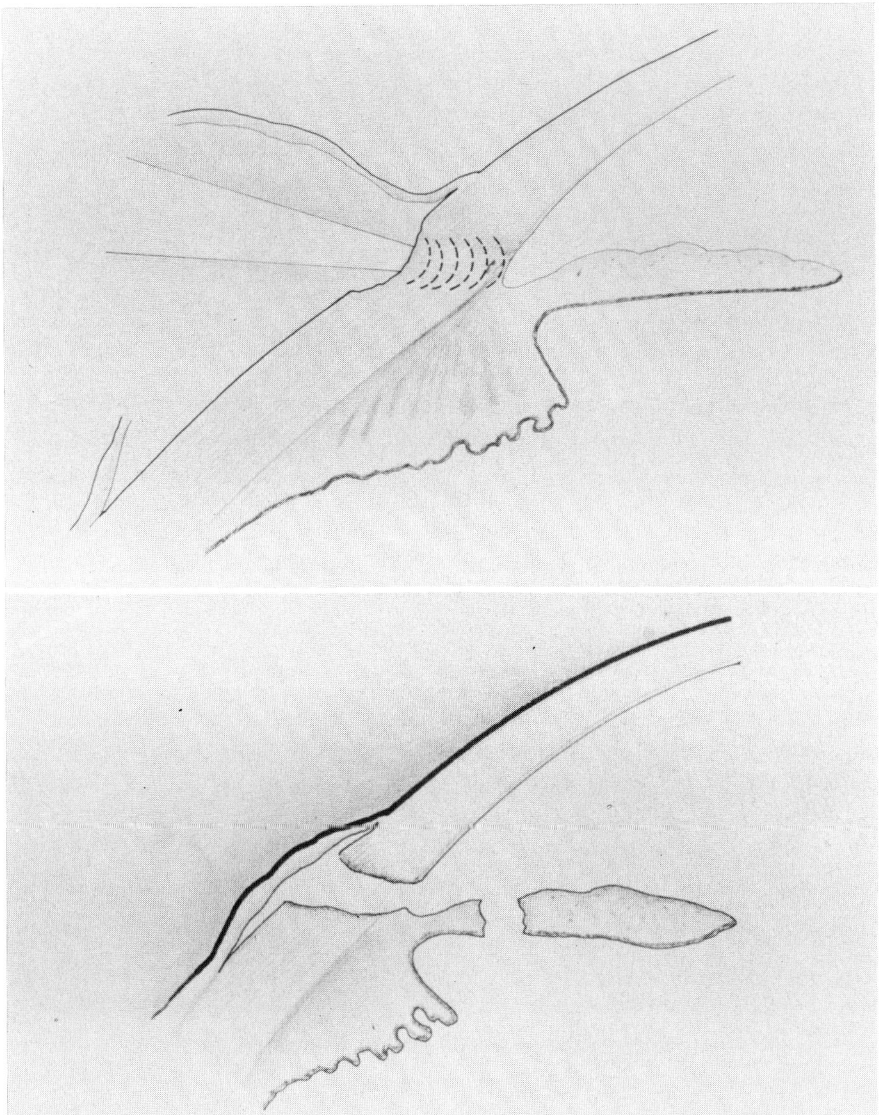

Fig. 20-17. A, External CO_2 laser sclerotrabeculostomy procedure. Conjunctiva has been dissected to limbus, and CO_2 laser beam has been applied directly to limbal area until it was vaporized into the anterior chamber with subsequent release of aqueous fluid. **B,** Appearance of eye following external laser sclerotrabeculostomy showing patent iridotomy and fistula between subconjunctival space and anterior chamber.

A

B

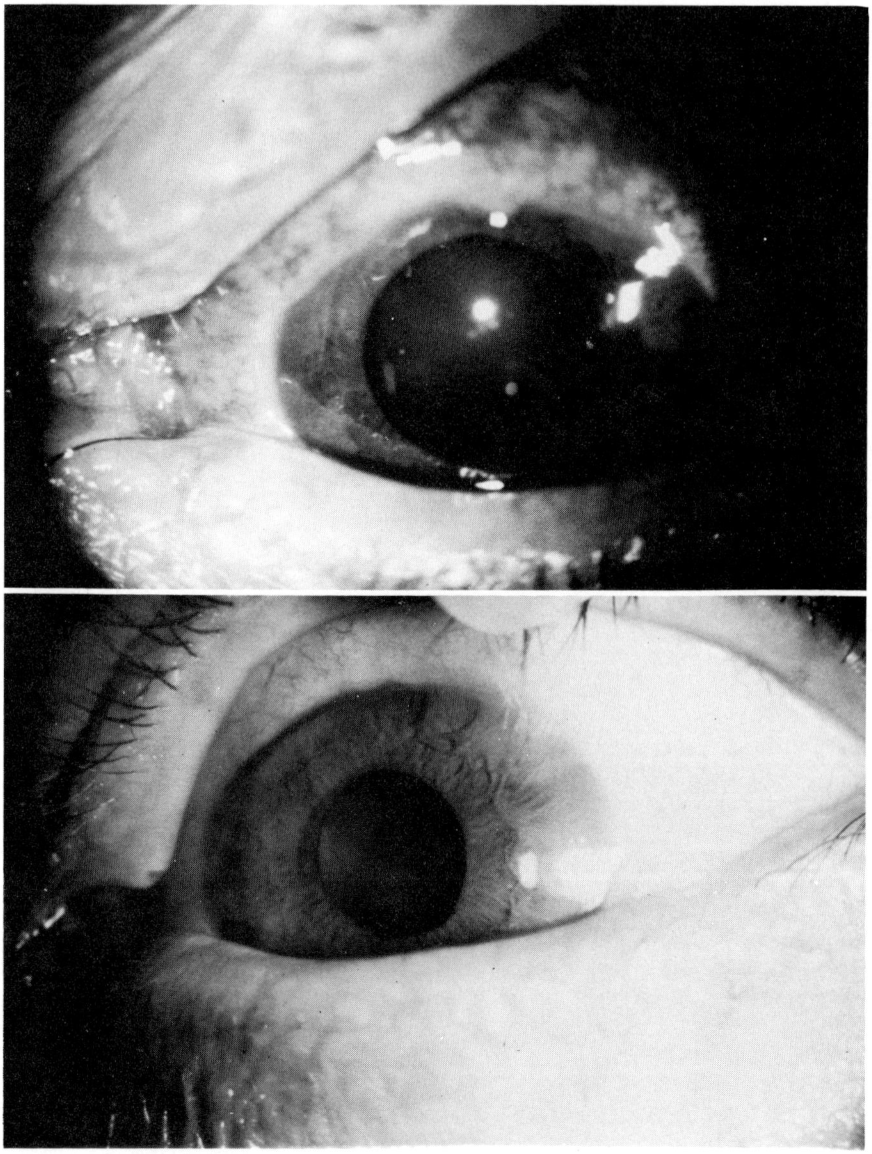

Fig. 20-18. A, Photograph of eye before external CO_2 laser sclerotrabeculostomy. Pressure is 58 mm Hg, with marked hyperemia and injection caused by extensive rubeosis iridis and neovasular glaucoma. Entire trabecular meshwork was blocked by 360 degrees of mound synechiae; patient was experiencing severe pain and could only detect hand movements before laser procedure. **B,** Three weeks after external CO_2 laser sclerotrabeculostomy with normalization of pressure to 12 mm Hg and production of healthy subconjunctival bleb. Patient's discomfort disappeared, and eye maintained vision of hand movements. Interestingly most of rubeosis iridis disappeared within several weeks following laser therapy.

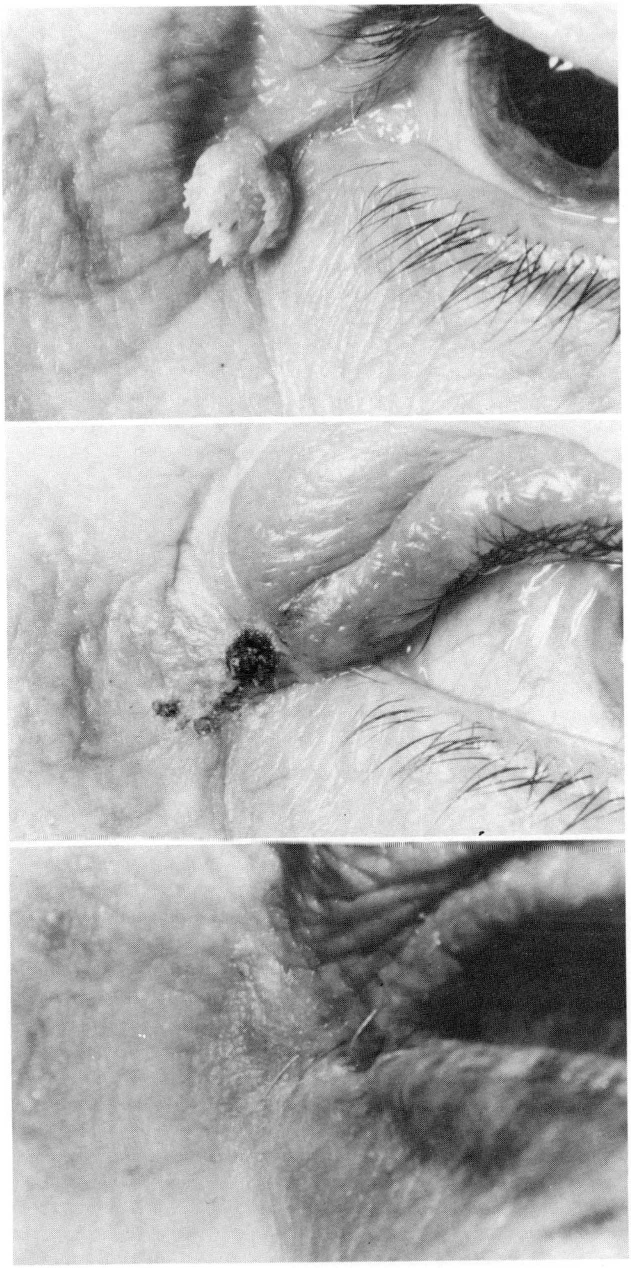

A

B

C

Fig. 20-19. A, Keratotic growth near inner canthus before CO_2 laser photovaporization. **B,** Appearance of keratotic area immediately after photovaporization. **C,** Appearance of area of photovaporized keratotic growth 3 weeks after therapy.

Table 20-1. Photovaporization of extraocular lesions

Lesion	*Number*	*Result*
Senile keratoses	8	+ + + +
Conjunctival papillomas	6	+ + + +
Pterygii	5	+
Corneal neovascularizations	3	0
Conjunctival nevi	4	+ + + +
Conjunctival varicosities	3	+ + +

+ + + + indicates best result.

the conjunctiva or lids have been removed expeditiously by CO_2 laser photovaporization (Table 20-1). It is imperative that a tumor specimen be obtained before vaporization to confirm the pathologic diagnosis and to plan the postoperative management of the patient. Pterygii respond poorly without the additional use of Grentz rays or some other local x-radiation. Telangiectic vessels, lymphoceles, and various melanotic or solid growths on the conjunctiva can be removed without bleeding and with total extirpation of the tumor.

SUMMARY

Although other high-powered lasers such as the argon or the frequency-doubled neodymium-YAG can produce excellent photovaporization results, photovaporization with the CO_2 laser appears to be an excellent method for removing lesions, with a minishaving technique for reducing the tumor mass. Intraocular and extraocular photovaporization with any of the high-powered lasers, particularly the CO_2, will become a vital part of our armamentarium, especially with lesions that demand marked hemostasis, bacteriostasis, lymphostasis, and exquisite cutting ability during the surgical procedure.

ACKNOWLEDGMENT

I would like to acknowledge the invaluable assistance of Beth Ann Hughes, Ruth J. Helmich, Paul Saivetz, and Virginia H. Cantarella.

REFERENCES

1. Auth, D.C.: Techniques for burn wound debridement, J. Trauma, **11:**926, 1979.
2. Baker, S.S., and others: Carbon Dioxide laser blepharoplasty, Ophthalmology. (In press.)
3. Beckman, H., and Fuller, T.A.: Carbon dioxide laser scleral dissections and filtering procedure for glaucoma, Am. J. Ophthalmol. **88:**73, 1979.
4. Beckman, H., and others: Limbectomies, keratectomies, and keratostomies performed with a rapid-pulsed carbon dioxide laser, Am. J. Ophthalmol. **71:**1277, 1971.
5. Bellina, J.H.: Gynecology and the laser, Contemp. Obstet. Gynecol. **4**(3):42, 1974.
6. Bellina, J.H.: Carbon dioxide laser in gynecology, Obstet. Gynecol. Annu. **6:**371, 1977.
7. Campbell, C.J., and others: Ocular efforts produced by experimental laser. II. Carbon dioxide laser, Am. J. Ophthalmol. **66:**604, 1968.
8. Fine, B.S., Fine, S., and Peacock, G.R.: Preliminary observations on ocular effects of high-power, continuous carbon dioxide laser irradiation, Am. J. Ophthalmol. **64:**209, 1967.
9. Goldman, L., and Rockwell, R.J.: Lasers in medicine, New York, 1971, Gordon & Breach.
10. Jako, G.J.: Laser surgery of the vocal chords: an experimental study with the carbon dioxide laser on dogs, Laryngoscope **82:**2204, 1972.
11. Jako, G.J., and Polanyi, T.G.: Carbon dioxide laser surgery in otolaryngology. In Kaplan, I., editor: Laser Surgery, Jerusalem, 1976, Academic Press, Inc.

12. Kaplan, I., and Peled, I.: The carbon dioxide treatment of superficial telangiectases, Br. J. Plast. Surg. **18:**214, 1975.
13. Kaplan, I., and others: The treatment of erosions of the uterine cervix by means of the carbon dioxide laser, Obstet. Gynecol. **41:**795, 1973.
14. L'Esperance, F.A., Jr.: Ocular photocoagulation: a stereoscopic atlas, St. Louis, 1975, The C.V. Mosby Co., p. 317.
14a. L'Esperance, F.A., Jr., Mittl, R., and James, W.A., Jr.: Carbon dioxide laser trabeculostomy for the treatment of neovascular glaucoma, Ophthalmology **90:**821, 1983.
15. Levine, N.S., and others: Clinical evaluation of the carbon dioxide laser for burn wound excisions: a comparison of the laser, scalpel, and electrocautery, J. Trauma **15:**800, 1972.
16. Miller, J.B., Smith, M.R., and Boyer, D.S.: Intraocular carbon dioxide laser photocautery. II. Preliminary report of clinical trials, Arch. Ophthalmol. **97:**2123, 1979.
16a. Miller, J.B., Smith M.R., and Pincus, F.: Intraocular carbon dioxide laser photocautery. I. Animal experimentation, Arch. Ophthalmol. **97:**2157, 1979.
17. Patel, C.K.N.: Interpretation of carbon dioxide optical laser experiments, Phys. Rev. Lett. **12:**588, 1964.
18. Peyman, G.A., and Raichand, M.: Full-thickness eye wall resection of choroidal neoplasms, Ophthalmology, **86:**1024, 1979.
19. Stellar, S., and others: Lasers in surgery. In Wolbarsht, M.L., editor: Laser applications in medicine and biology. Vol. 2, New York, 1974, Plenum Press.
20. Strong, M.S.: Laser surgery in the larynx: early clinical experience with the continuous carbon dioxide laser, Ann. Otolaryngol. **81:**791, 1972.
21. Ticho, J., and others: Carbon dioxide laser filtering surgery in hemorrhagic glaucoma, Glaucoma **1:**114, 1979.

21

Laser treatment of macular disease: recurrence of subretinal neovascular membranes after treatment

Robert C. Watzke

Two weeks after a membrane has been successfully treated with argon blue-green, argon green, or krypton red photocoagulation, pigment will begin to appear in the membrane, and the surrounding serous detachment will regress or at least stabilize. Although vision may have been temporarily worsened by treatment at this time, it will usually be at the pretreatment level. If hemorrhages were present before or have occurred during treatment, they are usually smaller after 2 weeks. An isolated hemorrhage within and surrounded by a photocoagulation scar does not mean an unfavorable prognosis.

A fluorescein angiogram done 2 weeks after argon photocoagulation will show such diffuse leakage into the inner retina that it is virtually useless (see Chapter 17). However, a fluorescein angiogram taken 24 hours after krypton red photocoagulation will show blocked fluorescence in the early transit, presumably a result of closure and necrosis of outer retina, pigment epithelium, and choriocapillaris without inner retinal edema (Fig. 21-1).

As remodeling and atrophy of the pigment epithelium occurs, the scar begins to show transmission defects and late hyperfluorescence, particularly at the margin. This "edge hyperfluorescence" is uniform and fades gradually, as shown by a later angiogram (Fig. 21-2). It probably results from leakage of dye from open vessels in the choriocapillaris at the margin of the scar. It should not be confused with marginal leakage caused by a recurrent subretinal membrane.

CENTRAL RESIDUAL VESSELS

It is common to see central hyperfluorescence and leakage at the 1-month angiogram (argon) or 2-week angiogram (krypton) (Fig. 21-3). This is probably caused by residual necrotic neovascular tissue and does not require immediate retreatment. Most central staining resolves as the scar remodels and becomes atrophic. If central hyperfluorescence and leakage persists after 1 month, and there is continued serous detachment with no other visible cause, the central scar should be retreated.

Text continued on p. 262.

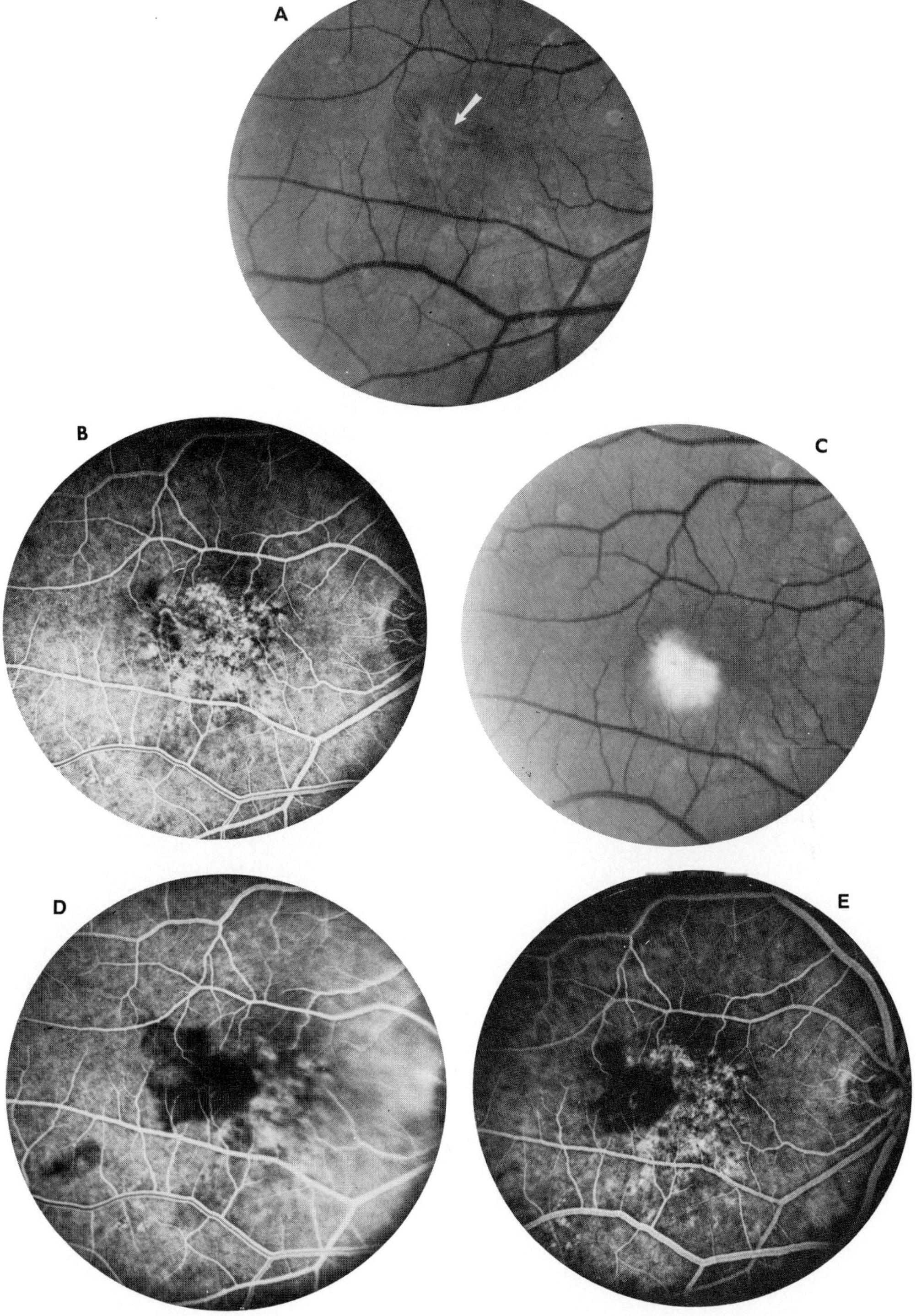

Fig. 21-1. **A,** Subretinal neovascular membrane *(arrow)* temporal to fovea in 54-year-old man. **B,** Early angiogram shows neovascular tissue with many drusen elsewhere. **C,** View after treatment with intense krypton red laser photocoagulation. **D,** Early angiogram 24 hours later shows complete blockage of treated area. **E,** In midphase there is central leakage of fluorescein from inner retinal vessels over zone of blocked fluorescence.

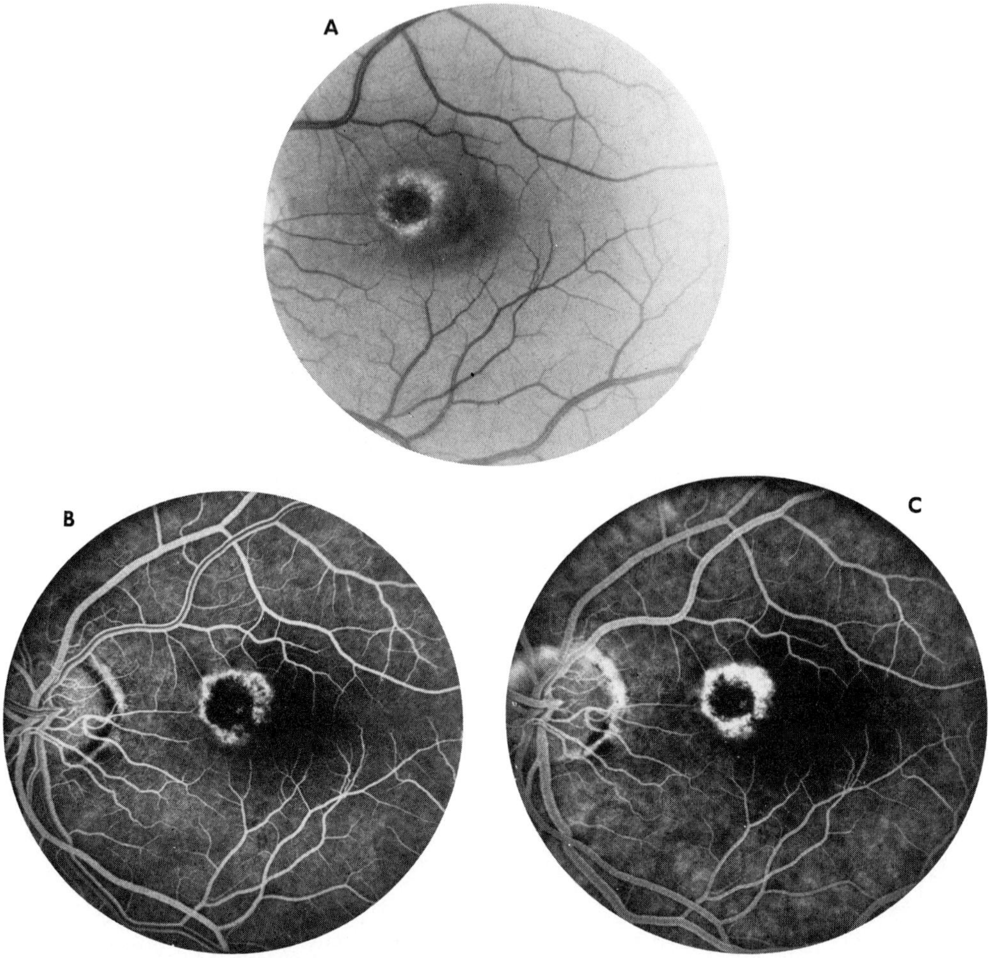

Fig. 21-2. A, Treatment scar of patient after successful argon blue-green photocoagulation. There is marginal hyperfluorescence in **B,** early, and **C,** late angiogram because of pigment epithelial atrophy and leakage from choriocapillaris.

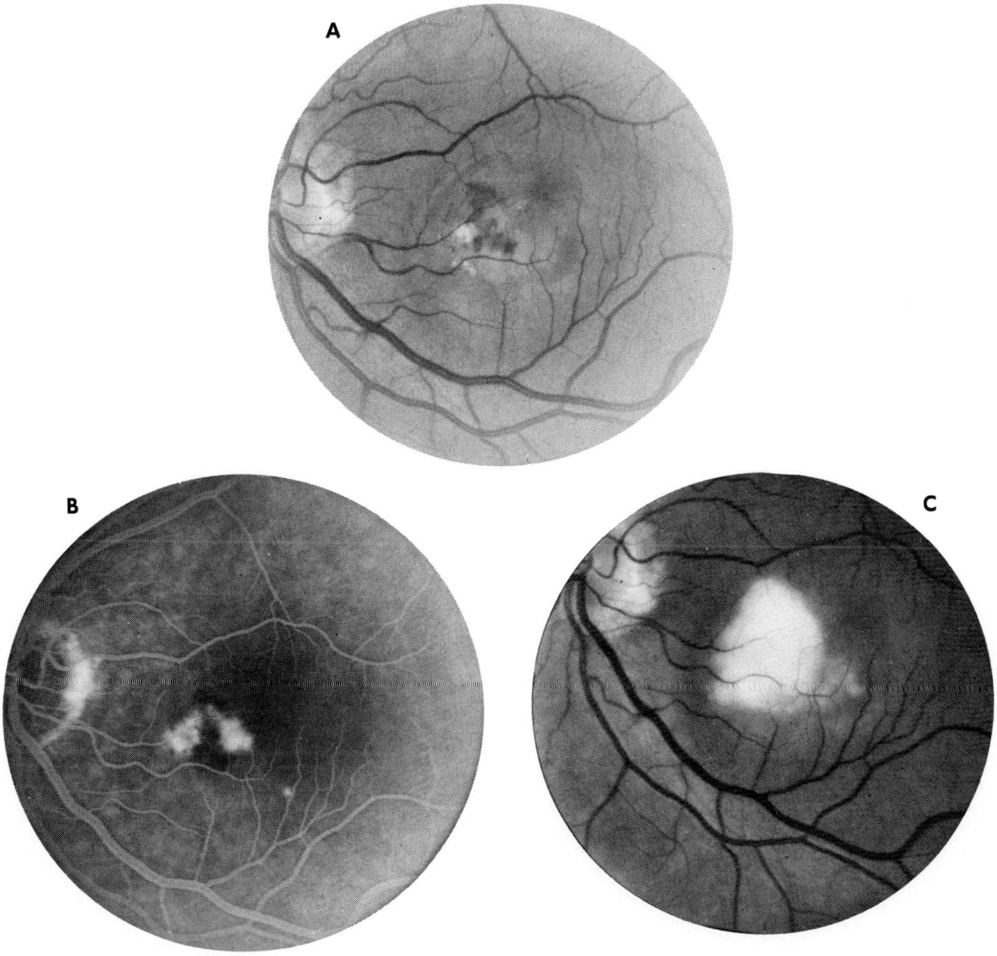

Fig. 21-3. A, Subretinal membrane with serous detachment and hemorrhage outside avascular zone. **B,** Pretreatment angiogram shows membrane to be treatable with argon blue-green photocoagulation. **C,** After treatment with intense argon blue-green therapy. *Continued.*

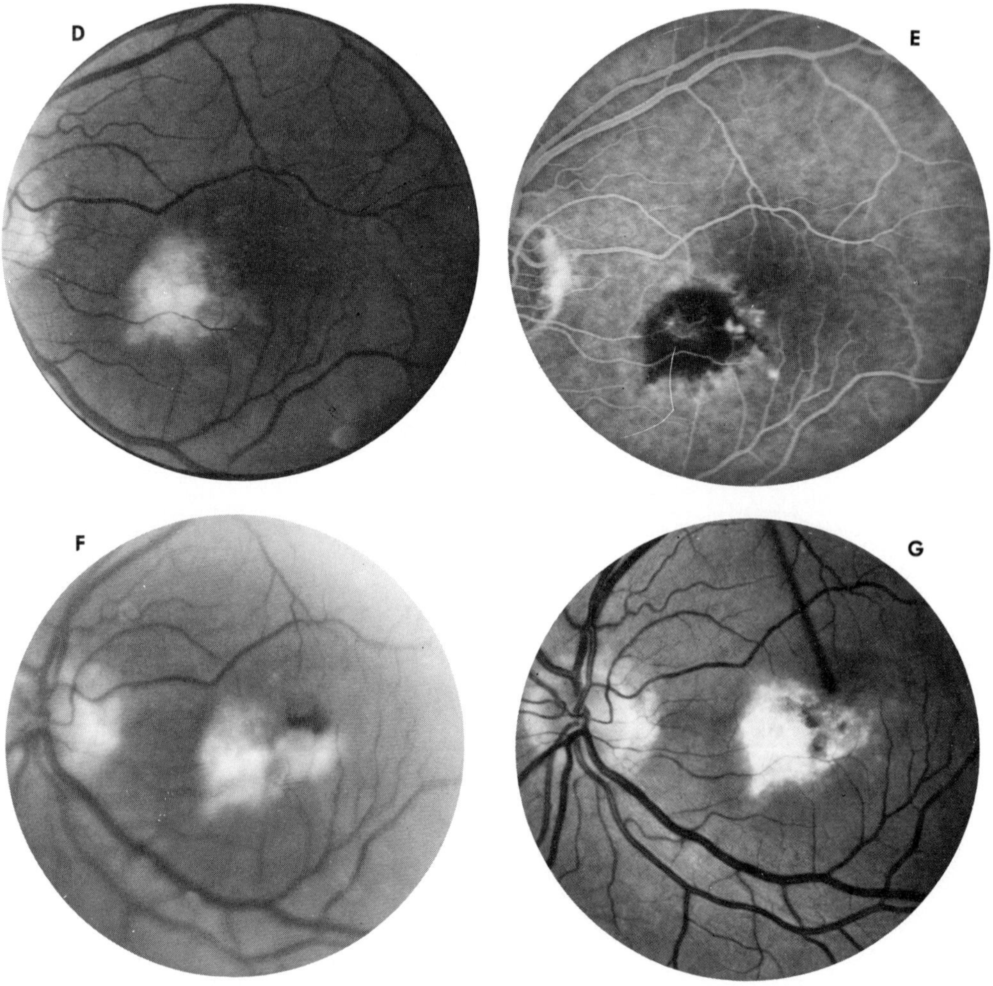

Fig. 21-3, cont'd. D, One month later scar is forming. **E,** There is hyperfluorescence and leakage from tissue in center of scar and at inferotemporal margin. **F,** Marginal area was later photocoagulated with krypton red laser after it had bled a few days before treatment. **G,** Two months later there is no serous detachment, and vision is 20/40.

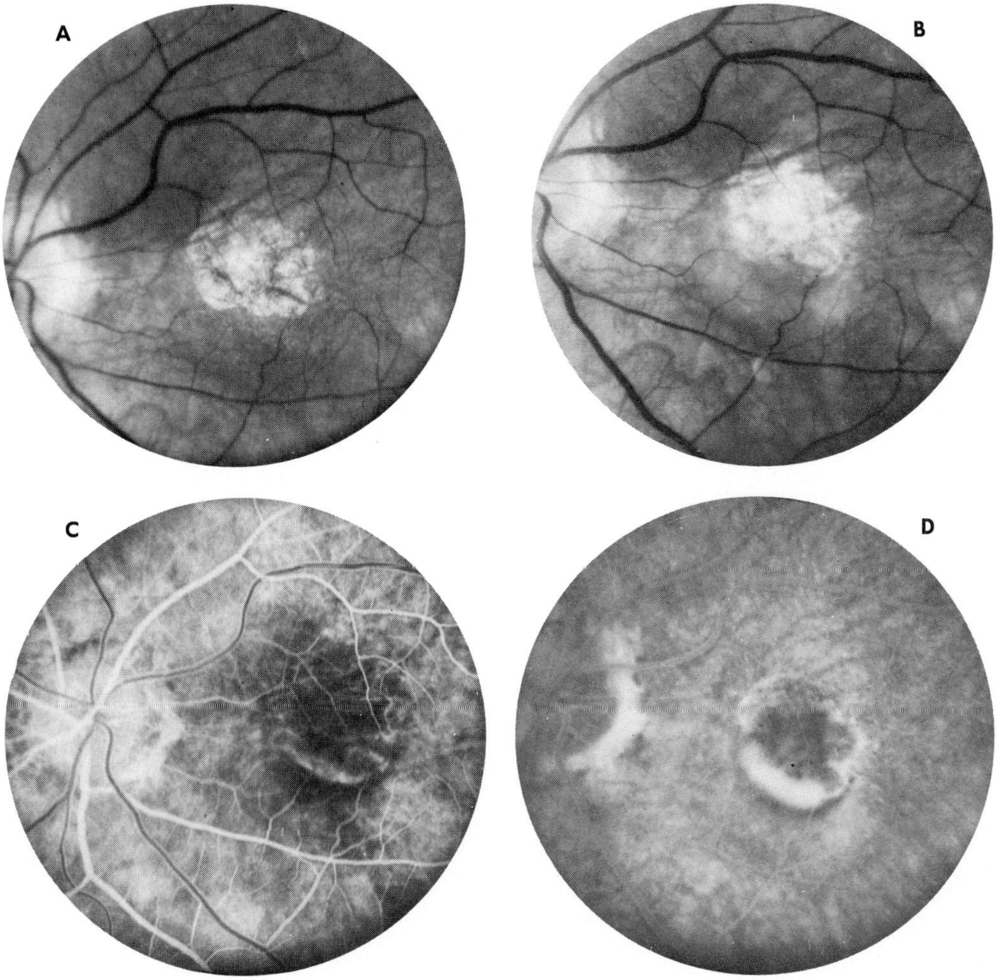

Fig. 21-4. A, Central scar 2 months after krypton laser photocoagulation to subretinal membrane near center of fovea. Vision is 20/50 (eccentric). **B,** Five months later vision is 20/200, and there is a serous detachment at lower margin of scar. **C** and **D,** Hyperfluorescence and leakage at inferior margin caused by recurrent neovascular membrane. Patient was not retreated.

MARGINAL RECURRENT SUBRETINAL MEMBRANES

The most common type of recurrent or residual subretinal neovascular membrane is regrowth and extent of neovascular tissue from the edge of the treatment scar. This is why it is so important to cover all of the membrane and pigment with intense photocoagulation. Despite this, the physician may see as early as 2 weeks or even several years later a pigmented nodular swelling, with serous detachment and retinal hemorrhage at or extending from the edge of the photocoagulation scar. An angiogram will show a hyperfluorescent spot from which fluorescein leaks that is much more intense and extreme than the normal edge hyperfluorescence (Fig. 21-3).

Marginal recurrence is the common response of vessels that have been inadequately treated. These vessels will usually be seen on the first angiogram; however, marginal vessels can occur at any time at the margin of the treatment scars. The edges should therefore be carefully scrutinized.

These vessels should be retreated with the appropriate laser as soon as they are diagnosed, or the final visual result will be no better than if treatment had never been done.

LATE RECURRENCE

The long-term stability of laser photocoagulation scars has not been documented. Since treatment has usually been done for eyes in which subretinal neovascular membranes are part of the degenerative disease, new areas of neovascular membranes at the margin of apparently stable and atrophic scars is occasionally seen after several months or years (Fig. 21-4). Patients must be counseled to check their vision frequently, to watch for changes in their paracentral scotomas, and to look for metamorphopsia on an Amsler grid. Although laser photocoagulation is effective for treating one phase of macular degeneration, it does not cure the basic disease.

22

The future of glaucoma filtering operations

Harry A. Quigley

With the increased interest in laser treatment for the glaucomas, many may think surgical operations are headed for obsolescence. In this brief discussion I will suggest that surgery is far from dead as a needed step in glaucoma treatment. Furthermore, new information and research approaches are raising hopes that the surgical cure of glaucoma may be an answer for many glaucomatous eyes in the near future.

HAS THE LASER KILLED THE FILTER?

After the introduction of laser trabeculotomy by Krasnov[5] and initial laboratory and clinical trials by Worthen and Wickham[13] and Ticho and Zauberman,[11] Wise and Witter[12] reported initial success with what is now known as laser trabeculoplasty. In the 5 years since this treatment was introduced and modified, it has proved useful in many patients. However, the many studies on this subject by many large centers make it clear that the present argon laser trabeculoplasty (ALT) is not the cure for glaucoma. In patients who would otherwise have gone on to filtering surgery in the past, a substantial proportion now have their intraocular pressure (IOP) reduced to levels that are considered safe. It will be some time before we determine whether the visual function of these patients has benefited more from this approach than from the filtering surgery they would have had. Unfortunately no study ever randomly assorted eyes to ALT and filters to determine this point. Instead we have data that show that IOP can be lowered to a level generally considered safe for extended periods. This may or may not be the best choice for these patients.

The successful ALT patient who was on maximum medical therapy before laser treatment is almost always still taking drops or pills later to hold IOP down. It can be argued from the data of many surgical series that a much higher percentage of filtered patients can cease taking any medicine for at least the length of follow-up reported. Kass and co-workers have recently pointed out that the compliance with medical therapy is far less than what we hope patients will do. Thus there is the strong possibility that if ALT and filters were compared, this factor would give surgery an advantage in long-term visual field preservation. We are constantly working on more effective laser treatments to change this continued need for medication, but it remains true at present.

It is also true that the patient who undergoes ALT or filtering surgery incurs a significant risk to vision from the treatment itself. The IOP elevation that occurs transiently after ALT and the unknown long-term risk to the eye represent its greatest potential threats. Filtering surgery exposes the patient to the risks of anesthesia, hypotony and cataract hastening, and early and late endophthalmitis. Clearly ALT compares favorably when considering these infrequent but devastating surgical problems, which is why it has taken a deserved place between failed medical treatment and surgery.

At our institution, however, filtering surgery continues to be required in many eyes. Some are those eyes that rarely respond to laser therapy; in others it is impossible. Among this group are children, patients with major primary or secondary angle closure, uveitic patients, and those with past ocular surgeries. In addition, we continue to experience a failure of ALT to control a substantial minority of difficult glaucoma patients. Some authorities, particularly Watson and Cairns of Great Britain, even argue effectively that we should be using filtering surgery much earlier in glaucoma management. Likewise, a national trial of initial ALT compared to initial medical therapy is beginning. As we reconsider all of our treatment concepts, we should take stock of what works now and what new information we need. I propose that ALT is an important new step but is far from ideal, and surgery is still necessary in many eyes. What improvements in filtering surgery should we make, and how are we to implement these changes?

WHY DOES FILTERING SURGERY FAIL?

In the comparison of ALT and surgery I suggested that both were reasonably successful, but there are greater risks from surgery. In order for us to run these risks with our patients, the success rate of surgery must be quite high. Unfortunately this is far less than perfect, especially in those eyes that need it most. These are the same ones that do not respond well to ALT—eyes in young patients, inflamed eyes, and those previously operated on and complicated. In the last few years a number of new approaches to filtering surgery have been undertaken. The idea behind several of these[6,8,10] is to use an artificial device to carry fluid out of the anterior chamber to the subconjunctival space or beyond. In considering the potential usefulness of these devices, we must look at why filters fail.

In our laboratory[1] we obtained a number of specimens of tissue from eyes that had undergone both successful and failed glaucoma surgery. We were able to confirm the impression that is gained from reoperating on failed eyes in the operating room. The difference between the successful and failed blebs was the greater thickness and density of collagenous connective tissue in the subconjunctiva of the failures. Some blebs that are elevated, solid structures have walls as thick as the cornea. Whereas fluid can move through such tissue slowly, the rate of fluid movement is simply not rapid enough to prevent IOP elevation. Blebs that are successful in maintaining low IOP share clear spaces in the subepithelial conjunctiva that are relatively free of extracellular matrix components. These microcystic spaces can be observed at the slitlamp and serve as a good sign of functional filtration. Thus the difference between success and failure is to keep the subepithelial conjunctiva—or the zone to which aqueous is shunted in seton operations—from becoming a dense connnective tissue.

The chief cell type responsible for our problems is the fibroblast. Histologic studies of experimental filtering operations show that the fibroblast responds to the filtering opening by rapid proliferation and by synthesis of extracellular "glue" chiefly glycosaminoglycans and collagen.[7] The problem is not the surgeon's inability to make a satisfactory hole from anterior chamber to subconjunctiva; the problem is that as aqueous fluid arrives at Tenon's capsule area, it is blocked from further exit.

The chief difficulty to be attacked, therefore, is to circumvent the body's normal healing response, which is carried out by fibroblasts. It should be immediately obvious from this discussion why filters fail more commonly in certain groups whose normal healing response is intact or even constantly activated. The young or inflamed eye and those eyes with past scarring simply have too strong a stimulus to fibroblast proliferation and synthesis to allow the development of the appropriate conjunctival setting for a good bleb.

These facts should also point to a potential problem with some of the new seton operations. If the seton tube leads simply from the anterior chamber to the subconjunctiva, then the failure by scarring at this usual locus for failure is unaffected. The presence of plastic materials not only leads to problems with erosion through the tissues, but can generate a foreign body reaction that contributes to the chance of fibroblast stimulation and ultimate failure. Other seton systems have been devised that carry aqueous off to the spaces more posteriorly—to encircling elements or to posterior implants. Further experience with such devices will show whether they are prone to failure for the same reasons as other filters—scarring by fibroblast healing. It would be most helpful if the developers of new procedures would subject their methods to comparisons with other procedures in a controlled fashion.

WHAT CAN BE DONE TO KEEP FILTERS FROM FAILING?

A number of potential attacks on the failure mechanism could be productive. First, we could attempt to stop the fibroblasts from proliferating in the early phase of healing. This would mandate the use of drugs that are useful as anticancer agents because of their ability to prevent cell division. Second, we could try to prevent fibroblasts from synthesizing collagen effectively. Third, we could inhibit synthesis of glycosaminoglycans. Finally, we could attempt to dissolve formed extracellular matrix. In a sense we have always tried to do this with an agent that does most of these things to some degree—corticosteroids. However, if this class of drug could have solved our problem, it would already have done so. Let us consider potential approaches in each of these categories.

A number of agents are already available that suppress cell division. Our problem is to select that agent or combination that can hurt the fibroblast worst, while allowing the conjunctival and corneal epithelium to heal after surgery. Also, the selection of any new agent must be accompanied by the strictest possible attention to ocular and systemic toxicity. Any drug placed on the cornea or under a bleb will contact internal ocular structures at concentrations possibly similar to those applied. The retina and lens must be able to tolerate exposure to the therapy without unacceptable adverse reaction. By testing drugs on cultured cells, Blumenkranz and co-workers[2] found 5-fluorouracil to be effective and relatively nontoxic for this purpose. The drug can be injected directly into the eye to counter intraocular proliferative disorders. Initial studies on 10 primates and a series of human eyes[4,9] have led to enthusiasm for this drug's possible usefulness in glaucoma surgery. Remaining questions include how to deal best with the poor healing of conjunctiva and cornea when the antidivision-type drug is given, and what systemic toxicity is possible. Animal studies of systemic drug levels and effects on bone marrow and other organ systems should be undertaken. Our research group has recently begun testing methotrexate and other agents of this class in a glaucoma filtering, surgical model system in primates.

A second approach of potential benefit is to destroy the effective synthesis of collagen by the fibroblast. Mason, Hohman, and I[7] researched the drug cis-hydroxyproline with this intent. The molecule is the incorrect stereoisomer of a precursor of collagen, trans-hydroxyproline. We hoped that we could achieve substantial concentrations of the agent at a time when maximum uptake by fibroblasts was occurring, leading to defective collagen synthesis. There was, however, no prolongation of the life of experimental filtering blebs in eyes treated in masked fashion with this drug compared to controls. A second agent aiming at a similar portion of the healing response shows more promise. Beta-aminopropionitrile inhibits the cross-linking of collagen and prevents it from achieving maximum normal fiber diameter and strength. Administering this agent to animals that had filtering surgery did produce prolongation of bleb life to some degree.[7] The agent has been used systemically in human beings for other disorders and is now being tried in human eyes with glaucoma surgery.

The inhibition of mucopolysaccharide (glycosaminoglycan) synthesis is, as far as I know, still untried as a method. Although one could attack all intracellular synthetic pathways in a nonspecific fashion, this would likely injure innocent bystanding cells and produce unwanted toxicity. It is attractive to also consider the possibility of dissolving already formed glycosaminoglycans in the extracellular matrix. Since these molecules form a sizable proportion of the matrix and help to bond the other components together, debulking the bleb of their presence could be an advantage. The available agents have thus far seemed too toxic and too liable to dissolving adjacent structures.

The search for a biochemical aid in filtering surgery should not be directed at only one agent. As with anticancer therapy, the best approach may well turn out to be combination chemotherapy, with an antidivision agent aided by a collagen synthesis inhibitor and other drugs.[3] This might also allow the use of a highly toxic agent at a low enough concentration to be safe, although at a dose that by itself it would be insufficient.

The delivery of new agents to improve filtering surgical success is likely to involve a number of routes. In some cases we have used systemic drugs; systemic steroids now are used in some filtering surgical patients, and we have delivered beta-aminopropionitrile systemically to primates. This is the least satisfactory choice. We wish to suppress healing reponse of approximately 25 square millimeters of conjunctiva—to immunosuppress the entire body for this purpose should be our last choice. Injection under the conjunctiva is an efficient means of delivery to the involved site. However, repeating such injections is likely to be necessary, and this becomes not only uncomfortable for the patient and inconvenient (daily office visits), but also might contribute to bleb scarring by the repeated trauma and occasional hemorrhage. Eyedrop delivery is a good choice but presupposes that the agent successfully penetrates the epithelial tissues in effective concentration. This mode also exposes the conjunctival and corneal epithelium repeatedly to agents that might influence their normal function. Steroids can inhibit epithelial healing and predispose to superinfection when delivered by this route, and the bathing of the anterior ocular surface with 5-fluorouracil has given rise to significant problems. The ideal system would be the subepithelial implantation of enough drug(s) to avoid the need for repeated dosage by another route. The Ocusert pilocarpine system demonstrated the feasibility of such methods, and we have placed some of our experimental drugs in the primate glaucoma model system in flat pellets of synthetic matrix to be buried in the sclera under the bleb site. This leaves foreign material present, which is undesirable, as already noted. However, if it replaces repeated drop or injection delivery for a sufficient time to establish bleb formation, this factor might be outweighed.

SUMMARY

Trabeculectomy and its variations are far from obsolete in glaucoma management, and many eyes remain with a need for IOP control that is unsatisfied by medical therapy and ALT. Filtering surgery has the great potential advantage of eliminating the need for medication in many successfully treated eyes. However, its present success rate is insufficient to outweigh the infrequent but substantial risks in its use. Improvements in filtering surgery are being attempted by a number of experimental approaches. The approach that appeals to me most is the frontal assault on the chief cause for filtering surgery failure—fibroblast-initiated scarring in the episcleral area.

REFERENCES

1. Addicks, E.M., and others: Histologic characteristics of filtering blebs in glaucomatous eyes, Arch. Ophthalmol. **101:**795, 1983.
2. Blumenkranz, M.S., and others: Fluorouracil for the treatment of massive periretinalproliferation, Am. J. Ophthalmol. **94:**458, 1982.
3. Brancato, L.J., and Yablonski, M.E.: Effect of dexamethasone and D-penicillamine on filter surgery, Invest. Ophthalmol. Vis. Sci. **24**(suppl.):87, 1983.
4. Gressel, M., and Parrish, R.K.: Fluorouracil and healing of posterior lip sclerectomies in owl monkeys, Invest. Ophthalmol. Vis. Sci. **24**(suppl.):87, 1983.
5. Krasnov, M.M.: Laseropuncture of anterior chamber angle in glaucoma, Am. J. Ophthalmol. **75:**674, 1973.
6. Krupin, T., and others: Long-term results of valve implants in filtering surgery for eyes with neovascular glaucoma, Am. J. Ophthalmol. **95:**775, 1983.
7. Mason, R.P., Quigley, H.A., and Hohman, R.M.: Experimental glaucoma filtering surgery in primates, Invest. Ophthalmol. Vis. Sci. **24**(suppl.):87, 1983.
8. Molteno, A.C.B., van Rooyen, M.M.B., and Bartholomew, R.S.: Implants for draining neovascular glaucoma, Br. J. Ophthalmol. **61:**120, 1977.
9. Parrish, R.K., and others: 5-Fluorouracil and glaucoma filtration surgery—a clinical study, Invest. Ophthalmol. Vis. Sci. **24**(suppl.):2, 1983.
10. Schockett, S.S., Lakhanpal, V., and Richards, R.D.: Anterior chamber tube shunt to an encircling band in the treatment of neovascular glaucoma, Ophthalmology **89:**1188, 1982.
11. Ticho, U., and Zauberman, H.: Argon laser application to the angle structures in the glaucomas, Arch. Ophthalmol. **94:**61, 1976.
12. Wise, J.B., and Witter, S.L.: Argon laser therapy for open angle glaucoma: a pilot study, Arch. Ophthalmol. **97:**319, 1979.
13. Worthen, D.M., and Wickham, M.G.: Argon laser trabeculotomy, Trans. Am. Acad. Ophthalmol. Otolaryngol. **78:**371, 1974.

23

Special features and modifications of laser trabeculoplasty: where are we today?

Richard J. Simmons
John V. Thomas*
James A. Savage*
C. Davis Belcher III*

All of those involved in glaucoma treatment and research owe a debt to Dr. James Wise, who recommended laser trabeculoplasty for open-angle glaucoma and suggested parameters that were immediately effective and safe. Although further modifications and knowledge have been added, the basic recommendations were very sound, accurate, and reproducible. We think, therefore, that Dr. Wise should be clearly thanked for giving us this therapy which offers great benefits to glaucoma patients. Naturally details of its use, the benefits, potential complications, and correct pattern of usage should be evaluated thoroughly and be familiar to all who employ the technique, but discussions of complications and correct use do not and cannot detract from the marked advance that this technique represents.

Since the initial report of argon laser trabeculoplasty as a successful treatment for open-angle glaucoma,[26] our group has treated more than 1400 eyes with this therapeutic modality. The experience discussed in this chapter also involves our colleagues, Stephen R. Deppermann and Thomas M. Richardson.

With time it has become apparent that laser trabeculoplasty may produce beneficial effects in a variety of situations. We have learned that the procedure may have certain serious complications and that certain techniques may be used to minimize them. It is the purpose of this chapter to examine our present understanding of trabeculoplasty and its place in glaucoma therapy.

TECHNIQUE

Instrumentation

Many different brands of argon laser machines are available at present. Two of the brands we use are the MIRA MF 2050 and the Coherent System 900 argon laser. The krypton laser has also been found to be equivalent in effectiveness to the argon green or blue-green laser in performing trabeculoplasty.[16] Although the neodymium (Nd)-

*M.D.s, Glaucoma Consultation Service, Massachusetts Eye and Ear Infirmary, Harvard Medical School and the New England Glaucoma Research Foundation, Boston.

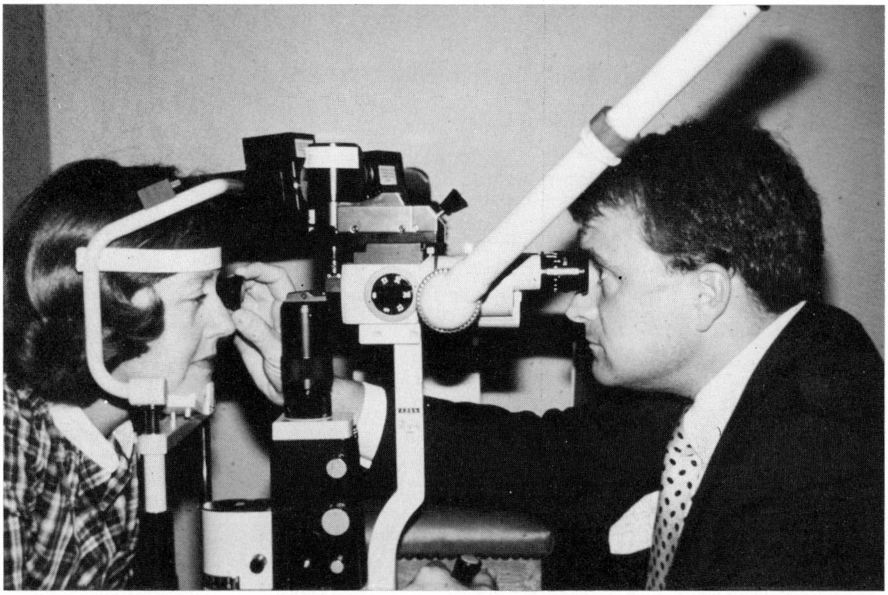

Fig. 23-1. Correct positioning of patient and surgeon for laser therapy. Patient leans forward so that forward excursion of slitlamp body is unimpeded by his body. For comfort, surgeon rests the elbow on book or specially prepared arm rest, such as shown.

YAG laser has multiple uses in the anterior segment, its value in performing trabeculoplasty using the thermal mode has not been sufficiently explored. It is important not to equate ''trabeculopuncture'' lesions, which would be produced by the Nd:YAG laser in its ''disruptive'' mode, with the thermal changes induced on the trabecular meshwork with the argon laser.

Fig. 23-1 shows positioning of patient and physician during laser treatment.

Laser settings and laser energy delivery

We continue to use laser settings for trabeculoplasty similar to those proposed by Wise[26]: a spot size of 50 μ (sharply focused), exposure of 0.1 second per application, and 100 applications, with some variations. Although Wise suggested using a power level of 1000 mW, we have varied the power from 700 to 1000 mW, depending on the degree of pigmentation of the meshwork. The laser applications are evenly spaced on the trabecular meshwork, approximately 3.6 degrees apart, resulting in approximately 50 applications per 6 clock hours of angle (see boxed material). The aiming beam is focused very sharply before each application to achieve a more consistent spot size. The desired end point on pigmented meshwork is creation of a blanched spot with a small gas bubble. Large explosions with many bubbles and scattering of copious pigmented debris due to use of excessive power settings in heavily pigmented angles should be avoided by reducing power when the explosions are noted. In eyes with little or no pigment on the trabecular meshwork, the desired end point for laser applications is a visibly blanched spot. In some instances the laser power must be increased to as high as 1800 to 2000 mW to achieve this reaction.

Argon laser trabeculoplasty technique

Visualization	Use coated goniolens. Identify landmarks with careful prelaser gonioscopy.
Sequence	Treat inferior angle first, where landmarks are most clearly identified.
Distribution	Evenly space applications, approximately eight per clock hour, so that 50 applications per six clock hours result.
Desired response	Create blanched spot or formation of a small gas bubble in the area of the trabecular meshwork. Avoid explosions.

Before performing trabeculoplasty, the precise gonioscopic identification of angle structures is essential. In some eyes certain angle landmarks may be confused with others, such as a pigmented Schwalbe's line mimicking the trabecular meshwork (Fig. 23-2). Careful gonioscopy should be done before treatment with the slitlamp, using 25X magnification to accurately identify angle landmarks.

At present we are treating half the circumference of the meshwork at each session and waiting 4 to 6 weeks between sessions. We have arbitrarily chosen to treat the temporal angle first and then the nasal angle. It is easiest to begin treating the 6 o'clock position of the meshwork, where angle landmarks are usually most clearly visualized.

Clearly trabeculoplasty can be modified in many ways in terms of laser settings, site of treatment, number of applications, and amount of angle treated per session.[23] We have made few modifications from our original technique, since changing the parameters from time to time might limit our ability to evaluate long-term results in a large group of patients. Furthermore, many investigators have established currently employed settings as being effective, and therefore we have been reluctant to compromise a patient's chance for beneficial results from these parameters.[5,9,24-26]

Laser techniques in eyes with narrow angles

In eyes with potentially closable angles and open-angle glaucoma, it is probably best not to perform both an iridectomy and trabeculoplasty at the same session. It is preferable to do the iridectomy first, wait for approximately 4 weeks, and then proceed with trabeculoplasty 1 or more months later.

A more common situation is an angle that does not have the potential for closure, in which the convexity of the peripheral iris makes visualization of angle landmarks and therefore delivery of laser applications difficult. In such cases trabeculoplasty may be facilitated by first performing peripheral iridoplasty (gonioplasty) to widen the inlet of the angle and permit accurate delivery of trabeculoplasty burns.[11,13] Gonioplasty can be done by using trabeculoplasty settings and applying an oblique burn to the crest of the peripheral iris roll. If the power is excessive and causes an explosion and crater rather than contracture of the iris, then the beam may be defocused or the power reduced. Usually one application will widen approximately one-half clock hour of angle.

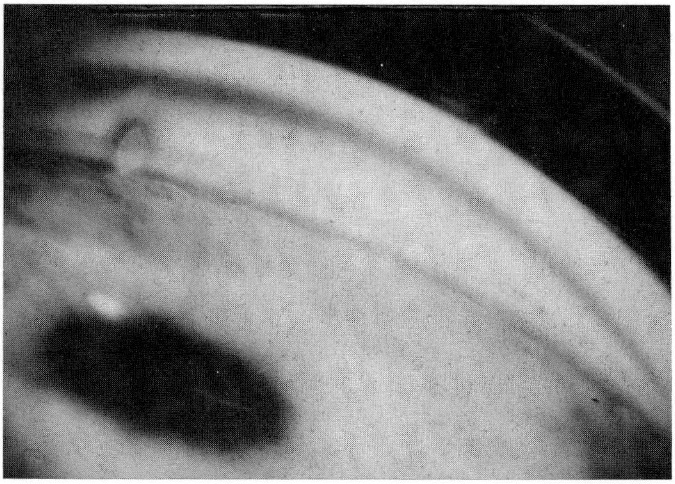

Fig. 23-2. Gonioscopy view of angle with irregularly pigmented Schwalbe's line, which may be confused with trabecular meshwork and result in inaccurate treatment.

INDICATIONS

Indications for argon laser trabeculoplasty include the following:

1. Presurgical glaucoma patient—maximum tolerated medical therapy
2. Medication intolerance—*not* to replace tolerated medications, when they are available
3. Noncompliance
4. Very high prelaser tension—response proportional to initial tension
5. Advanced glaucoma and low-tension glaucoma—disc and field deterioration at "normal" or "low" tensions
6. Following failed glaucoma surgery
7. Before planned cataract surgery
8. Patient age—in young patients there is less pressure lowering and greater likelihood of postlaser pressure spike
9. Trabeculoplasty as initial therapy for glaucoma for developing areas—not advocated at this time in situations where socioeconomic factors such as availability of care and medications are optimal
10. Retreatment—can be beneficial in some eyes but need to observe closely for postlaser pressure spike; be prepared for urgent surgery
11. Particular types of glaucoma
    Pseudoexfoliation and pigmentary glaucoma—excellent results
    Secondary glaucomas—variable results but can be tried since some success has been seen

The presurgical patient

The main and widely accepted indication for laser trabeculoplasty is the management of the glaucoma patient who is losing visual field and/or showing progressive glaucomatous cupping of the optic disc despite maximum tolerated medical therapy. Although filtration surgery and other glaucoma surgical procedures have undergone improvement in precision and sophistication of technique with use of microscopic instruments and sutures, their potentially serious complications cannot be overlooked.[3,15] These surgical candidates undergo less risk with laser treatment than with conventional surgery.

Intolerance to medication

A second important indication for laser trabeculoplasty is to help facilitate the discontinuation of poorly tolerated medications. For example, miotics may incapacitate younger patients and those with cataracts. Another frequent intolerance to medication is seen with the use of carbonic anhydrase inhibitors, which may produce serious side effects such as anorexia, weight loss, and fatigue. Before trabeculoplasty we attempt to have the patient use all medications, including miotics, epinephrine or dipivalyl epinephrine, timolol, and carbonic anhydrase inhibitors. In a practical sense, however, medications are only given to the extent that the patient tolerates them.

At present the use of laser trabeculoplasty as a substitute for available and tolerated medications is not indicated. In most instances some indication of progression, such as visible disc damage or progressive field loss, should be noted before trabeculoplasty is employed. Following laser therapy maximum tolerated medical therapy is continued. If a substantial reduction of intraocular pressure (IOP) is achieved with trabeculoplasty, previously tolerated medications may be gradually discontinued if a clinically significant lowering of IOP continues to be maintained.

Noncompliance

Noncompliance in the use of medication is another indication for trabeculoplasty. In some instances it is difficult to distinguish the noncompliant patient from the patient in whom medications simply are not effective, but in recent years attention to the widespread nature of noncompliance has made using the laser in such patients more common. When such a patient shows progression of visual field or disc cupping with maximum tolerated medical therapy, laser trabeculoplasty is indicated. In this instance the lasting effect of the laser may protect the patient from his poor compliance.

High prelaser intraocular pressures

It has been suggested that since the average drop in IOP obtained with trabeculoplasty ranges from 7 to 10 mm Hg, the procedure will not be of sufficient benefit in eyes whose pretreatment IOP is 30 mm Hg. or greater.[24] However, we have found that the lowering of IOP is proportional to the prelaser IOP (Table 23-1 and Fig. 23-3). It is reasonable, therefore, to expect that a patient with high initial IOP may have a substantial reduction of pressure from trabeculoplasty and perhaps be able to avoid conventional glaucoma surgery.

Advanced glaucoma

Some eyes are so severely damaged from glaucoma that the optic nerve is totally or nearly totally cupped and vulnerable to even small elevations of IOP. These eyes can continue to lose visual field at normal pressure ranges, such as 15 or 16 mm Hg. Some have thought that laser trabeculoplasty is a futile gesture in such instances, since the expected reduction in pressure would be so slight. We believe that it is reasonable to try trabeculoplasty in such cases, since in some of these eyes the IOP may be reduced to the single numbers.[18] In a series of 180 patients we found that it can be possible to achieve very low tensions with laser trabeculoplasty[10] (Table 23-2).

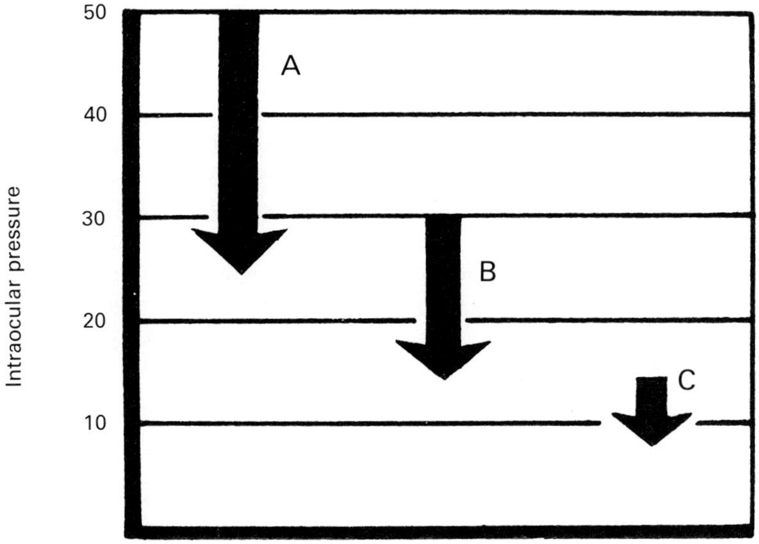

Fig. 23-3. Diagram of differential drop in IOP from laser trabeculoplasty, depending on initial pressure. Sequence of *A, B,* and *C* depicts greater response to laser trabeculoplasty that can be expected with higher prelaser pressures. (From Simmons, R.J., and Thomas, J.V.: Laser treatment of open angle glaucoma. Interview with Benjamin Boyd, Highlights of Ophthalmology, tri-weekly letter, IX:17-18, X:1, 1982.)

Table 23-1. Average Δ IOP* in relation to prelaser IOP in successfully treated eyes

Prelaser IOP (mm Hg)	*Eyes (number)*	*Average Δ IOP (mm Hg)*
≥ 50	3	−25.0
≥ 40-49	6	−21.3
≥ 30-39	45	−13.9
≥ 20-29	134	− 7.6
≥ 10-19	65	− 4.2

From Thomas, J.V., Simmons, R.J., and Belcher, C.D.: Argon laser trabeculoplasty in the pre-surgical glaucoma patient, Ophthalmology **89:**187, 1982.
*Change in IOP after trabeculoplasty.

Table 23-2. Argon laser trabeculoplasty (LTP) in advanced glaucoma: 180 patients, 231 eyes—80 eyes with pre-LTP tension ≤ 19 mm Hg (average follow-up, 19.1 mo); 151 eyes with pre-LTP tension ≥ 19 mm Hg (average follow-up, 25.5 mo)

	Final post-LTP tension (mm Hg)		
	10-12	*6-9*	*0-5*
Eyes with pre-LTP tension ≥ 19 mm Hg	5%	3%	None with 6-mo follow-up
Eyes with pre-LTP tension ≤ 19 mm Hg	28%	12%	None with 6-mo follow-up

However, a note of caution is appropriate here, since a postlaser pressure spike could be disastrous in the presence of a severely cupped and vulnerable optic nerve. Therefore, in such eyes we recommend that only two to three clock hours of angle be treated per session to minimize the magnitude of a spike in IOP following trabeculoplasty. As with any other case, we would wait approximately 4 weeks between treatment sessions. With shorter time intervals IOP elevations appear to be more frequent. Other precautions that may be taken to prevent or decrease the chance of a postlaser pressure spike include pretreatment with extra antiglaucomatous drops, carbonic anhydrase inhibitors, and even oral hyperosmotics. Even patients who are not able to tolerate carbonic anhydrase inhibitors on a continuing basis may be temporarily pretreated with these medications as an added precaution against possible postlaser pressure spikes. Applying laser burns more anteriorly on the trabecular meshwork may be especially effective in this regard.

Following failed glaucoma surgery

Laser trabeculoplasty is effective for eyes in which conventional glaucoma surgery has failed to control IOP. In such eyes, if progressive optic nerve cupping or field loss occurs, laser trabeculoplasty can be beneficial.

Before planned cataract surgery

In patients who have significant cataracts and glaucoma, with the glaucoma under borderline control with medical therapy, laser trabeculoplasty is indicated. Since laser trabeculoplasty is more effective in phakic eyes than in aphakic eyes, it should be employed before rather than after cataract surgery. The type of cataract surgery—intracapsular cataract extraction without lens implantation, extracapsular cataract extraction without lens implantation, or extracapsular cataract extraction with posterior chamber lens implantation—does not appear to influence the magnitude of pressure reduction obtained with trabeculoplasty.[1] The angle is treated in two sessions, with 4 weeks between sessions. It is best to wait 8 weeks after the second session of trabeculoplasty before performing cataract surgery.

Patient age

Laser trabeculoplasty is relatively contraindicated in patients under 40 years of age. It has been our and others' experience that the pressure lowering effect of trabeculoplasty is substantially less in this age-group than in older patients. Also, a higher frequency of postlaser pressure spikes is seen in patients under age 40.[20]

Trabeculoplasty as initial therapy for glaucoma

An issue that needs to be explored is whether laser trabeculoplasty is indicated as initial therapy for open-angle glaucoma. The recommendation that trabeculoplasty be done only if glaucoma remains uncontrolled despite maximum tolerated medical therapy is appropriate for countries where socioeconomic factors are favorable. However, in developing countries it is difficult to effectively manage glaucoma with medical therapy. In conjunction with colleagues in Egypt we have evaluated the role of trabeculoplasty as an initial form of glaucoma therapy in patients who had not received prior medical therapy. It was found possible to avoid medical and/or surgical therapy in 83% of patients treated with trabeculoplasty.[21] It should be stressed that in environments where medication is available and affordable, there is insufficient evidence at present to justify trabeculoplasty before medical therapy.

Retreatment

Available data on the issue of retreatment are scant, and further investigation is necessary. In our experience of argon laser trabeculoplasty retreatment of 22 eyes in 21 patients, wide variability in results has been seen. Patients have fallen into three groups; those with IOPs markedly better, those with little or no change, and those who were made markedly worse. The latter group is striking and mandates caution as well as careful discussion in choosing retreatment. Taking the average of all 22 eyes, tension after retreatment was slightly decreased, from 24.3 to 23.7 mm Hg (see boxed material below). However, three of the eyes (13.6%) had a lasting elevation in pressure greater than 9 mm Hg following retreatment, whereas an equal number had an improvement in pressure of more than 9 mm Hg. Fifty-four percent of the eyes had worsening of visual fields, and 54% had subsequent glaucoma surgery performed. In some cases this surgery took the form of an emergency glaucoma filtration operation because of a postlaser pressure spike in an eye with advanced cupping and visual field loss.[2]

Argon laser trabeculoplasty (LTP)—retreatment

Subjects

21 patients (average age: 62.2 years)
22 eyes
22 phakic
2 aphakic
17 primary open-angle glaucoma
3 pseudoexfoliation
2 pigmentary glaucoma

Results

Average tension before to LTP I—28.2 mm Hg
Average tension after LTP I—24.3 mm Hg (average 14.9 months of follow-up)
Average tension after LTP II—23.7 mm Hg (average 4.4 months of follow-up)
Increase in tension—10 mm Hg (3 eyes: 10-37 mm Hg)
Decrease in tension—10 mm Hg (3 eyes: 10-33 mm Hg)

Visual fields before and after LTP II

Worse—12 (54.5%)
Same—10 (45.6%)
Better—0

Subsequent glaucoma surgery

Surgery required—12 (54.5%)
Surgery not required—10 (45.6%)

It is especially important to take measures to avoid potential postlaser pressure spikes in eyes undergoing retreatment. At present we agree with Wise's suggestion that retreatment be reserved for those who had an initial pressure lowering response to trabeculoplasty with a gradual return of IOP to baseline.

RESULTS

Several investigators have shown laser trabeculoplasty to produce an average reduction of IOP of approximately 7 to 10 mm Hg in phakic, primary open-angle glaucoma. In our experience conventional glaucoma surgery has been avoided in 87% of phakic eyes and 62% of aphakic eyes. Even though aphakic eyes appear to respond less often and less well to laser trabeculoplasty, the procedure should be done in such eyes before surgical intervention. Failure of trabeculoplasty to lower IOP does not appear to adversely affect the results of subsequent glaucoma surgery.

In general the secondary open-angle glaucomas are difficult to manage; however, in some eyes in this group beneficial and at least temporary improvement in IOP can be obtained.[12] Trabeculoplasty can be effective in pseudoexfoliation and pigmentary glaucoma. The efficacy of laser trabeculoplasty is not well established in glaucoma because of angle recession or uveitis. It is not clear whether there is a relationship between the extent of angle recession and the effectiveness of trabeculoplasty. Before final judgment can be passed regarding the true efficacy of trabeculoplasty in these rarer forms of secondary glaucoma, more experience with treating larger numbers of cases and long-term follow-up will be necessary.

In eyes that have partially closed angles due to previous angle closure with formation of peripheral anterior synechias, trabeculoplasty may be beneficial in increasing outflow through the remaining areas of open angle.

COMPLICATONS

A mild iritis is common after trabeculoplasty and resolves spontaneously or with the use of topical steroids. Other complications include hemorrhage from the meshwork (Fig. 23-4), peripheral anterior synechiae formation (Fig. 23-5), and posttreatment elevation of IOP (see boxed material on p. 278). Hemorrhage occurs rarely and is not a serious problem. Synechiae usually occur as small, tentlike areas, but on occasion may be rather broad. We have had the clinical impression that synechiae may develop more readily in black patients. Therefore, it is recommended that gonioscopy be performed weeks to months after treatment.

The major complication following laser trabeculoplasty is the occurrence of posttreatment IOP spikes (see boxed material). The occurrence of a pressure spike does not necessarily indicate failure of treatment. The vast majority of eyes that have a postlaser pressure spike are known to have a lowering of IOP with continued follow-up.[19]

Varying degrees of visual field loss following trabeculoplasty have been noted by a number of observers[4,8,14,27] and are, in our opinion, probably a result of postlaser pressure spikes, which cause optic nerve damage. The pressure spike following laser therapy can be acute and occur within an hour or two after treatment, and many last from 12 hours to 1 to 3 weeks. This elevation of pressure may extinguish a small central island of vision or produce peripheral field loss. If a marked elevation of pressure occurs, oral hyperosmotics are given on a temporary basis. In patients with severe glaucomatous optic nerve damage, it is important to check IOP 1 to 2 hours after the procedure and also within 24 to 48 hours.

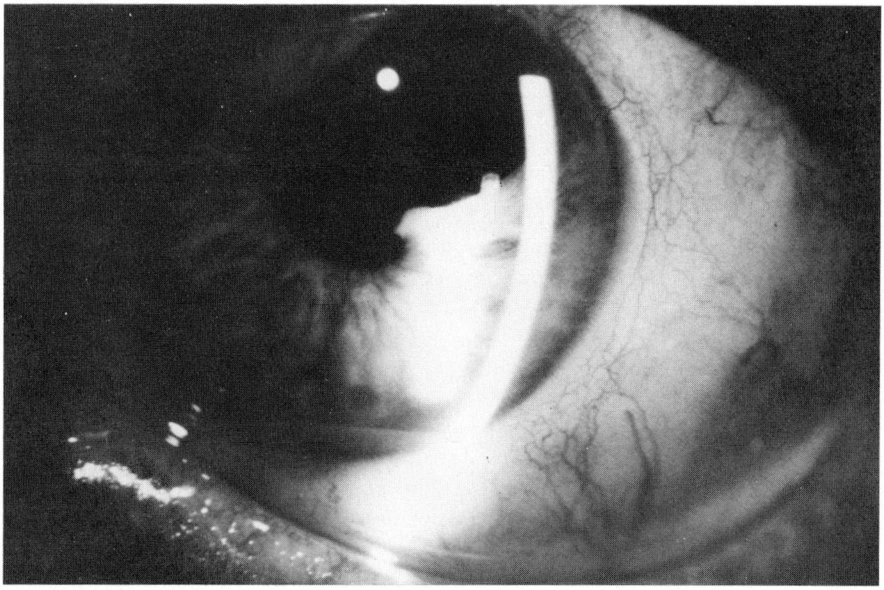

Fig. 23-4. Photograph of eye with small hyphema following laser trabeculoplasty. (From Belcher, C.D., Thomas, J.V., and Simmons, R.J., editors: Photocoagulation in glaucoma and anterior segment disease, Baltimore, 1984, Williams & Wilkins, p. 77.)

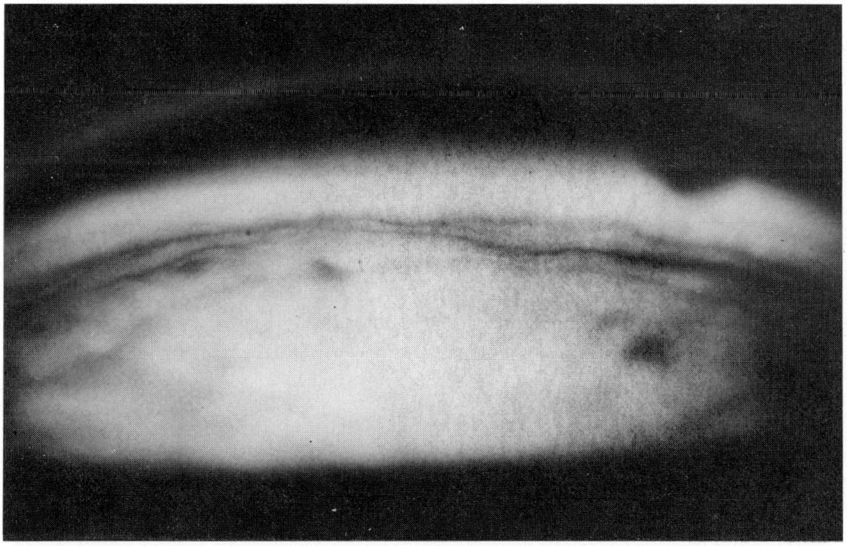

Fig. 23-5. Gonioscopic view of peripheral anterior synechiae following laser trabeculoplasty. This case illustrates that synechiae can be broad rather than localized and tentlike.

Complications of argon laser trabeculoplasty

Mild iritis	
Hyphema	Minor and very infrequent
Peripheral anterior synechiae	Usually localized and peaked; can occasionally be broad, occluding 2 to 6 hours of the trabecular meshwork (gonioscopy recommended at follow-up visits)
Postlaser pressure rise	The most worrisome of complications Does not indicate failure of the procedure Usually is temporary but may be lasting Observe badly damaged and susceptible eyes closely Treat with oral hyperosmotics, intensive miotics, timolol, epinephrine, and carbonic anhydrase inhibitors A few of these patients will need emergency surgery
Dangerous situations	Eyes with prior pressure spike following laser Young patients: less than age 40 Severely damaged and susceptible eyes in which even a moderate pressure rise could have significant consequences with respect to the central visual field and fixation Trabeculoplasty retreatment
Avoidance	Treatment in divided session: usually 180 degrees, then 180 degrees a month later; in very susceptible eyes limited treatment of angle (two or three clock hours per session) Placement of burns: Treatment at site A—less frequent tension rise, less severe tension rise Treatment with extra drops, carbonic anhydrase inhibitors, and oral hyperosmotics after detecting tension rise or before laser trabeculoplasty

Table 23-3. Comparison of one treatment session and two treatment sessions

Parameter	*One treatment session (139 eyes)*	*Two treatment sessions (102 eyes)*
Average Δ IOP after treatment (mm Hg)	−7.8	−6.3
Success (%)	84.9 (118/139)	86.3 (88/102)
Eyes with elevated IOP after treatment	25.2 (35/139)	25.4 (26/102)
Eyes with IOP elevation ≤ 5 mm Hg above baseline	42.9 (15/35)	65.4 (17/26)
Eyes with IOP elevation > 5 mm Hg above baseline	57.1 (20/35)	34.6 (9/26)
Eyes with IOP elevation > 10 mm Hg above baseline	37.1 (13/35)	11.5 (3/26)

From Thomas, J.V., Simmons, R.J., and Belcher, C.D.: Argon laser trabeculoplasty in the pre-surgical glaucoma patient, Ophthalmology **89:**187, 1982.

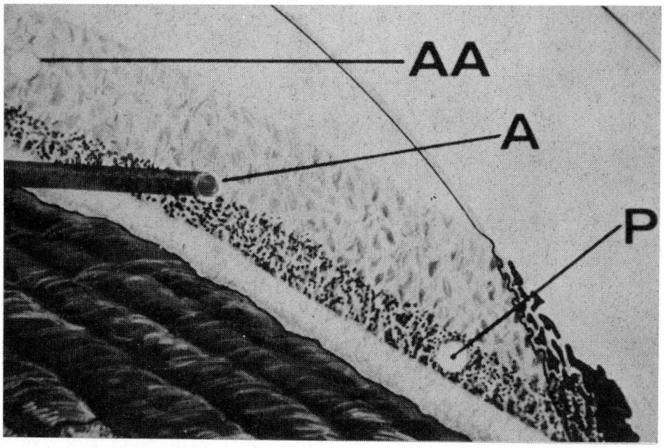

Fig. 23-6. Diagram showing various sites used for laser applications in trabeculoplasty. (*A*, Anterior; *P*, posterior, *AA*, far anterior.)

Postlaser pressure spikes have been found to be less in magnitude when one half of the circumference of the trabecular meshwork is treated at each of two sessions than when the entire circumference is treated at one session (Table 23-3). For this reason we have recommended since March 1980 that it is safer to perform trabeculoplasty in divided treatments.[18] Using the same logic, in eyes with severely damaged and susceptible optic nerves present, it is reasonable to treat even less than 180 degrees of the meshwork at any one session in an attempt to further minimize the magnitude of potential postlaser pressure spikes.

Another important aspect of the technique pertinent to lowering the frequency and magnitude of pressure spikes is the location of the laser applications on the meshwork. In our experience the frequency and magnitude of postlaser pressure spikes is less if the laser applications are made at the junction of the functional, frequently pigmented and nonfunctional, frequently nonpigmented trabecular meshwork than if they are applied more posteriorly.[17] In addition, peripheral anterior synechiae seem to occur less when laser burns are applied in this location.[22] We are currently investigating the results of treatment in an even more anterior location than the anterior edge of the functional, usually pigmented trabecular meshwork (Fig. 23-6).

Some have raised the question of the advisability of deferring treatment of the second half of the circumference of the meshwork if excellent pressure reduction is achieved following 180 degrees of treatment. At present we prefer to wait before treating the second half if the IOP has been reduced to an ideal level. Wise, however, who has extensive experience with this laser modality, believes that the entire angle should be treated in all cases for maximum, lasting benefit.

CONCLUSION

In conclusion it is appropriate to note that 3% of eyes treated with trabeculoplasty have had permanent elevations of IOP above baseline and required conventional glaucoma surgery.[18] It should be kept in mind that early investigations of the effect of laser energy on the trabecular meshwork of experimental animals[6,7] resulted in the creation of glaucoma and that even with currently accepted laser settings, it is possible to make glaucoma worse.

REFERENCES

1. Brown, S.V.L., Thomas, J.V., and Simmons, R.J.: Effect of type of cataract surgery on intraocular pressure reduction obtained with laser trabeculoplasty. (Manuscript in preparation.)
2. Brown, S.V.L., and others: Argon laser trabeculoplasty—retreatment. Manuscript in preparation.
3. D'Ermo, F., and others: A critical analysis of the long-term results of trabeculectomy, Am. J. Ophthalmol. **88:**829, 1979.
4. Drance, S.M.: Personal communication.
5. Forbes, M., and Bansal, R.K.: Argon laser goniophotocoagulation of the trabecular meshwork in open angle glaucoma, Glaucoma **4:**100, 1982.
6. Gaasterland, D., and Kupfer, C.: Experimental glaucoma in the rhesus monkey, Invest. Ophthalmol. **13:**455, 1974.
7. Gaasterland, D., and Kuwabara, T.: Effects on monkey eyes of argon laser glaucoma treatment, ARVO Abstracts, Invest. Ophthalmol. (suppl.), 1980.
8. Hoskins, H.D.: Personal communication.
9. Schwartz, A.L., and others: Argon laser trabecular surgery in uncontrolled phakic open angle glaucoma, Ophthalmology **88:**203, 1981.
10. Sharpe, E.D., and others: Manuscript in preparation.
11. Simmons, R.J., and Simmons, R.B.: Gonioplasty. In Belcher, C.D., Thomas, J.V., and Simmons, R.J., editors: Photocoagulation in glaucoma and anterior segment disease, Baltimore, 1984, Williams & Wilkins.
12. Simmons, R.J., Thomas, J.V., and Agulto, M.B.: Special problems in the secondary glaucomas. Paper presented at The Glaucoma Society of the XXIV International Congress of Ophthalmology, Oct. 28-29, 1982, San Francisco.
13. Simmons, R.J., and others: Laser gonioplasty for special problems in angle closure glaucoma. In New Orleans Academy of Ophthalmology: Symposium on glaucoma, St. Louis, 1981, The C.V. Mosby Co.
14. Spaeth, G.L.: Personal communication.
15. Spaeth, G.L., Joseph, N.H., and Fernandes, E.: Trabeculectomy: a re-evaluation after three years and a comparison with Scheie's procedure, Trans. Am. Acad. Ophthalmol. Otolaryngol. **79:**349, 1975.
16. Spurney, R.V., and Lederer, C.M.: Krypton laser in laser trabeculoplasty, Arch. Ophthalmol. (In press.)
17. Thomas, J.V.: Laser trabeculoplasty. In Belcher, C.D., Thomas, J.V., and Simmons, R.J., editors: Photocoagulation of glaucoma and anterior segment disease, Baltimore, 1984, Williams & Wilkins.
18. Thomas, J.V., Simmons, R.J., and Belcher, C.D.: Argon laser trabeculoplasty in the pre-surgical glaucoma patient, Ophthalmology **89:**187, 1982.
19. Thomas, J.V., Simmons, R.J., and Belcher, C.D.: Complications of argon laser trabeculoplasty, Glaucoma **4:**50, 1982.
20. Thomas, J.V., and others: Intraocular pressure elevation following laser trabeculoplasty. Paper presented at the XXIV International Congress of Ophthalmology, Oct. 31, 1982, San Francisco.
21. Thomas, J.V., and others: Laser trabeculoplasty as initial therapy for open angle glaucoma, Arch. Ophthalmol. (In press.)
22. Traverso, C., and others: Presentation at Wills Eye Hospital Annual Clinical Conference, July 1982, Philadelphia.
23. Weinreb, R.N., and others: Influence of the number of laser burns administered on the early results of argon laser trabeculoplasty, Am. J. Ophthalmol. **95:**287, 1983.
24. Wilensky, J.T., and Jampol, L.M.: Laser therapy for open angle glaucoma, Ophthalmology **88:**213, 1981.
25. Wise, J.B.: Long term control of adult open angle glaucoma by argon laser treatment, Ophthalmology **88:**197, 1981.
26. Wise, J.B., and Witter, S.L.: Argon laser therapy for open angle glaucoma: a pilot study, Arch. Ophthalmol. **97:**319, 1979.
27. Worthen, D.M.: Personal communication.

24

Chronic open-angle glaucoma: new findings and possible new treatments

David G. Campbell
John W. Boys-Smith*
Wendell D. Woods‡
Nancy Tanchel§
John M. Ruderman||
Angela Vela¶
Donald G. Aiken**

SEGMENTATION OF PIGMENTATION

Although there are many theories on the etiology of chronic open-angle glaucoma, none is universally accepted, and there is much disagreement and bewilderment. Grant's laboratory work has led to the general belief that most of the increased abnormal resistance to outflow in chronic open-angle glaucoma, as well as the normal resistance to outflow, resides within the trabecular meshwork, particularly in the juxtacanalicular region. These experiments, conducted on perfused enucleated human eyes and measuring the facility of outflow before and after removal of the trabecular meshwork, *do not rule out the possibility* that collapse of Schlemm's canal may also play an important role.

Gonioscopy

There is also no universal agreement that any gonioscopically visible abnormality exists in open-angle glaucoma. If the intraocular pressure is elevated and the clinician can find no abnormality on gonioscopic examination of the trabecular meshwork, the diagnosis of chronic open-angle glaucoma is made. However, there have been reports that the angles of patients with chronic open-angle glaucoma have more pigmentation than normal angles, and these have been confirmed in our recent studies.

---

*M.D., Department of Ophthalmology, Tulane University School of Medicine, New Orleans.
‡Ph.D., Glaucoma Research Laboratory, Department of Ophthalmology, Emory University School of Medicine, Atlanta.
§Department of Ophthalmology, Emory University School of Medicine, Atlanta.
||M.D., Glaucoma Research Laboratory, Department of Ophthalmology, Emory University School of Medicine, Atlanta.
¶M.D., Department of Ophthalmology, University of Texas School of Medicine, Galveston.
**M.S., Glaucoma Research Laboratory, Department of Ophthalmology, Emory University School of Medicine, Atlanta.

Several years ago one of us noticed that many chronic open-angle glaucoma patients, particularly those having obvious dispersion of pigment within the anterior segment, exhibit a peculiar segmentation of pigmentation within the trabecular meshwork. If confirmed, this finding might indicate that some areas of the trabecular meshwork function better than other areas and that chronic open-angle glaucoma may be a segmental disease exhibiting areas of variable degrees of pathology.

A new pigment-scale gonioscopy lens

To evaluate this possibility, a special gonioscopic lens was created to document accurately the degree of pigmentation within the human trabecular meshwork. Such a lens incorporating a pigment scale was developed in our laborabory.[1] Human pigment was isolated from the posterior surface of human irides and plated out in various concentrations on filters. A scale of five different gradations of pigment was made. This was then scientifically matched by lacquers and incorporated into a three-mirror lens with the aid of the Ocular Instrument Co., Bellevue, Wash. The scale was placed in a position such that scale and angle could be seen simultaneously under the same lighting condition, allowing reproducibility of readings.

Using this gonioscopic scale, eyes with chronic open-angle glaucoma were compared to normal control eyes.[2] Significantly we found that patients with chronic open-angle glaucoma have more variation and segmentation of pigmentation than do control eyes. In addition, chronic open-angle glaucoma patients were found to have more overall pigment, confirming previous studies. These findings lend support to the hypothesis that the pathology of chronic open-angle glaucoma may be segmental rather than evenly distributed throughout the trabecular meshwork (Fig. 24-1).

Patients with pigmentary glaucoma were uniformly found to have no segmentation of pigmentation. Assuming that the trabecular meshwork was normal in such eyes before the dispersion of pigment, these findings indicate that in young and normal eyes all of the trabecular meshwork is functioning well. In turn, normal trabecular function would account for the even distribution of dispersed pigment within the eyes.

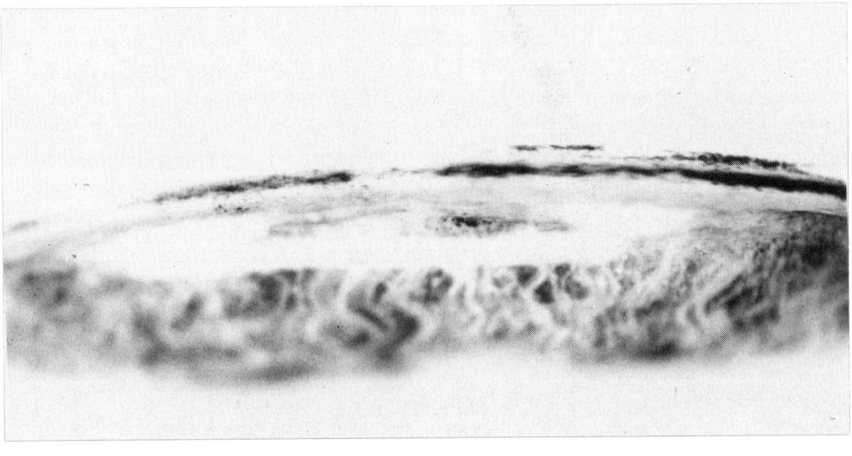

Fig. 24-1. Photograph of trabecular meshwork of enucleated human eye with chronic open-angle glaucoma. Note segmentation of pigmentation, with light areas *left* and *central*.

Correlation between regions of hyperpigmentation and collector channels

Further investigations in our laboratory have shown a correlation between the location of collector channels and the areas of darker pigmentation.[4] Injections and casts of Schlemm's canal, correlated with the location and level of pigmentation in the trabecular meshwork, showed that areas of hyperpigmentation were closely related to the presence of collector channels, often prominent ones. These studies may indicate that the segmented areas of hyperpigmentation are areas of high flow and that areas of lesser pigmentation are areas of decreased flow.

Further studies are needed to elucidate this phenomenon. Specifically studies are needed to determine whether there is a difference in the electron microscopic appearance of the trabecular meshwork in darker versus lighter areas of trabecular meshwork in patients with chronic open-angle glaucoma. Accurate counts of the number of collector channels in chronic open-angle glaucoma patients must be compared to those in normal eyes to see if these patients have fewer or less functional channels.

INTERNAL TRABECULOTOMY

One of the more surprising aspects of adult nonfiltration trabecular surgery is that it generally does not work. Occasional initially favorable results do not seem to be lasting. If what we currently understand about chronic open-angle glaucoma is true—the increased resistance to outflow in the eye lies within the trabecular meshwork or within the consequences of a primary or secondary collapse of Schlemm's canal—then opening the trabecular meshwork to the posterior wall of Schlemm's canal should be curative. Unfortunately, however, no lasting success has been achieved.

Many different attempts have been made to open the trabecular meshwork permanently. Perhaps the first such approach was the placement of a goniotomy incision within the adult trabecular meshwork. Another attempt involved the use of external trabeculotomies to perform trabeculotomy ab externo. A third involved cannulating a suture into Schlemm's canal, grasping the two ends and pulling this suture into the anterior chamber, thereby disrupting the trabecular meshwork. Others have tried to puncture the trabecular meshwork permanently with either argon or YAG laser applications. None of these attempts, although theoretically sound, has been universally effective in creating a long-standing cure for chronic open-angle glaucoma.

Two problems

There are two reasons why these attempts do not work. First, our laboratory studies show that if one merely cuts into the trabecular meshwork, the cut edges do not retract but immediately close again because of the natural forces within and around the trabecular meshwork. Thus the cut edges seal and presumably heal almost instantly. It is this tendency for closure, plus healing and scarring, that seems to cause most surgical failures. A second problem with trabecular surgery is the difficulty in achieving a penetraton of the trabecular meshwork of the proper depth—through to Schlemm's canal but not so far that the back wall is damaged.

Possible solutions

Modern advances in technology can alleviate both of these problems, although with difficulty. We have successfully and permanently opened the cut edges of the trabecular meshwork by placing a row of small argon laser applications on each cut edge. We achieve the proper depth of incision or penetration by the prior placement of a smooth-tipped 6-0 nylon suture into Schlemm's canal.

Current investigational trabeculotomy techniques

In our investigations[3] to date we have employed and evaluated the following techniques. Chapter 3 outlined four major advances that allow safe access to and surgery on the trabecular meshwork. The first advance involved the use of the chamber-deepening procedure to provide a wide and safe entrance into the angle. The second advance entailed the use of sodium hyaluronate in the anterior chamber to hold the deepened configuration, to help stop hemorrhage, and to contain hemorrhage within a local droplet, maintaining surgical view. The third advance used irrigating surgical instruments to help maintain the deepened chamber and provide sudden elevation of intraocular pressure, if necessary to stop unwanted hemorrhage. The final advance was the use of direct visualization techniques with reliable high magnification loupes (4 to 6×), since accurate angle surgery cannot be performed without direct visualization under high magnification.

Using these techniques and advances to gain safe surgical access to the angle in the laboratory, we evaluated the following techniques to open a significant portion of the trabecular meshwork permanently. First, a 6-0 smooth-tipped nylon suture is passed into Schlemm's canal via an external approach using an operating microscope. Initially we tried grasping both ends of this suture externally, with approximately four to five clock hours of separation, and pulled on each end, causing the suture to rupture into the anterior chamber. The point of rupture proved to be unreliable, and we abandoned this approach.

Next we tried placement of the suture followed by YAG laser applications to the trabecular meshwork overlying the suture. We found that we could separate the tissue of the trabecular meshwork and expose the suture in this manner, but high power settings were necessary. Further laboratory investigations are necessary before human trials of this procedure can begin, but it may well be that it will be safely used in the future.

In our current investigations 6-0 nylon suture is threaded through Schlemm's canal, and a sharp irrigating goniotomy knife is used to make an incision to the suture. This incision, which is made by approaching the suture from across the anterior chamber—that is, from the opposite limbus using a Barkan goniotomy lens and 4 to 6× loupes for visualization—is extended for approximately four clock hours. The eye is then taken to an argon laser, where the cut edges are treated with 50 spots of 100 μ each, causing permanent retraction. The suture is then removed, exposing the undamaged back wall of Schlemm's canal to the anterior chamber. In the laboratory there is a dramatic increase in the facility of outflow in enucleated human eyes.

At present, it is not known whether any of the approaches described will effect a permanent in vivo cure for chronic open-angle glaucoma. Problems remaining to be solved include the lack of absolute control of hemorrhage, poor visibility, and an inability to pass the suture into Schlemm's canal for a sufficient length. As technology improves, it is hoped that further efforts in this area will lead to the establishment of direct and curative trabecular surgery for patients with open-angle glaucoma.

REFERENCES

1. Boys-Smith, J.W., and others: A new gonioscopy lens for the gradation of trabecular meshwork pigmentation, Invest. Ophthalmol. Vis. Sci. **25** (suppl.):173, 1984.
2. Campbell, D.G., Boys-Smith, J.W., and Woods, W.D.: Variation of pigmentation and segmentation of pigmentation in primary open-angle glaucoma, Invest. Ophthalmol. Vis. Sci. **25** (suppl.):122, 1984.
3. Ruderman, J.M., and others: Internal trabeculotomy: a new approach to trabecular surgery, Invest. Ophthalmol. Vis. Sci. **25** (suppl.):44, 1984.
4. Tanchel, N.A., and others: Correlation of segments of trabecular meshwork pigmentation and collector channels, Invest. Ophthalmol. Vis. Sci. **25** (suppl.):122, 1984.

25

Laser trabeculoplasty before and after aphakia and pseudophakia

James B. Wise

Cataract and glaucoma are a common and frustrating combination and have been the subject of numerous articles and opinions over the decades. In the past the options have included continued medical glaucoma therapy before and after cataract surgery; glaucoma filtering surgery followed by later cataract surgery; cataract surgery followed by later cyclodialysis or other procedures, excluding filtration surgery; and combined cataract and filtration procedures. Frequently all of these options failed, and the surgeon was reduced to the last resort of cryosurgery of the ciliary body. The advent of laser trabeculoplasty, with its demonstrated long-term results,[1,2] introduces a new option for this problem. The introduction of effective extracapsular cataract surgical techniques, intraocular implant lenses, and the neodymium-YAG laser has also greatly altered the perspective. This chapter analyzes the interplay of these factors to determine the most effective way of dealing with the problem of glaucoma and cataract.

When laser trabeculoplasty was introduced[2,3] essentially all cataract surgery consisted of intracapsular cataract extraction (ICCE), except for a few surgeons performing phacoemulsification plus capsulotomy or capsulectomy. Although laser trabeculoplasty has worked very well in phakic eyes, the success rate in these aphakic eyes was considerably less.[3] Table 25-1 presents the results in 36 aphakic eyes followed for 6 months or more and emphasizes the continued relatively poor results obtained with laser trabeculoplasty in eyes that have had ICCE. These results are to be contrasted with 12 patients who also had an ICCE, but with the addition of a pupil-supported implant lens (Table 25-2). Similar results were obtained in eyes that had undergone phacoemulsification with pupil-supported lenses (Table 25-3) and phacoemulsification with posterior chamber implant lenses (Table 25-4). The results of the various implant lens groups were so similar that they can be combined (Table 25-5). The difference in the results between eyes receiving ICCE and eyes with implant lenses is striking, particularly in the control rates at 2 and 3 years and in the overall surgical rates. It should be noted that no anterior chamber lenses were present in these groups. Only a few eyes with glaucoma and anterior chamber lenses have been seen. In virtually all of these eyes there was so much uveitis and corneal edema that the eyes were not considered to be candidates for laser trabeculoplasty.

Laser trabeculoplasty is frequently used in eyes that have early or moderate cataract, either to control medically uncontrolled glaucoma or to eliminate the need for miotics

Table 25-1. Laser trabeculoplasty after intracapsular cataract extraction

	6 mo	*12 mo*	*24 mo*	*36 mo*
Eyes (number)	36	36	23	17
IOP <21 mm Hg (number)	23	19	13	8
IOP <21 mm Hg (%)	64	53	57	47
Surgery (%)	25	28	39	47

Table 25-2. Laser trabeculoplasty after intracapsular cataract extraction and pupil-supported implant lens

	6 mo	*12 mo*	*24 mo*	*36 mo*
Eyes (number)	12	11	7	5
IOP <21 mm Hg (number)	9	9	6	5
IOP <21 mm Hg (%)	75	82	86	100
Surgery (%)	0	0	0	0

Table 25-3. Laser trabeculoplasty after phacoemulsification and pupil-supported implant lens

	6 mo	*12 mo*	*24 mo*	*36 mo*
Eyes (number)	20	13	9	5
IOP <21 mm Hg (number)	15	9	7	4
IOP <21 mm Hg (%)	75	69	78	80
Surgery (%)	5	0	0	20

Table 25-4. Laser trabeculoplasty after phacoemulsification and posterior chamber implant lens

	6 mo	*12 mo*	*24 mo*	*36 mo*
Eyes (number	17	16	8	2
IOP <21 mm Hg (number)	13	11	6	2
IOP <21 mm Hg (%)	76	69	75	100
Surgery (%)	0	0	0	0

Table 25-5. Laser trabeculoplasty after intracapsular cataract extraction or phacoemulsification and pupil-supported or posterior chamber implant lens

	6 mo	*12 mo*	*24 mo*	*36 mo*
Eyes (number)	49	40	24	12
IOP <21 mm Hg (number)	32	29	19	11
IOP <21 mm Hg (%)	65	73	79	92
Surgery (%)	2	0	0	8

Table 25-6. Cataract surgery after laser trabeculoplasty—no IOL (controlled at time of cataract surgery; data at last visit, from 1-47 mo postoperatively)

	Eyes	
Parameter	*Number*	*(%)*
IOP <21 mm Hg	6/9	(67)
Cryosurgery	1/9 eyes	(11)
Poor control	2/9 eyes	(22)

Table 25-7. Cataract-IOL surgery after laser trabeculoplasty (62 PC-IOL, 15 pupil-IOL; controlled at time of surgery; data at last visit

	Eyes	
Parameter	*Number*	*(%)*
IOP <21 mm Hg	70/77	(91)
IOP >21 mm Hg	7/77	(9)
Glaucoma surgery	None	

so that the patient is not visually disabled from their side effects. As time goes by, the cataracts can progress, and cataract surgery becomes necessary. In nine such eyes (Table 25-6) ICCE alone was performed. One eye required glaucoma surgery, two eyes have rather poor glaucoma control with advanced cupping, and six eyes have maintained their preoperative level of control. The results were rather different when the cataract surgery was combined with an implant lens. Fifteen eyes with pupil-supported lenses and 62 eyes with posterior chamber implant lenses were analyzed. The results were virtually identical, and so the two series were combined (Table 25-7). Of these 77 eyes controlled by laser trabeculoplasty at the time of cataract surgery, 91% have maintained that control, and the other 9% are well enough controlled that so far none of the 77 eyes has had any further glaucoma surgery.

Access of vitreous to the anterior chamber fundamentally alters the difficulty of glaucoma control. Filtering procedures cannot be used except with the addition of total vitrectomy at the time of filtering surgery, resulting in an increased risk of retinal detachment. Laser trabeculoplasty is less effective in these eyes (see Table 25-1) and is ineffective in eyes containing loose vitreous in the anterior chamber (Fig. 25-1). Furthermore, with an open capsule the aphakic eye can develop severely blurred vision or retinal vasospasm from epinephrine derivatives or blurred vision from timolol. The presence of vitreous in the anterior chamber therefore drastically reduces the options available in the treatment of glaucoma. In the phakic eye all modalities of glaucoma treatment remain available, including laser trabeculoplasty, filtering surgery, and the use of epinephrine and timolol.

If extracapsular cataract extraction (ECCE) alone is done, leaving the capsule intact, the "phakic" state is preserved (Fig. 25-2). Unfortunately nearly all posterior capsules will ultimately become cloudy, with recurrent, severe blurring of vision. The iris will usually become adherent to the bare capsule, with formation of iridocapsular membranes. If a capsulotomy is done either surgically or with the neodymium:YAG laser,

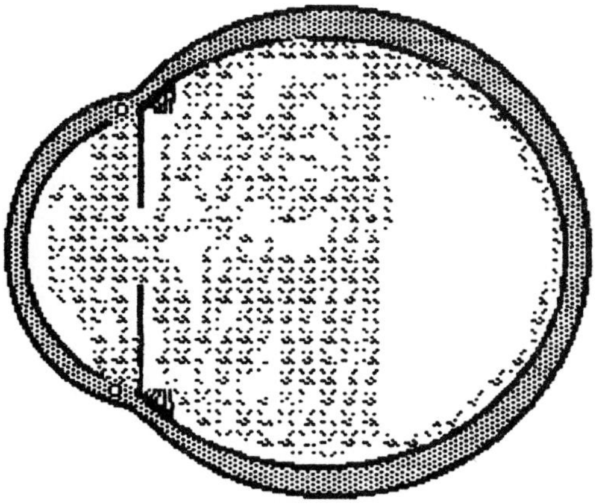

Fig. 25-1. Vitreous permanently obstructs trabecular meshwork. Later vitrectomy is not effective.

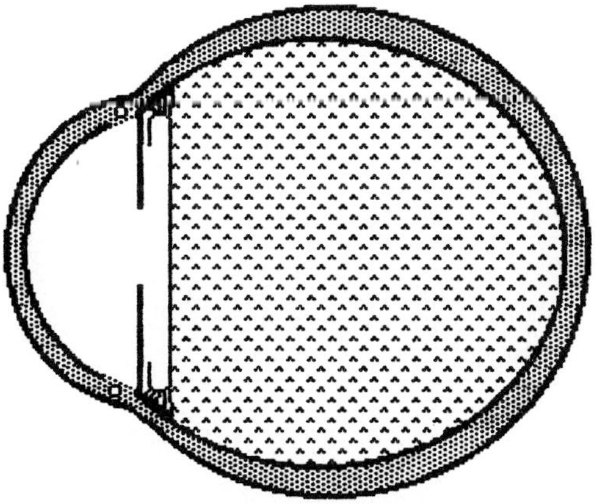

Fig. 25-2. Intact capsule keeps vitreous away from the trabecular meshwork.

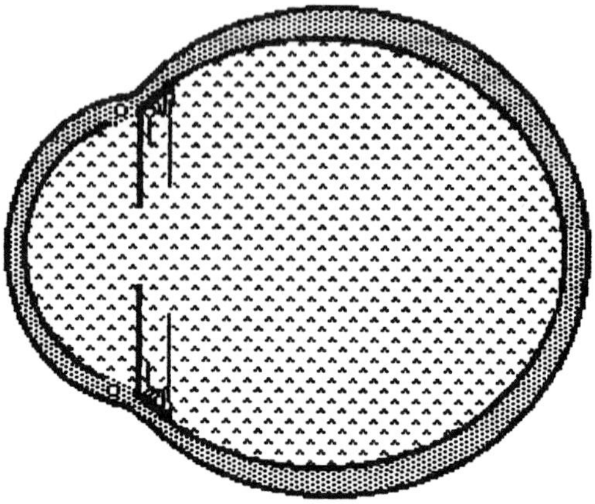

Fig. 25-3. Capsulotomy allows vitreous to coat meshwork, causing "aphakic" glaucoma.

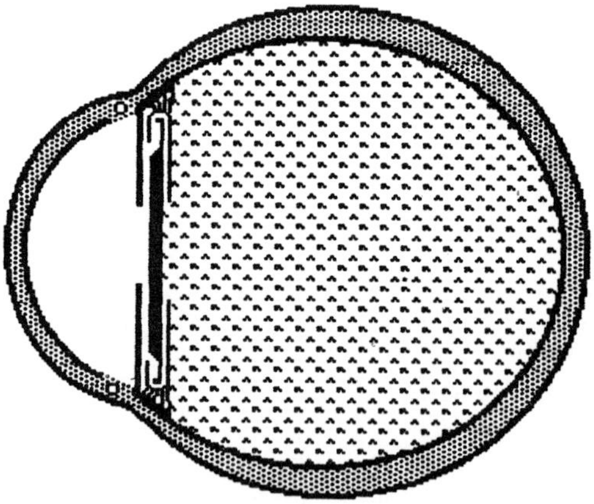

Fig. 25-4. Posterior chamber lens allows clear pupil with capsulotomy but maintains "phakic" state by keeping vitreous back.

vitreous can enter the anterior chamber, and the "phakic" glaucoma is converted to the refractory aphakic type (Fig. 25-3). If capsular integrity is to be maintained, the patient must be subjected to repeated operations to surgically polish the capsule. Until a method of reliably preventing capsular opacification is discovered, ECCE with intact posterior capsule will only defer access of vitreous to the anterior chamber but not reliably prevent it over the long term, except at the severe visual cost of capsular opacification.

Although implant lenses are inserted primarily for optical reasons, they also serve as a barrier across the pupil and keep vitreous out of the anterior chamber. As noted, the glaucoma control percentages are much better if laser trabeculoplasty is done in eyes containing either pupil-supported or posterior chamber lenses, and control is better maintained if later cataract surgery is done with pupil-supported or posterior chamber lenses rather than by ICCE alone. However, pupil-supported lenses are not well tolerated if miotic therapy is still required. Also, they frequently will greatly interfere with examination of the retina because of reflections from their supports and frozen, nondilatable pupils (Table 25-8).

The posterior chamber implant lens avoids these difficulties. As it does not depend on pupil support, the pupil can be freely dilated. As the iris sphincter does not squeeze its supports, even the strongest miotics can be used. By serving as a barrier, a posterior chamber lens allows a central capsulotomy to be performed, either surgically or with the neodymium:YAG laser, without the risk of vitreous entering the anterior chamber (Fig. 25-4). If the glaucoma still remains uncontrolled, a standard filtering procedure can be done, without the fear of corneal contact present with pupil-supported lenses. Except for occasional blur from timolol or epinephrine, the posterior chamber, pseudophakic eye appears to behave exactly as the original phakic eye did in its response to glaucoma medications, glaucoma surgery, and laser trabeculoplasty (Table 25-9). When one adds the remarkable visual benefits of the posterior chamber lens to its beneficial effects on glaucoma control, the routine use of posterior chamber lenses in patients with

Table 25-8. Therapeutic options: pupil-IOL vs. intracapsular cataract extraction (ICCE) alone

	Pupil-IOL	*ICCE*
Laser trabeculoplasty	Yes	50% failure
Filtering surgery	No	No
Use of timolol	+/−	+/−
Use of epinephrines	+/−	No
Use of miotics	+/−	Yes

Table 25-9. Therapeutic options: posterior chamber (PC)-IOL vs. ICCE alone

	PC-IOL	*ICCE*
Laser trabeculoplasty	Yes	50% failure
Filtering surgery	Yes	No
Use of timolol	Yes	+/−
Use of epinephrines	+/−	No
Use of miotics	Yes	Yes

glaucoma and cataract is strongly suggested. The only shortcomings are the greater tendency of the glaucomatous eye to give lens precipitates and form adhesions. Close follow-up and the use of topical corticosteroids will manage these problems effectively.

The marked limitation of therapeutic options and the marked reduction in efficacy of the remaining options in glaucoma therapy after ICCE suggest that ICCE is the worst operation one can do in an eye with cataract and glaucoma. Because of their damaging effects on the already compromised trabecular meshwork and their tendency to cause uveitis and pupillary block, anterior chamber implant lenses are equally bad, and their use in eyes with glaucoma and cataract is discouraged.

Certain modifications of standard extracapsular surgery and phacoemulsification are advisable in the glaucomatous eye. If the pupil will not dilate, the iris should be split down into the pupil, allowing easy access to the posterior chamber. Squeezing the nucleus through a small pupil can be done, but the stretched iris tends to wash around, to prolapse, and to get into the aspiration tip. Later the atonic sphincter can adhere to the capsule and then crawl under the implant lens.

After anterior capsulotomy and removal of the nucleus, the incision should be closed with 3 to 5 temporary sutures of 7-0 silk, so that the irrigation will hold the posterior capsule far back and allow leisurely, complete removal of all the cortex. This is particularly easy with the longer incision of elective ECCE, since the irrigation-aspiration tip can be inserted at the nasal and temporal ends of the incision to give good access to the 12 o'clock area. Before inserting the posterior chamber implant, the anterior chamber and the cavity of the lens capsule should be reformed with sodium hyaluronate (Healon), allowing easy "in the bag" placement of the lens without any corneal contact. A flexible-loop (Sinskey or Kratz type) lens is preferable. The posterior capsule is left intact. Suture of the iris is unnecessary, but the iris leaves should be carefully repositioned. After placement of the 10-0 nylon or polypropylene suture, the Healon is removed with the irrigation-aspiration tip, with the irrigation bottle lowered to avoid posterior displacement of the implant. The suture is then tightened, tied, and trimmed. The 7-0 silk sutures are cut with a razor fragment under careful microscopic observation to avoid the 10-0 suture. Miotics should be given for several weeks postoperatively to avoid adhesion of the iris to the capsule, with creeping of the iris under the implant. Topical steroids should be given somewhat longer than usual, and the eye monitored for possible steroid glaucoma. If capsular clouding occurs, the neodymium:YAG laser should be used, with focusing behind the capsule through a magnifying lens of the Abraham type to avoid any nicking of the implant.

REFERENCES

1. Schwartz, A.L., and Kopelman, J.: Four year experience with argon laser trabecular surgery in uncontrolled open-angle glaucoma, Ophthalmology **90:**771, 1983.
2. Wise, J.B.: Long-term control of adult open angle glucoma by argon laser treatment, Ophthalmology **88:**197, 1981.
3. Wise, J.B., and Witter, S.L.: Argon laser therapy for open-angle glaucoma: a pilot study, Arch. Ophthalmol. **97:**319, 1979.

Round table discussions

PROBLEM CASES IN ANGLE CLOSURE

DR. DAVID G. CAMPBELL

Campbell: We'll cover a few points about angle closure. I have a patient with angle closure on whom I'll bring out a few points which might be of interest to some of you. May I have the first slide, please. I would like to present this patient, who is a 70-year-old white female. She is a mild hyperope, and she has slightly narrow angles. You can see from the photograph that her central anterior chamber depths aren't too bad; they are about two corneal thicknesses centrally. She was doing well, in good ocular health, until one day when she developed rather sudden pain and halos in the right eye. Her IOP was found to be 70 mm Hg, and on gonioscopic examination she had a completely closed angle. She was seen 2 hours, rather quickly, after this pain began and she was treated for acute angle closure glaucoma. I would like to ask Dr. Harry Quigley to make a few comments now about the treatment of acute angle-closure glaucoma. Harry, is it as it has always been? Do we have any new wrinkles, any new things that can help us?

Quigley: David, I think there are a couple of things you can mention. I don't think the medical treatment has changed very much at all, although I would assume everyone also adds beta-blockers to their acute management because they are good aqueous formation suppressants. I assume that everyone adds steroids almost immediately, as soon as they see a patient with angle closure, because the patient is going to need antiinflammatory medication, and it's something to start at that point. There have been reports by Dr. Anderson that one can push on the central cornea, either with a goniolens or with a Q-tip, and by this means push the iris back and physically open the angle. Our approach has been more to take the patient directly to the laser and not push on the cornea for fear that by manipulating the cornea we are going to mess it up further in terms of the view. The critical factor is to get the cornea as clear as possible, as soon as possible, so that you can do the laser iridotomy. We do a laser iridotomy as immediately as we can with the patient, hopefully having lowered the pressure medically first, since that usually helps you with the cornea. But, if a couple of hours have gone by and the pressure still hasn't gone down with the medicines that were delivered, we go ahead and try to make a laser hole, which rather promptly drops the pressure. Be sure that you treat the other eye at the same sitting; don't give the patient time to think about whether they want to have their other eye treated; just go ahead and cure that eye right then. I think that's a good approach. I would see the patient back after a laser iridotomy very quickly, when the iridotomy has been done for an acute attack. The reason is that these eyes have much more inflammation in them and much more of a tendency to accumulate pigment around the hole. In addition, you often are shooting through a hazy cornea, which gives you difficulty producing a large-sized opening, and because they could go right back into an attack immediately if the hole that you have made is small and is plugged, I think it best to see them within 1 to 3 days again for a possible retreatment. You tend to need more treatment sessions in people who are treated in the middle of an acute attack. David, we have an experimental protocol right now in patients on whom an argon iridotomy was unable to be performed. Dr. Alan Robin of our institution is the principal investigator of utilizing the YAG laser to produce iridotomies in such eyes as a means of avoiding surgical iridectomy. That has been successful in some, and unsuccessful in others, in producing an iridectomy nonsurgically, as it were, with the laser. That work is continuing, and I think the YAG laser still needs to be evaluated as an experimental instrument only, due to the great dangers of anterior segment treatment doing damage to the lens and other things. Finally, if you have the angle fall open and the attack is broken, immediately reexamine for PAS in the angle for two reasons: First, you can find that way what the prognosis for such a patient is. If the angle has fallen widely open you can smile and say, "Well, that looks as if we caught things in time," as with your patient 2 hours after the attack. One might consider the possibility, if there are PAS present and the attack has been of relatively short duration by history, of using energy delivery to the hump of the PAS just short of the angle in hope of pulling that PAS out of the angle. I have no idea if that produces functional angle underneath PAS that's been so pulled away, but I know that some PAS of recent onset can be so yanked out of the angle by hitting the base of them with the laser.

Campbell: Are there any other comments from the panelists about the treatment of acute angle closure. Dr. Beckman?

Beckman: Yes, I guess I have two comments to add to that. One would be that if you do see one of these right away, don't applanate them, because if you put fluorescein in the eye, it makes it hard for you to see to do the laser iridotomy. So, basically, if I think I'm dealing with an angle-closure glaucoma and I think I am going to abort it with the laser right away, I really try to use a pneumotonometer and avoid getting fluorescein staining onto an eye which may have bullous keratopathy. Or even just the fluorescein film itself can actually reflect back a lot of the laser into your eye as you are trying to work, and it makes an eye with poor visibility even a worse visibility. The only other comment that I would make would be that all angle-closure glaucoma is not pupillary block. After you create the iridotomy, if the pupil doesn't come down right away, you may be dealing with a nonpupil block, primary angle-closure glaucoma and you must recheck the pressure, because sometimes an iridotomy does not reduce it.

Campbell: Well, let's find out what happened here. This patient was treated only 2 hours after the attack began really, and responded well to standard medical therapy of pilocarpine and Timoptic and some Diamox. The pupil constricted, and the pressure came down to 15 mm Hg, and gonioscopy revealed that the angle was entirely open except for 2 hours superiorly where there were 2 hours of synechial closure. The iris was rather convexed. It looked a little bit like a classic relative pupillary block, angle-closure glaucoma attack. The next day, then, the patient was taken to the laser where, as you can see, an uncomplicated laser iridotomy was placed in the 10 o'clock region. Two days later the patient was seen again. She had been told to maintain her pilocarpine, and when she was reexamined, her pupil was 2 mm on pilocarpine, and the angle was once again gonioscoped and was seen to be open for 10 hours with, of course, the 2 hours of synechial closure remaining. A good bit of the previously seen convexity to the iris was now gone. In other words, the relative pupillary block was gone. However, the angle was still somewhat narrow in its periphery. The pilocarpine was discontinued, and the patient was seen a few days later. At this time the pupil was now 4 mm, and the intraocular pressure had elevated to 25 mm Hg. The patient was taking no other glaucoma medications. At this time the gonioscopy revealed that the iridotomy was still open but that the posterior portion of the trabecular meshwork—for the entire 10 hours that it had been previously opened—was now covered. I would like to ask Dr.Simmons at this point what he feels about this case in regard to both diagnosis and treatment.

Simmons: I think if the iridotomy is still open at that time, I would be very much concerned about plateau iris, and that would be my bet at the moment. This is a disease about which Dr. Shaffer and Dr. Chandler shared observations on the first few cases known to ophthalmology.

Campbell: Dr. Shaffer, any comments about the diagnosis here and treatment?

Shaffer: It's such a wonderful story about Paul Chandler. He is a great advocate of iridectomy, of course, and did a lot to teach us in the 1940s and 1950s that we needed to perform iridectomies. A patient came in with an acute angle-closure glaucoma at Harvard. He showed the patient to the residents and said, "Well, take this patient to the operating room, and we'll do an iridectomy, and the patient will be cured." About 2 weeks later the patient came back with the iridectomy, and he said, "Now, we have a cure; we'll dilate this pupil." Bang! The pressure went up to 60 mm Hg. He thought that can't be; we haven't done a good iridectomy. He took the patient back and performed another iridectomy, and again the pressure went up to 60 mm Hg. This was the first finding of the plateau iris; it was actually recognized by Paul Chandler. Would it be proper to branch out just a little? I remain a little bit concerned about the long-term future of laser iridectomies. Again, you have to think in terms of time with any of these things. Jim, here, was doing 35% . . .

Wise: Remember, Dr. Shaffer, that these are people who are referred to me from all over, and it is just astonishing how many referral uncontrolled glaucoma patients actually have a considerable element of angle closure. It's a selected group.

Shaffer: I'm not criticizing it at all; I think you are probably absolutely right. But, remember, I went through the era where they really didn't know what iridectomy was doing. Ten years after iridectomies almost half of them, for some reason, have a mild, chronic, open-angle glaucoma that has to be treated. And a surprising number of them, after 10 or 15 years, get cataracts. I am just not at all sure that the same thing won't happen after another 10 or 15 years with these little openings. So, that's one question. The second question I would like to ask of Jim, and it concerns our having considerably more complaints from patients of halation, that little pencil of light in the peripheral field. A big iridectomy doesn't seem to cause it, but we have some patients who must really be sensitive souls, and they complain bitterly about this little pencil of light. Have you noticed that?

Wise: No, I really haven't Dr. Shaffer. Where are you putting the iridectomies?

Shaffer: The one in particular that I am thinking of is right smack at 12 o'clock and so far out you can hardly see it. Yet the patient frets and fusses.

Wise: I try to put mine quite far out and usually succeed in doing so. As far as the question of late cataract after surgical iridectomy, of course you are doing something rather different there. You are making an incision; you are temporarily dropping the IOP to zero; you have sutures; and so on. So I don't know that a laser iridectomy and a surgical iridectomy would be comparable to this. I can say that laser iridectomies stay open apparently indefinitely and, Dr. Beckman, who has the longest follow-ups of anyone here since he is the one to first do them, can come in. . . . How long, Dr. Beckman, are your iridectomies staying open?

Beckman: Basically, once an iridectomy is open for 6 weeks, it generally stays open forever. How reliably one of them stays open depends on how big you make it and how little inflammation you cause. I am going to talk about that tomorrow or Sunday. This almost goes into my Round Table so, Dave, if you don't mind, I think I'll ask the question now because I don't know the answer to this. I do know that there are a whole bunch of cases that the laser iridotomy has allowed observation in that the surgical iridectomy never allowed observation. I mentioned it before you told me what the case was. I know that there are a percentage of cases in which you do an iridotomy and then come back the next day and the pupil is dilating more. It will take the exact same course as this. You can pour pilocarpine into the eye, but no matter how much you pour into the eye, the pupil will dilate more—until you go from a 2 mm pupil to a 4 mm pupil to a 6 mm pupil—and the pressure will start to rise. Now, there may be such a thing as plateau iris, but most of these cases aren't plateau iris. They are the result of some kind of an abnormal iris neurogenic activity or something that I don't really understand. I know that you have theoretically cured the pupillary block because you have a patent iridectomy, and since my iridectomies are all more peripheral than that, it is not the lens which is coming up and closing it. Mine are open, and they are open to what I think is posterior chamber, and I know that no matter what I do the pupil keeps getting bigger. Some of these patients are treated with oral steroids, and the process reverses. I know that you can't just drill an iridotomy and then walk away from it and come back the next day and know 100% that it is cured.

Shaffer: What had been the pressures as the pupil dilated?

Beckman: It gets higher and higher. I grew up under the theory that one of the reasons that the pupil froze in mid-dilatation was that the pressure was so high that it was causing some kind of atrophy of the sphincter muscles, so you couldn't get the pupil down. That is not so. As an end point for penetration into the anterior chamber, I use the moment the pupil constricts, and it will constrict immediately on penetration. Sometimes, it doesn't; when it doesn't constrict, I become very leery. If the pupil has been resistant to pilocarpine before laser, I become leery. I use prior pilocarpine for two reasons. I put it in because I am interested in obtaining a small pupil for purposes of making a taught iris, and two, I really want to see if pilocarpine is going to bring the pupil down. If it doesn't bring the pupil down, I am leery for the reason that I suspect that I am dealing with something that may not be just pupil block; it may be what this is—and I don't think it has a thing to do with the anatomic relationship between the root of the iris and the trabecular meshwork.

Campbell: Let me try to clarify. I think Dr. Beckman is talking about a type of glaucoma, and this comes down to the question of how many primary angle-closure glaucomas are there. I personally classify and recognize at least three. The first is the most routine, relative pupillary block angle-closure glaucoma that is cured by peripheral iridectomy and is also benefited in general by pilocarpine. The second group that we recognize is the group that this patient I believe falls into, which is what Drs. Shaffer and Simmons call "plateau iris" angle closure. This group of patients is also cured or benefited by pilocarpine, but a peripheral iridectomy is not completely curative. We'll come back to the cure for this patient in just a minute. But there is a third type of primary angle closure that perhaps Dr. Beckman is seeing and that I see, and this is caused by a forward movement of the lens within the eye. In this group all the rules are reversed. An iridectomy does not help because relative pupillary block is not the main problem. Pilocarpine does not help; in fact, it makes it worse by allowing that lens to come further forward. And in this group mydriatic cycloplegic therapy can sometimes be effective by moving the lens posterior. That's roughly the way I break it down to avoid, I hope, a lot of confusion. Let me come back to this case and ask Dr. Simmons how he would treat this case at this point. We now have an angle that is beginning to get covered up again with medication.

Simmons: I would put miotics in the eyes as the first step. The angle is closed; the pupil is enlarging. That will usually open the angle in the presence of a plateau iris, so that should be the first step. I think it very fortunate that Dr. Campbell, who of course has had a lot of experience with this condition, did not put in something like atropine at any point in the course. It used to be thought at one time to be a good idea to put atropine in the eye after surgical iridectomy for angle-closure glaucoma. But that can be almost the kiss of death in a plateau iris eye because it closes the angle, so miotics would be the first step here.

Campbell: Dick, do you feel that there is any role for peripheral iridoplasty in the cure of this type of glaucoma, and where do you place peripheral iridoplasty in your therapeutic regimen?

Simmons: The first step is the miotic. I didn't want to steal something that you were about to lead into. However, the definitive therapy of plateau iris is peripheral iridoplasty or gonioplasty to direct the laser beam to the peripheral roll of the iris. This will flatten the peripheral iris; in the presence of a miotic pupil you can usually flatten it and permanently prevent the syndrome of angle closure due to plateau iris from recurring. It does this by permanently flattening the peripheral iris roll for which I think Bob Shaffer coined the name "plateau iris." It is sort of like flattening the edge of the plateau, so instead of being at more or less a right angle, it now becomes a plane and then cannot close. It is important after doing this procedure to follow the patient with gonioscopy, because it is possible that in some cases more peripheral iridoplasty would be needed. If you keep looking at the angle and it shows some narrowness in an area, or loss of effect of the laser iridoplasty, then apply more.

Campbell: All right. Well, this patient was told what her problem was, and I asked here if she would like to consider a lifetime of pilocarpine or if she would rather have me try a peripheral iridoplasty to see if this would be beneficial to her. She said she would really rather try the peripheral iridoplasty than put up with the pilocarpine, which she hadn't liked very much. So she did have a peripheral iridoplasty. I use a 500 or even sometimes 1000 micron spot size to the periphery of the iris. One treats in a circle for 360 degrees, leaving a little space in between the treatments, and as Dr. Simmons has described in the past, one sees peripheral iris fall back dramatically. In her situation, even without pilocarpine, it did open up her angle, and in fact in most areas the scleral spur could be seen as well. A rather dramatic change. I think you can see just a little fall-off in the peripheral iris out here due to the treatment. So, for the time being at any rate, her pressure is now normal once again, and she is doing well. Dr. Simmons' admonition about watching this patient is certainly well taken, and it is possible that at some point in the future she may require pilocarpine therapy. Dr. Wise?

Wise: This procedure has a rather interesting history. The first person to do a laser peripheral iridoplasty, I believe, was Hugo Hager. He did one of the very, very early papers on treatment of glaucoma. What he did was he went around and treated the peripheral iris; he took patients with open-angle glaucoma and treated the peripheral iris with what amounted to peripheral iridoplasty and tightened the root of the iris, and in doing so he controlled about 30% of the cases of open-angle glaucoma. This is one of the places where I got the idea for tightening up the trabecular meshwork by treating it directly.

Campbell: Dr. Quigley?

Quigley: David, I don't think you are dealing with plateau iris here until you redilate the pupil and the pressure goes back up to 60 mm Hg. There are many too many people who have had intermittent attacks, and you pick them up after they have had 10 attacks. You did in fact break the pupillary block component, but now she goes back up to 25 mm Hg due to the fact that she has had past angle damage or has a combined mechanism. We looked at a group of almost 200 people who had laser iridotomies, gonioscoping them, and judging the approach both before and after. Two thirds of them distinctly looked deeper after the iridotomy. On one third of them I really couldn't tell that they were dramatically deeper, much as you are describing here. The patient comes off pilocarpine, comes off steroids, and you look in the angle, and it still looks a little narrow. Yet, when we dilated those people we didn't see a single example of plateau iris in that particular group. So I wonder if we shouldn't be much more strict in limiting the diagnosis of plateau iris to those people who have a recurrent attack when we redilate the pupil. You have to follow a glaucoma patient with a dilated exam anyway; you're going to have to use a dilated exam. So you might as well do a mydriatic provocative test some point a week after the iridotomy, telling the patient there is the possibility the pressure is going to go up, but certainly not recommitting to a laser procedure unless you are sure that you are dealing with plateau iris, which I think is much less frequent perhaps than might be imagined.

Campbell: Oh, it's not terribly frequent. Your point is well taken in that the open angle here might not be functioning normally. At least up to this point, however, her pressure has come down to a normal range off medicines, and the angle does appear to be normal at this point. Thank you.

GLAUCOMA AND CATARACT

DR. RICHARD J. SIMMONS

Simmons: We'll touch upon a few problems encountered with cataract and glaucoma. The first case is a patient mentioned by Jim Wise the other day. He has a direct line to our computer and he is always kibbitzing on it, so he knew about this very interesting patient who is 65 years of age and had a serious glaucoma in his right eye with double Bjerrum scotomas and total cupping. The left eye was amblyopic. The patient had had an old trabeculectomy in the right eye, which had failed, followed by a bleb revision, which was of benefit. Pressures were stabilized at around

10 to 12 mm Hg. Gradually the pressure edged up towards 14 mm Hg. Jim Wise had pointed out, and I strongly agreed, that patients with very advanced glaucoma have to be managed in a different way from the ordinary glaucoma case. We think one of the ways to keep Dr. Quigley's lamina cribrosa from collapsing is to have an unusually low pressure for the advanced glaucoma case. We attempted to do that in this case. We performed an extracapsular cataract extraction from below. At the same time the pressure had gradually crept up from 10 to 14 mm Hg. We thought the bleb was getting more restricted. Therefore, we did a filtration procedure from below. The patient, however, had been through the mill and had declining filtration from above; a cataract extraction from below; and had a second filtration procedure from below. The patient was, in fact, filtering from the lower bleb, which persisted after the extracapsular extraction. The sector iridectomy had been done some time before by another surgeon, who had done the original glaucoma procedure. In short, this was the situation. The other eye was amblyopic. Having just been to a couple of meetings and having been told that you can do 6000 YAGs without complication, we proceeded with this one, which by chance happened to be the first YAG that we did. We opened up the posterior capsule and had immediate improvement in vision. The patient went home happy. Unfortunately the patient returned a couple of days later. The vitreous had herniated right through the hole in the membrane and was obstructing the sclerostomy inferiorly, which had been keeping the pressure at very low levels.

I have a question for the panel. Obviously something was amiss here. It is less likely to happen if the posterior capsule had been opened widely? Is the small hole in the posterior capsule apt to induce the vitreous to extrude through and follow this pathway? And, why did the vitreous go to the inferior sclerostomy? Dr. Wise looks restless there. Jim?

Wise: The inherent evil nature of vitreous is the problem.

Simmons: You've got it! I think that's pretty true. Can there be any sort of relative block, Dr. Campbell, which might induce vitreous to follow this path, whereby if we had made a wide opening in the posterior capsule, would this have changed things?

Campbell: Well, I don't know, Dick. I've lost two filters that were working well superiorly following cataract extraction in one-eyed people. I was very unhappy about it. It was in the days that I was doing intracapsular surgery following filtration surgery, and it was one of the reasons I switched to extracapsular surgery—to keep that posterior plane intact and not allow the vitreous to come forward and do this. I guess it would be easier for the vitreous to fall into a filter at the bottom than in the two cases just described, where it moved superiorly. I wonder if in this situation, when vitreous begins to herniate forward, if it is not a very bad thing for a person to rub his eye. We all rub our eyes from time to time, and I wonder if a little bit of a rub in a situation like this doesn't just push that vitreous, pretty quickly sometimes, down into the filter. But that's speculation.

Simmons: Hugh Beckman?

Beckman: Dick, let me ask you a couple of questions. One, do you remember what you used to create the capsulotomy? How many millijoules, how many shots?

Simmons: I don't remember. I think it was around 2.5 to 3.0, but I can't remember.

Beckman: The next question would be when was the first time after you did the YAG, the capsulotomy, that you took the pressure?

Simmons: The pressure was taken the same day, and remained at the same level, but 3 days later. . .

Beckman: No, it was the same pressure the same day?

Simmons: Pressure was low the same day before the patient left, but 3 days later the pressure was elevated to about 45 mm Hg with corneal edema.

Beckman: The reason that I asked you was that I have never seen the vitreous come pouring out of the capsulotomy, but I have seen the pressure go up within 1 to 4 hours in maybe 25% to 30% of patients.

Simmons: Yes.

Beckman: But I wondered if maybe when the pressure went up that it just pushed the vitreous into the path of least resistance, like with Healon or something. I thought maybe the pressure came first and pushed the vitreous out through that capsulotomy into the path of least resistance, which was the bleb.

Simmons: Yes, and I think the audience should be aware that we are all seeing, those of us on the panel, pressure rises after capsulotomy that is with an open angle and without this screwball syndrome I first described with this case. Harry?

Quigley: We've certainly documented a pressure rise, which is due to a decrease in outflow facility in almost two dozen eyes after capsulotomy. As a matter of fact, it's the most dramatic fall in tonographic outflow facility that we have ever seen in any study we have ever done on anything.

Simmons: Wow.

Quigley: And, in that study by Arlo Terry, Walter Stark, Ed Maumenee, and myself, the outflow facility fell to half of what it had been pre-Yag capsulotomy. And again, that's independent of whether vitreous came forward, but it's a substantial minority of the cases. If you do a capsulotomy either with or without the presence of an intraocular lens, the vitreous gel appears to dissolve and come forward around the corner of an intraocular lens or, as here, right on through. I would imagine you had debris plugging up most of the rest of the angle—debris from the extracapsular clump that you broke up. Therefore, as Hugh pointed out, the only path out of which water was going at all at that point was your bleb. So, the vitreous being loose and present in the AC, it just followed the only way out.

Simmons: Jim?

Wise: Well, really, again vitreous just seems to have a tendency to go where you don't want it at all times. David Paton once did a study in which he did a large number of microsurgical intracapsular cataract extractions and demonstrated that in 55% of them they had a broken vitreous face with loose vitreous in the anterior chamber—in spite of the fact that he had used meticulous surgical technique to avoid this. I have had people years ago where I aspirated fluid vitreous and had the intraocular pressure literally at negative levels before doing intracapsular extractions. Then, I immediately made the pupil small with Miochol and kept it that way, and low and behold, loose vitreous came through. That vitreous simply must be kept out of the anterior chamber. It is not a matter of saying, "If I do this or I do that the vitreous will stay back." The vitreous will not stay back, and what you do with these people is you polish their capsule. You cannot afford to open the capsule and allow the vitreous to get in there if you have a filtering bleb. You have to polish the capsule, and if it clouds, you have got to polish it again and again and again. The only way you can get around this is to put in a posterior chamber lens and do the capsulotomy behind it.

Simmons: Harry?

Quigley: Well, I'll stick my neck out as a noncataract surgeon just to point out that some recent data suggest that polishing the capsule probably doesn't—did you mean to suggest that it prevents opacification, Jim? There is good histological evidence recently published by Peter McDonnell and Dick Greene from Wilmer in *Ophthalmology* that opacification comes from anterior capsule left behind.

Wise: No, that is not what I said. Harry, you must not have been listening.

Quigley: That's why I asked what you meant.

Wise: I said that you have to polish it again and again and again.

Quigley: To do what? To accomplish what?

Wise: That what you wind up with these people. Didn't you hear me say you polish, and it will cloud, and you polish it again and again and again. That is exactly the case. You can polish a capsule till the world looks level, and it will still cloud again. But, the point is that if you open it the vitreous will plug your bleb in a considerable percentage of cases. So, if you have an extracapsular cataract operation alone, and the capsule clouds, and you have a filtering bleb, you are going to just have to polish the capsule. And when it clouds in 6 months or a year or two, you are going to have to polish it again and again and again. That is just part of the deal if you do this operation.

Quigley: Oh, I understand. Have you done that?

Wise: In a number of cases. In one case, after I polished the capsule three times, I finally did a capsulotomy, whereupon the bleb failed, and I wound up having to do cryosurgery on the patient.

Simmons: I have a few other goodies, so I don't want to spend a lot of time on this. This is an easy case. It is a reason why I think one should use a posterior chamber lens if you are going to do extracapsular surgery in the presence of a filtering bleb. I now do it; I think it is more conservative than to be faced with this type of situation. We have encountered other situations where the vitreous has come forward after YAG and obstructed filtration operations, so it can be grave. Now, if we look at this patient who came in in 1982—the patient had prior surgery by another ophthalmologist, and the doctor had not done an iridectomy. He put in an AC lens and, as you would expect, there was aphakic pupillary block, and it had been of 1-week duration. The angle was closed. You could deepen this chamber with mydriasis and see that the angle was closed. The tension at this time was only 20 mm Hg. We did laser iridectomies and relieved the pupillary block, and the chamber deepened. However, after that the angle was closed 270 degrees. Laser gonioplasty, also called peripheral iridoplasty, was used to contract the peripheral iris after the pupil was brought down to a very small miotic pupil, thereby opening peripheral anterior synechia and opening the angle 360 degrees. This case illustrates that synechiae can be reversible and that peripheral iridoplasty can reverse certain early synechiae. But the story was not over; the iridectomy closed and pupillary block recurred. This was broken again with mydriasis, and the iridectomy was reopened. The angle then remained open thereafter. The case illustrates several things. In addition to the fact that gonioplasty can be effective, it illustrates that aphakic pupillary block in the presence of an anterior chamber IOL can recur and that this is a main danger. Now, if the gonioplasty had not been effective, Dr. Campbell, would you have picked up the syringe on the left and employed it in some manner?

Campbell: Well, I would have done what Dr. Simmons has shown me to do, and that is, if the angle had remained closed and remained synechially closed at this point, and if laser treatment to the periphery of the iris could not cause the iris to fall away from the trabecular meshwork, and if there was every reason to think that this synechial closure hadn't been existent for too long—and in this case I guess it hadn't—we are thinking about weeks to months, and that is favorable. I would consider taking the patient to the operating room to perform a chamber-deepening procedure, and if a significant amount of synechial closure remained after that—and that procedure can sometimes in itself cause a few synechiae to come away—then would have considered the procedure that I told you all about and which I know Dick has used in the past as well, which is goniosynechialysis.

Simmons: I think, Dave, if you could show us that procedure in your short film, I think it is really of value because, technically, this synechiolysis is very difficult. Dave has developed a very neat method, better than the method I had previously employed for peripheral anterior synechiolysis, and I think you would all enjoy seeing his film.

Campbell: This is about a 7-minute film showing the procedure that I described to you yesterday. What one does here is, if one has reason to think he has a patient with a lot of synechial angle closure, and it hasn't been there for too long, one puts an inferior and superior rectus bridle suture on it so that one can rotate the eye and also hold that eye in the proper position. The first thing one does is to make a paracentesis wound inferiorly into the anterior chamber to do the chamber-deepening procedure. One lets fluid out of the anterior chamber with either a Wheeler or Zeigler knife and shallows the anterior chamber to about two corneal thicknesses. One then presses on the limbus to force the fluid that is in the posterior chamber up into the anterior chamber, and I go around a couple of times and have a little fun, as you can see. Then, replace the knife into the anterior chamber. Once again, shallow the anterior chamber to a depth of about two corneal thicknesses. This is part of the chamber-deepening procedure. Then, using Healon, one does the actual chamber deepening. The lens is placed posteriorly, generally to a depth of about six to eight corneal thicknesses, depending upon the eye. But this presses the lens back out of danger. It also causes the peripheral iris to fall back posteriorly. One then gonioscopes the patient to be sure that there is the significant synechial closure that you are supposedly after. Then, one makes incisions at 3 o'clock and 9 o'clock for the synechialysis spatula. Now, this incision is important. It has to be small on the outside and wide on the inside. There are two reasons for that. The first is that if it is small on the outside, you won't lose your anterior chamber quickly, and if it is wide on the inside, the synechialysis spatula will pass without causing wrinkling of the cornea. Having made the incision, one then deepens the anterior chamber again, and now one takes the synechialysis spatula, which is an irrigating spatula, and this has a curve on it so that it will vault the lens and yet remain under the cornea. One then places a Barkan surgical goniotomy lens on the eye, and using a headlight—and I like to use either 4X or 6X loupes for good visualization of the angle—one then in an anterior to posterior motion places that synechialysis spatula across the anterior chamber. The Healon does two things for you: it holds the chamber deep—and reliably so—and it not only helps coagulate any bleeding that occurs, but it localizes any bleeding that occurs in the angle, thus preventing an obscuration of the surgical view. Now, here is an indirect lens, and we are looking at the angle down through an operating microscope. This is a special cutaway lens that was made for us for this procedure. But, it is tough to operate backwards, and I have given up the use of this lens, and we are looking into a double-mirror lens system at the present time. One half of the angle has been opened, and we are going to go after a few hours of synechiae on the other side, and you will be able to see through an indirect mirror just how this is done. Again, a wider incision on the corneal side than on the external side. The chamber is deepened again; the irrigating cyclodialysis spatula is very important, having the irrigation at the tip. Again, it prevents unwanted flattening of the anterior chamber, and it allows you to stop bleeding instantly by elevating the pressure in the eye if you need it. Now, here we are with some synechiae formation, and in an anterior-to-posterior motion, the spatula simply lyses the synechiae, and in this case we didn't get any bleeding as we pulled the synechiae off the trabecular meshwork. At the end of the case, you have to get the Healon out of the eye, and you do that by placing a cannula across the anterior chamber, and the Healon will usually squirt out in a bolus around the needle. I then close the two incisions on each side with a buried 10-0 nylon suture, and that completes the case. Dick, I'll turn it back to you.

Simmons: Thank you very much, Dave. Really interesting. I would like to ask Bob Shaffer—Bob, you have taught us and we know that in some eyes where there is angle closure the meshwork becomes damaged, and in others where there has been angle closure it seems to function when opened. Is there some way to determine or guess which will function and what is going on there? Can you comment on that phenomenon?

Shaffer: I doubt it. It seems to me that Dr. Chandler had done quite a few of these and didn't feel that he had improved the facility of outflow very often, especially after a few months of closure. But Dave is showing that it can work.

Simmons: Harry Quigley, what goes on when the angle closes temporarily, and what happens histologically when an angle becomes functionless so that opening it would not produce improvement in outflow?

Quigley: I have seen traumatized angles and also angles in eyes with chronic narrow-angle glaucoma, and when there is no flow, it ordinarily is collapsed together. Now David ought to show us angle histology from eyes such as this and also what tonographic outflow facility does from before to after the procedure to show that outflow facility in fact has improved. That would be evidence that the procedure has actually done something good. But, one would guess—and it is just a wild guess—that things are going to fuse together and there will be nonfunctional angle underneath a long-standing synechiae. I think that is what David said when he said he wouldn't do it on a case that had long-standing synechiae.

Simmons: Yes. So the duration is certainly an important factor in this. Hugh?

Beckman: I just want to clear up one thing on this case that we did. Was there synechial closure on the case you presented?

Simmons: This case? Oh yes. The pupillary block was relieved repeatedly, and the angle remained closed by synechiae.

Beckman: Closed by synechiae?

Simmons: Yes.

Beckman: Eventually it remained closed . . .

Simmons: And then laser peripheral iridoplasty, that is gonioplasty, was used to direct the laser to the base of the synechiae, and they were peeled off the angle so that the angle opened under our eyes, as shown in the slide I had projected.

Beckman: And that worked?

Simmons: Yes. The facility of outflow improved to around 0.20. Some cases can reverse. The patient on the right had a synechiolysis after pupillary block and aphakia in 1975. That patient had a history of flat chamber, as best we could reconstruct from the history, of 3-months duration. Nobody had done anything about it, and finally the patient was sent in, and iridectomy was done to relieve the block. Then the synechiae were stripped with synechiolysis, and the facility of outflow in that patient was 0.23. It definitely improved and definitely opened. We were kind of startled that anybody who had been closed for 3 months could function, but that patient retained a pressure of 15 mm Hg for many years thereafter. I was very interested in Dave Campbell saying he might even go up to a year in certain cases, but in the short-duration cases of 8 days or 8 weeks, it certainly is important to consider it. Harry?

Quigley: One of the things Dave and I have talked about is whether or not he is actually doing a cyclodialysis either advertently or microinadvertently. And, if not, it might well be that you are also improving this so-called uveal scleral outflow pathway, that is, access of aqueous humor to the ciliary body face by pushing this down, so that the trabecular meshwork might be scarred shut, but you are still getting aqueous out by the unconventional outflow pathway.

Simmons: Yes, we have looked for cyclodialysis clefts in these, and I think in the 1950s in particular, Bob Shaffer said he did—and I know Drs. Chandler and Grant, in trying this, created some clefts inadvertently. Particularly when techniques were used where you couldn't see the angle well. Dave Campbell and I think that now being able to visualize it bettter, it helps with that problem, but still you must guard against those.

Quigley: You would take a functioning cyclodialysis to control the pressure, wouldn't you? Nothing wrong with it.

Simmons: Well, anything that works. But I guess it would be nice to restore the angle if it can be opened. Also, there are some other cases related to glaucoma in aphakia that are very difficult. This patient had congenital cataracts. The cataracts were taken out from above at an early age years before, and the patient's other eye developed glaucoma. The eye was lost after recurrent elevated pressure. She had a prosthesis, and she is 23 years of age. In this eye, when she came in, she had pressures that were bouncing into the 30s from the 20s. The upper third of her angle was closed; the remainder of the angle was open and looked rather dirty, with debris lying on it obscuring landmarks. There is scarring at the limbal region above; there is a sector iridectomy. What in the world can one do for this difficult patient? She has nystagmus; this is her only eye; she has 20/200 vision; she says she is getting recurrent blurring and halos in this remaining eye. What is available for a patient like this? Bob Shaffer?

Shaffer: That's a mean one to ask. We see too many eyes like this, and I don't know what you do with them. You try a trabeculectomy. We are now getting these implants and trying them, but I have put many different implants in over the years, and they all get a nice little envelope of connective tissue around them after a month or two and up goes the pressure. I am skeptical. The Molteno valve is the one that has the most promise now. He has done 200 to 300 of these claims good results, but I just bet that they scar down.

Simmons: Jim Wise?

Wise: I have taken care of several cases of terrible glaucoma in children. First of all, I don't believe that trabeculectomies ever work in children. They have such a tremendous ability to fibrose and scar that they will heal up any and all trabeculectomies. What I have found to be fairly effective—and I have had at least an 80% success rate with this—is to do a full-thickness filtering procedure. At the time I do it, I will balloon up Tenon's capsule with saline and then have the assistant hold up the edges of conjunctiva while I will sit there and painstakingly cut away all the Tenon's capsule from beneath the flap to create an exceedingly thin flap, composed—as nearly as I can get it—of conjunctiva alone. I mean these are flaps where you can just see right through the thing and see the scissors with unbelievable clarity. Then, when I have cut this incredibly thin flap with a full-thickness filtering procedure, I will go ahead and sew it down. They will typically have flat chambers for quite a while. Sometimes a couple of weeks, but they tend to work; this is the only way I know of. I have managed to make bilateral filtering procedures work in a 7-year-old black child; I managed to make one of these work in a kid who had had something like four trabeculectomies elsewhere. This is the only procedure I feel will work in these children—a superthin flap, full-thickness filtering procedure.

Simmons: I am glad that something can work. This is a real patient, and the patient is waiting for me when I get back from here. I want all the advice I can get. Dave Campbell, have you had success with eyes of this sort? Twenty-three years of age.

Campbell: Well, it looks as if—at what age was the cataract extraction done?

Simmons: Young, when she was a child.

Campbell: But somehow the superior conjunctiva is all scarred down?

Simmons: Aphakic, yes, from the cataract surgery done years ago.

Campbell: Well, of course, once the conjunctiva superiorly becomes scarred, it's almost impossible—I won't say it's totally—but it's almost impossible to get that conjunctiva to accept successful filtration, and a very bad sign on the photograph on the right is that kind of light gray color to the superior conjunctiva, indicating to me that there is a layer of collagen underneath the conjunctiva, and it is going to be very difficult to get this conjunctiva to filter. I think we will have to ask Dr. Beckman what he would do in light of his recent lecture. There are a couple of new advances coming along that I think we hope are going to help—biochemical adjuncts to prevent scarring in filtration blebs—and two approaches are being investigated. One done by Dr. Parrish down in Miami is to inject an antimetabolite 5-FU into the subconjunctival space on a daily or twice daily basis to inhibit fibroblastic growth within the filtration site. I think he might tell us that this might help us a little bit in this situation. Other investigators are looking at collagen cross-linking blocking agents such as BAPN, and I think we have to hope that perhaps some of these agents will help us in the future.

Simmons: Dr. Beckman, how about your therapy?

Beckman: I certainly think what Dave said is very applicable. This might be a case where 5-FU might work, particularly if you have some decent conjunctiva. Actually, for laser cyclocoagulation, these cases have been the best group—the aphakes. You are talking about a period of over 10 years with almost an 85% success rate with really reasonably minimal complications. Although everyone is reluctant to do anything on a 23-year-old's only eye that is slipping, I believe a cyclocoagulation might be indicated.

Simmons: Harry and then Jim Wise.

Wise: I just want to make a quick comment, and that is that when I talked about the thin flap procedures, I thought this patient was phakic. If this is an aphakic patient, no filtering procedure will work.

Simmons: It's aphakic, yes.

Wise: No, what I was speaking about phakic patients, not aphakic.

Simmons: Harry, wrap it up with the answer.

Quigley: No, I haven't got the answer, but we're one of the laboratories; I guess the other laboratory is doing laboratory work on inhibitors, and we have tried to fool the fibroblast into making faulty collagen with 6-hydroxyproline in research done by Roger Mason in my lab. That did not work in an animal model; however, what did work in an animal model very mildly was use of the drug David mentioned—beta-aminopropionitrile. There is now a trial about to be reported on that. We hope that we will have something that is going to prevent the fibroblasts from ruining these operations, because that is where we are losing them. No one wanted to say it, so I'll say it: cyclocryotherapy is a way of lowering the pressure in this person's eye. It is also a threat to her vision, and if there is nothing else going to keep her from going blind from glaucoma, cyclocryotherapy will work, but with a big risk.

Simmons: Hugh, last word?

Beckman: I think when most suggest cyclocryotherapy or cyclocoagulation, I know they are getting splinters under their fingernails from scraping the bottom of the barrel. But, there is—you know, Jackson Coleman's technique—which if it is as good as he reported at the Academy, it really is very promising with therapeutic ultrasound.

Simmons: So, it is going to take new procedures to make these cases do satisfactorily in general. It is a very difficult case, and conventional procedures are unlikely to be very successful. Let's hope for luck in this case. Thank you.

PROBLEM CASES

DR. ROBERT N. SHAFFER

Shaffer: You have had so much heavy emphasis on therapy—and a lot of it on laser therapy—to a point that you would conclude that if you had somebody in the waiting room, there is no point in examining them, just put them down behind the laser and shoot. So, I still think there is some small place at least for diagnosis, and that is essentially what these problem cases are about. You still have to look at the patient. So often in our dimly lit consultation rooms, we don't really pay attention to see if the patient looks healthy. Are they pale? Do they limp? Do they have a shuffle? Do they have any heterochromia and this sort of thing? I think we all check with slit-lamp examinations, but when you are using a slitlamp, you look first at one eye and then you look at the other, and you don't look at the two together. If there is just a little bit of heterochromia, it is very easily missed. So I would like to ask my panel of experts. Here is a patient, a 52 year old, with glaucoma diagnosed a year ago and referred to me by a doctor from San Francisco who repeatedly got pressures somewhere in the 30 to 40 mm Hg zone in both eyes. Therapy didn't seem to help a whale of a lot. He had perfectly normal discs, with perfectly normal fields, a slight exophthalmos, and takes thyroid, and in our office we got pressures of 20 mm Hg in the right eye—15 Shiøtz in the right and similarly in the left. Normal pressures higher with the Goldmann than with the Shiøtz. Normal facilities of outflow. In the first place, why was I getting a difference with Goldmann and Schiøtz measurements? Harry?

Quigley: The patient has low scleral ridigity, and probably on top of the fact that the Schiøtz scale reads low relative to applanation, that's a little out of line—5 mm Hg between the eyes. So the patient probably has low scleral rigidity.

Shaffer: Low scleral rigidity.

Quigley: Myope? Is the patient near sighted?

Shaffer: No. We sent this patient back to the referring doctor, and he again got high pressures. Why? Dr. Simmons?

Simmons: He's testing a patient in a position where the eyes are in semiupward gaze, which will raise the pressure in the presence of thyroid exophthalmos.

Shaffer: That is exactly right. This man always used a Schiøtz tonometer. He had one of these surgical chairs that lean them back halfway. I bet his target was actually behind the patient. With eyes straight the pressure was normal. With eyes up it would go up as far as 40 mm Hg if I really forced it. So, this is one of those things to keep in mind. We had one like that just this last week in the office. All right, here is a case of heterochromia. It is an obvious heterochromia. Which eye is the affected eye? One of these eyes has glaucoma and the other does not. I think I will ask Dave to discuss this. Dr. Campbell? I realize that this is an unfair question, but you have some hints here anyway. If one of these eyes has an increased pressure. . .

Campbell: We see on the right a pale-blue iris, and on the left an iris that is darker and seems to be transmitting a little more of the posterior pigment layer through it. I have been fooled, though, in trying to figure out without a little more help, which eye is the eye that has changed. I guess the left, I would say, is . . .

Shaffer: Because of the pupil size.

Campbell: Yes.

Shaffer: He is under therapy. He is on pilocarpine. You are quite right. It is the left eye that is at fault. And this will surprise you, I think, Dave, because this is a monocular pigmentary glaucoma. They are very rare, and I have only seen two or three. Have any of the others seen monoculars?

Quigley: I have seen asymmetrical, but not totally monocular.

Shaffer: Yes. The other one was just as clean as a whistle. It worries you because you are afraid you are missing a melanotic lesion somewhere in the eye. This man I followed for over 20 years so that I am sure that it is not anything except pigmentary. Dave?

Campbell: I have had called to my attention one patient who had monocular pigmentary glaucoma. It was a man who had had a lens extraction early in life in one eye, and he did not develop pigmentary glaucoma in the eye with the lens extraction, but in the other eye he did. I have had another patient in my practice who had almost pure unilateral pigmentary glaucoma, and that was in an eye that was myopic, whereas his other eye was emmetropic.

Shaffer: That's terrific. That proves the Campbell theory. Dr. Quigley?

Quigley: If you didn't have the patient on miotics, you could have a little bit of ptosis on that side, a little miosis and heterochromia, and it could have been a congenital Horner's on the left.

Shaffer: Don't be impatient. Exfoliatives can also produce pigmentation. This is exfoliation on the zonules. All right, here is another one. Which eye, Harry, is the affected eye here? One of them has glaucoma.

Quigley: Well, the pupil on the right certainly looks like it is not only larger, but pulled up and totally out of shape up there. If there hasn't been surgery . . .

Shaffer: It's an aphakic eye.

Quigley: On the right.

Shaffer: Yes.

Simmons: It has Fuch's heterochromia, and the cataract was taken out.

Shaffer: Yes. What would the angle look like?

Campbell: Fine new vessels.

Shaffer: Little tiny vessels in the angle. This is Fuch's heterochromia that has had the lens extracted. What a terrrific panel. OK, which is the affected eye here? Jim? Would you advise laser on that right eye?

Wise: No, I would like to know what all that pigment is histologically, though.

Shaffer: That's mascara.

Wise: No, no, in the dark-brown iris. Again, any time you have heterochromia, the abnormal eye can be either the dark eye or the light eye. If you have heterochromia in a brown-eyed person, it doesn't have to be total. That is, they can be dark brown on one side, and be a normal eye, and be light brown on the other. So it really is impossible to sit here and say which eye is in fact the abnormal eye. The right eye, however, is a little bit injected. If I were to pick one, I would say that it is probably that right eye.

Shaffer: Batting 100%. This was a traumatic eye with a big vitreous hemorrhage. This is the siderosis, if you will, from the hemoglobin.

Wise: Hemosiderosis.

Shaffer: How about this one?

Wise: Well I think here, again, you still have the dilemma that it could be either eye. On the right eye you have a very light-brown iris and a small pupil, and you might postulate that that eye was the abnormal eye and on pilocarpine. On the other side, on the left, the eye is darker. You could think of siderosis or melanoma or vitreous hemorrhage in the other side, particularly after trauma. I would bet on the left eye being the abnormal eye.

Shaffer: This one is pretty obvious in terms of heterochromia, but if there was much less heterochromia, it could be missed. Believe me, you'll be in trouble if you have to explain that in front of a jury. This was siderosis from an intraocular foreign body.

Wise: So it was the left eye.

Shaffer: Yes, it's the left eye. All right, what about this one? This is an open-angle glaucoma patient of Steve Kramer. He kindly loaned this slide to me. Let's let Dr. Beckman discuss this. The other eye did not have this browness.

Beckman: This is an open-angle glaucoma case?

Shaffer: It's open angle, and it is an unfair question. I will warn you ahead of time.

Beckman: It looks like an eight-ball hemorrhage.

Shaffer: It's an open-angle glaucoma

Quigley: Is this patient wearing something cosmetic on the cornea?

Shaffer: Let him keep going. I was going to say that the patient is on pilocarpine and epinephrine therapy. He is a myope.

Quigley: And you owe him a new lens.

Shaffer: And he needs a new lens. This is a staining from epinephrine of a soft contact lens.

This was a patient of mine followed for 25 years. He had a moderate increase in pressure but good optic nerves when I first saw him some 20 years ago. He had these peculiar bumps on the iris. They went right over into the angle; down below they were pigmented; up above they looked almost like dew drops—almost like little keratic precipitates. In the center of these brown nodules, most of them had tiny blood vessels which you could see. The angle looked like this, with partial covering of the trabeculum.

Quigley: Was he completely unilateral?

Shaffer: He was completely unilateral, yes. He had a few nevi on the other blue iris, but nothing spectacular.

Quigley: Café au lait spots on the rest of him anywhere?

Shaffer: No café au lait spots on the skin elsewhere, no.

Simmons: KP in the angle?

Shaffer: Well, these looked a little like KP up above, but they really didn't below, and they certainly didn't on the iris.

Simmons: Sarcoidosis?

Shaffer: He did not have sarcoidosis, no. So what had we better do with him? Dave, do you have a suggestion? Shall we just follow him along medically? The discs and fields are OK. We can wait.

Quigley: There are two other things that simulate it. One is iris nevus syndrome, and the other would be an iris melanoma that has seeded around several different spots and is very slow growing.

Shaffer: Yes.

Quigley: It would be rare for a metastatic lesion to the iris to be 25 years.

Shaffer: The iris nevus syndrome—there was no real closure of the angle due to this tissue and no pull-up of iris nor displacement of the pupil. Well, with fear and trembling we did an iridectomy the iridectomy being a biopsy. And lo and behold it was a spindle A melanoma! He has gone for 25 years now. Gradually the pressure got somewhat higher. We could not control the pressure completely. Then he developed a little bit of cataract, and at present only has about a 20/100 vision. I am afraid to feel his liver, but so far he seems to be all right.

Simmons: Are these multiple tumors, Bob?

Shaffer: Multiple ones all over the iris, yes. It is a worry. This dates back far enough that I had Dr. Zimmerman, Dr. Reese, and Dr. Hogan, all of them looking at this guy, and they all reassured me and told me not to do anything, and I'm glad I haven't. This next case is an interesting one in that this was a photograph I took in my office in 1947. It's not too bad a kodachrome after that long—it looks better than I do. This was a slightly raised brown lesion of the iris which goes into the angle, climbs up as far as Schwalbe's line internally. What would you do with such a lesion? Would you excise? Would you wait and watch? What would you do? Jim?

Wise: Well, there certainly was a time when such a lesion would have called for enucleation, and you saw this patient at that time. So, if you did not enucleate the eye, you were, as usual, ahead of your time.

Shaffer: You are pretty safe.

Wise: But it could either be a nevus or a melanoma. With presently available surgical techniques, if one were to feel that it were a melanoma you could do an iridocyclectomy, but I would think that this eye is better watched. As I say, it could be either a nevus or a spindle A melanoma. But it could very well sit there for the next 37 years.

Shaffer: I think you are very wise. What we did was to get photographs, and then we measured it very carefully. Every two years we remeasured. Year after year after year—absolutely no change in this thing. In 1972 he disappeared for about 5 years, and I didn't see him. When he came back, this is how he looked. The right eye was the blue eye with the lower temporal brown spot, and now it is brown everywhere. That's the way the iris looks now. Now you can see he has a cataract. He was quite happy, actually, because suddenly he was able to read without glasses with his right eye. Pressures were up to around 30 to 32 mm Hg, and over a period of about the last 4 or 5 years, gradually the pressure has gone up in the eye. The cataract has gotten worse and he has practically no vision in the eye now. What shall I do with him? What does he have?

Simmons: He's got a melanoma.

Shaffer: He has a melanoma for sure. What will we do about it?

Simmons: I'd take it out. He's got another good eye on the other side.

Shaffer: You'd take the eye out?

Simmons: Yes, it is only going to get glaucoma and get worse and worse.

Shaffer: OK.

Quigley: I think, before you make a decision, you want to have a look at his liver with noninvasive studies. You would want to do a chest x-ray. You would want to get liver enzymes and have a good internist look him over to be sure that there are not now present signs of metastases.

Shaffer: He has gone to the tumor clinic at the University of California, and there are no other signs whatsoever. Will you enucleate?

Quigley: If the eye is not painful, I would leave it there.

Shaffer: How about you, Dave? Should we leave it there?

Campbell: No, I would enucleate.

Shaffer: You would enucleate.

Campbell: Yes.

Shaffer: Jim?

Wise: Melanomas can change. That is, you can start out as a spindle tumor and then ultimately become an epitheloid tumor, which can kill you. Just as Dr. Simmons says, this eye is not going to do well. If you take out the cataract, it is still going to have glaucoma. It is still going to give trouble. Furthermore, the moment you open up the eye you run the risk of extraocular seeding of the tumor, and I think it belongs in a bottle.

Shaffer: Dr. Quigley?

Quigley: We will presume that you have transilluminated, and there is no sign that there is a ciliary body melanoma. It is purely involving the iris?

Shaffer: No, this is the angle picture, and it climbed up on the angle. But, so far as I could tell, there wasn't anything in the ciliary body.

Quigley: Some of the iris melanomas do get all over the angle, but as long as it is not a ciliary body tumor, those that were confined to the iris in a pathology series at Wilmer, there were only two that ever metastasized out of the eye. And in both of those there were attempts to control glaucoma surgically and preserve the eye that preceded the metastases of the iris melanoma. So, if the patient is comfortable, and he understands that he has even a very, very small chance that this might metastasize in the future, but wants his eye in his head, I don't see any reason to remove it.

Shaffer: I think you can jump either way on this one and be correct. If he gets his metastasis, then we have been wrong. We have not done anything about it; he has refused enucleation and he is still sitting tight. Dr. Beckman?

Beckman: Just to be a little avant garde, you could inject fluorescein and do a fluorescein angiogram to see how vascular this is. I suspect that is not going to be terribly vascular. But were it vascular, then you have a reasonable chance of getting hematoporphyrin derivative in. If you can get hematoporphyrin derivative in, then you might be able to do photoradiotherapy on this person. That would depend on, after much consultation with the patient as to the possible outcome of doing that, but certainly this is the kind of thing where photoradiation therapy is being investigated.

Shaffer: I am sure that you would be able to destroy a great deal of tumor just before you enucleated.

Here is a 70-year-old druggist with open-angle glaucoma in both eyes. The pressure is above standard, discs somewhat cupped, very mild arcuate defects, but the interesting thing was the very thickened conjunctiva in each eye. He had slight early cataracts, and vision was not much impaired at the time. This is the way both conjunctivas looked—both above and below. Jim?

Wise: Lymphoma of the conjunctiva.

Shaffer: Aren't you terrific! That's absolutely right. What did I do here?

Wise: On these, these fall into two categories. One is a pure lymphoma, where all the cells are pretty much normal at the same time—which is not thought to be malignant. It is a localized lymphoma of the conjunctiva, but it can cause some ungodly glaucoma. It will go away with radiation therapy, which is the treatment of choice. If, on the other hand, on biopsy it is found to be a multicellular type, then you are dealing with a systemic lymphoma, and the prognosis is entirely different. Most of these, however, are monocell type lymphomas and are not malignant. You just radiate them, and they go away.

Shaffer: At this time his health was perfectly normal. He had this pink, thickened conjunctiva. We gave him steroids, and this whitened up both eyes beautifully, but the pressure went sky-high, so we had to stop the steroids, and immediately the irritation and thickness recurred. His fundi looked like this. What do you think of that, Jim?

Wise: I think I would like to see a fluorescein angiogram.

Shaffer: I don't have it, I'm sorry. I don't know the nature of the fundus lesion, but the subsequent course made me wonder about it. Well, let's keep going. We eventually took out both lenses in each eye—combined extractions in each eye—excised that thick Tenon's capsule and then, at the examination in the hospital, lo and behold he had a 26,000 white count and 85% lymphs, so he had been converted into a malignant lymphatic leukemia. He is now on chemotherapy and not doing extra well. His pressures did well, and he has at least kept vision. I haven't seen him now for about a year, and I am just afraid he is on his way. This is the biopsy.

Here is a 28-year-old woman. At the age of 15 she had bilateral iridectomies for angle-closure glaucoma. What do you think of that, just stopping there? Dave? How many angle-closure glaucomas have you operated at age 15?

Campbell: Yes, that is most peculiar, isn't it? Dr. Simmons mentioned the syndrome of nanophthalmos this morning, and that comes to mind. That's the patient with a very tiny eye, high hyperopia, and in these eyes it really seems that the eye is simply too small for a normal-sized or just-under-normal-sized lens.

Shaffer: This was an 11 mm cornea.

Campbell: OK. The other . . .

Quigley: Is she Oriental?

Shaffer: She is not Oriental. She is Finnish. These surgeries were done in Finland.

Campbell: The other syndrome that I have seen is one that we have kind of talked about a little bit on and off during the meeting. That is, that there are some patients who develop a primary angle closure, if you will, where the lens just simply seems to move forward in the eye. I don't know why that is. I don't know whether we should call this ciliary block glaucoma or malignant glaucoma or something else, because I don't know why the lens comes forward. Nevertheless, it does, and the treatment here has to be mydriatic cycloplegic therapy. If these people are given pilocarpine, then the lens just comes forward a little more and only makes things worse. In this syndrome I have generally seen it be quite asymmetric. Usually one eye can have this happen, and then it can be many, many, many years before it will happen in the other eye. I have seen it all ages, from early childhood and right up through the age of 70 or so, so this would come to mind for someone with peculiar iridectomies at this very young age.

Shaffer: This is the way the iridectomy looked in one eye. There are synechiae up above there, but most of the angle was open to a grade 3. These were her field defects in both upper temporal areas. What do you think of them? Her pressures have been intermittently elevated in the years since then.

Campbell: Can we go back and look at the gonioscopic picture again, and then once more to the iridectomy?

Simmons: Has she had trauma?

Shaffer: No.

Simmons: Big vessels on the outside of the eye?

Shaffer: No.

Beckman: Did she ever have KP?

Shaffer: No KP at this time. However, that is a cogent question. What about those field defects? I am interested in your reaction to that on a person who has increased pressure.

Simmons: Wise has got the answer. I agree with Wise.

Shaffer: OK, go ahead Jim.

Wise: Well, this morning I found out about iris cysts from Dr. Simmons, and I'll bet this is . . .

Shaffer: If it was a schisis or something like that, it would be up above, wouldn't it? What do you want to do with this one? Is this a glaucoma field?

Wise: No.

Shaffer: No, this doesn't fit at all. This is the way her discs looked. Both of them looked normal. This could not be glaucoma loss. What do you want to do then to find out about that field loss?

Quigley: CT scan.

Shaffer: You want a CT scan?

Quigley: Yes.

Wise: I would want to look at the peripheral retina first.

Shaffer: Why don't you look with the ophthalmoscope? There it was. She had an atypical coloboma of the upper temporal choroid. Darndest thing, never saw one like it. It turns out that she is one of these patients who have intermittent pressure elevations in both eyes. It would go up for a while, and then suddenly the pressure would drop and she would get flare and cells in both eyes, and I think it was an atypical type of glaucomatocyclitic crisis. Can you correct me on that, or do you think that's probable?

Campbell: Yes, in putting that together, could those colobomas have been due to severe inflammation of the choroid and retina? Or did they look developmental?

Shaffer: The retinal lesions were congenital. I think what happened was that she had a rise of pressure, enough to produce some corneal edema. The surgeon who saw her thought it was angle closure and did iridectomies, which were probably unnecessary.

Quigley: The reason those fields look neurologic, Bob, is that they were exactly straight up the vertical midline in each eye. A binasal loss like that might be dolechoectatic vessels. That was what led me to my CT scan. I asked whether she was Oriental before, because many of the patients we see, at least on the east coast, who have glaucomatocyclitic crisis are Oriental in extraction.

Shaffer: That is very interesting. OK, let's go ahead here. Here is a young baseball player. He didn't duck, and he got hit in the eye. He got a hyphema that filled half the anterior chamber. He had quite a large angle recession. He had quite a bit of pain, a considerable iritis, was treated locally; pressures were elevated; gradually the eye whitened. He began to feel reasonably good, but by the end of 3 weeks the hyphema had disappeared, and there was practically no flare in the anterior chamber. The pressure was 60 mm Hg and the child was somewhat nauseated and had a lot of pain. Antiglaucoma therapy did not help at all. Diamox made him sicker. What do you think? Dick, you are ready to jump.

Simmons: Well, one of the things that I certainly would be concerned about here is not so much the long-range glaucoma from traumatic angle recession, but an acute glaucoma which can occur early if there is contusion and be self-limited. So I think that is one thing I would certainly think about in this case.

Shaffer: How do you treat hyphemas these days? We were always taught to bilaterally patch and put them to bed. Do you do that now?

Simmons: I do, temporarily, yes.

Shaffer: Does everybody? Jim?

Wise: I am happy to report that I have not had to treat very many hyphemas lately. There seems to be a considerable improvement in the incidence of kids getting hit with BBs, rocks, and so on. But I still think that they should be—at least as far as children are concerned—that they should be in the hospital and patched at least for a while.

Shaffer: It is probably safer from a malpractice point of view anyway. Hugh?

Beckman: Yes, but if you get what this might be, a possible erythroblastic glaucoma, then I think one has to look to do a washout, and indeed this might be the case where a washout might help.

Shaffer: That is a good idea. What about this treatment that Dr. Goldberg advises, the Amacar treatment—aminocaproic acid? Do you know about that, Dave?

Campbell: Yes, I am impressed by the figures, and I use it. If I have a young. . .

Shaffer: Tell them about it.

Campbell: Well, according to McGetrick and Goldberg, the adult dosage is 5 grams orally every 4 hours. I use it for about 5 to 10 days following a hyphema. I do admit patients with hyphema. I put them at bed rest. I might bilaterally patch them, or I might just put a patch on one eye. If I bilaterally patch them, I'll allow them to take the patch off to eat and to go to the bathroom and then to rest the rest of the time, depending on their personality. I like to put the iris at rest with atropine and decrease inflammation with steroids, and use Amicar to try to prevent rebleeding.

Shaffer: Yes. What is the reason for the Amicar? What is it physiologically? Well, it prevents clot dissolution, so the idea was that by using it it would prevent those little clots from loosening up and giving the eight-ball hemorrhage later. The statistics, at least from Goldberg's experiments, were quite impressive. The only trouble is it makes them sick as a dog. The other thing, though, that surprised me is that most of the large series show that it doesn't make a bit of difference whether you hospitalize, whether you patch, or whether you let them walk around. They do not have any increase in hyphemas. So I don't know. Well, this is the punch line on this child: 21 days later they discontinued steroids that the original doctor had put him on. This was Dunbar Hoskin's patient, and he was smart enough to discontinue everything in the injured eye and give steroids to the uninjured eye, and by golly, it was the uninjured eye that went up to 40 mm Hg. This was a steroid glaucoma which was continued because they gave him steroids for the first week or two, but then they didn't stop it. So, dont' forget, steroids over a period of time can get you into trouble.

I am going to take advantage of this next one. This is a favorite of mine. It's a good object lesson. It goes back to our pigmentary problems. Here is a 55-year-old woman from Marin county, and on a Sunday she fell against her kitchen table. She immediately had a little bit of discomfort, but by the next day she had real halos, considerable blur, and discomfort, went to the opthalmologist, who found a pressure of 55 mm Hg in that eye and an angle abnormality. He took the precaution of getting a consultation from a local clinic, who confirmed angle recession with some increased pigmentation. He did a thermal sclerostomy. Within 2 weeks it failed. He did a second thermal sclerostomy, which failed in 2 weeks. And, at that time, he thought he ought to share the load. We saw her at that time. This is what the eye looked like. What do you think of that for a traumatic eye? Harry, do you want to take a crack at it?

Quigley: Bob, I don't see any pupil. Is the pupil way up high?

Shaffer: Yes, it's way up high, It's pulled up there and actually there is some pigment under the conjunctive up above. It isn't too obvious. This is a kind of a diffuse pigmentation of the iris, not really elevated.

Quigley: Well, once again, I'd be thinking of the differential that we ran through before. That it was a diffuse infiltrating melanoma. That it could be one of the ICE syndrome variations, something like a Chandler's type. I'd want to know what the gonioscopy showed.

Shaffer: Gonioscopy showed grown tissue covering the angle. She had a malignant melanoma and had had two filtering procedures which released the melanoma under the conjunctiva. Three years later she was dead from metastases. Now, the point to it is that the misdiagnosis came from the failure to take a decent history. All I did when taking the history was to ask her, ''Have you ever seen halos before this injury?' She said, ''Oh, yes, several times in the past year I have noticed some halos.'' Then I asked her if her vision was affected after this fall. She said that no, it didn't affect her vision. You can't get that much damage from a blunt trauma and see well after it for a while. So basically it was just failure to take an adequate history. It would have kept the opththalmologist out of trouble when he was looking at an angle that happened to have a lot of peculiar pigmentation of it. So, my favorite philosopher—Charlie Brown—will close this session with the object lesson, ''Do people really talk to doctors?'' And Linus answers, ''Of course, every day.'' But the punch line is, ''Do the doctors listen?'' So, let's all listen. Thanks a lot.

MEDICAL THERAPY OF GLAUCOMA

DR. HARRY A. QUIGLEY

Quigley: As anyone could see at the Iris Parade about an hour and a half ago, they were casting pearls off the floats. So we'll try to cast some pearls off the podium this afternoon for those of you who are willing to listen. What I've put up on those slides is eight things that I often tell our folks in training, that I would like to stress for anyone who launches into the medical therapy of open-angle glaucoma. These are general rules, which I hope the other panel mmebers will either add to, subtract from, or argue with in terms of how they behave in treating patients with open-angle or other forms of glaucoma that require medical therapy.

The first of the general rules is that you are supposed to *pick the drug which is most likely to work* for that patient, and most likely to be used by the patient. An example of a drug that is not going to be used is the selection of 1% pilocarpine for a 22-year-old male. He's not going to take it; there isn't any question at all that that man is never going to take pilocarpine adequately four times a day, because it is going to ruin his vision. In that case, you would have to use some other drug for that particular patient.

Secondly, *start with a low dose*. One of the things that I frequently see in practice is a patient who is referred, and the physician's referral note says that this particular patient is allergic to epinephrine, has asthma, and can't take timolol; and so when I first chose pilocarpine and started it with the patient he got a terrible headache and just brought the bottle in absolutely irate and couldn't take it. What had happened was that a blue-eyed patient had been given a bottle of 4% pilocarpine. Now pilocarpine acts on people depending upon the degree of the pigmentation of their eyes. If you have light-blue eyes, 4% pilocarpine is quite unlikely ever to be necessary. You would probably want to start at ½% pilocarpine. The low-dose theory also applies, in my view, if you are using carbonic anhydrase inhibitors. One can start with low doses of Neptazane or Diamox and work your way up. There's a lovely study that Beth Friedland, John Mallonee, and Doug Anderson did; they showed that the peak blood level of Diamox that is obtained from a 65 mg tablet is about the same as the peak blood level with a 500 mg tablet, although the duration of action is less. So, number two, start with a low dose in order to maximize the chance that the patient is going to be able to tolerate the medicine. Lo and behold, sometimes the low dose will give you just as big an effect as a big dose.

Third, if you are going to start a new medicine or change the medicine that the patient is on, it is very important for you to *change them in only one eye at a time,* if that is feasible. Now, there are patients for whom telling them to do one thing in one eye and one thing in the other eye is so confusing that you quite rightly you would never choose to do that. But, since the two eyes, generally speaking, move up and down together in their diurnal and hourly fluctuations, it is a lovely way to control the observation of what effect you had with your change of therapy—to change the medicine in only one eye at a time. Thereby, you utilize one eye as a control for what is really going on as a drug effect.

The fourth role is *don't change the patient's medication and say, "Come back in three months."* We frequently see those notes in charts—"add pilo and RTC three months." You'll find actually what the immediate effect of pilocarpine is within the first hour and a half. That's true of most other drugs as well. At the end of 1 week you are going to have found out not only what the pressure-lowering effect is, but whether the patient is able to tolerate it. So you certainly want to find out with an initial patient whether you have gotten to maximum medical therapy or not in less than a month. One week, each new drug, moving up once a week.

Number five, you have a patient who is taking timolol and pilocarpine, and the pressure level is not controlled. If you decide to add an epinephrine product, and there isn't much effect, *don't leave the patient on the drug*. Discontinue that medicine instead of just adding it on, because the patient is not only paying in money, he is paying in carrying bottles around for something you have scientifically demonstrated didn't do him any good.

In recording what the effect of the medicine is that you are using on that patient, *stay aware of the last time the patient took the drop* or the pill. Now, that sounds rather simple, and of course it is very important that you know whether you are looking at the pressure 2 hours after the last delivery of medicine—which you would expect that to be the lowest pressure that you would be achieving—but it does something else for you. It allows you, by the patient's response, to get a vague idea of whether they are really taking the stuff or not. Someone who says briskly, "Yes, I took it at 6:45 this morning," and stares you right back in the eye probably, although not always, did take it at 6:45 this morning; whereas, someone who stumbles around and sort of says, "Er, well, yea, it was yesterday." By asking the question of "When did you last take the medicine?" you are actually finding out a little bit as best you can about compliance. Although I mentioned earlier in the meeting how poor our idea is actually of what people's compliance is.

Periodically reevaluate what you are doing with a well-controlled or apparently well-controlled patient. Someone who has worked their way up to three kinds of medicine might really be overmedicated in a sense, might really be taking more than they actually need. So periodically you might try stopping a medicine in one eye and seeing whether the patient in coming back is just as well controlled as they were.

Probably the most important thing on both of those slides is exemplified by the patient who comes back to me—and I wish I had a nickel for every time I have heard it—and says, "Doctor, I keep taking those drops very faithfully but my vision just doesn't get any better." This is a patient who heard the first time I explained but needs it reinforced for them over and over again that glaucoma medicines don't improve vision. They are intended to prevent vision from becoming worse. That last statement also includes such things as writing out schedules for people of medicine so that they understand what four times a day means—that it doesn't mean four times during the morning—and so that they understand how three different kinds of medicine should be taken throughout the day. You can ask them things like, "When do you get up in the morning, and when do you go to bed, and what is a convenient time for you to get together with your bottles of drops if you work the night shift?''

I think that is enough about general rules. I am now going to ask each of the panelists if they would comment, if they feel so moved, on a few questions that I think are fairly typical questions about medical therapy and that may be of interest to the people in the audience. Question number one is, if you have a patient who is controlled on either epinephrine drops or on timolol drops alone—that is, one or the other alone—and the patient now goes out of control so that you are still taking timolol or epinephrine alone, do you add the other one? To ask the question another way, are epinephrine and timolol additive to each other? Dr. Simmons, do you want to touch on that question? There have been some studies of that in Boston.

Simmons: Yes, I would like to have a real good definitive answer on that, but Dr. Epstein and Dr. John Thomas worked on this question and found that there was a temporary additive effect, but then it disappeared on continued combined therapy with timolol and epinephrine. They found in one report that the optimal regimen was to keep the patient on epinephrine constantly, and then give 2 weeks of added timolol during each month, leaving 2 weeks without it. We call this pulsed therapy. The differences in intraocular pressure involved were rather small, and I would like to see more detailed work on that and I would like to hear from others on it.

Quigley: Dr. Wise?

Wise: Well, I have a rather different point of view entirely. That is that I almost never use epinephrine. First of all, in the aphakic patient, it so often causes blurred vision and macular edema, and it has been shown that epinephrine—even in the phakic eye—causes fairly severe retinovasoconstriction after you put it on the cornea. I think most people don't consider how strong a vasoconstrictor epinephrine is. That injectable anesthetics, for example, contain 1 to 100,000 epinephrine, whereas 1% epinephrine drops is 1000 times stronger than that. I just don't like the idea of giving the patient recurring and severe anterior segment vasoconstriction, particularly for years. I also wonder whether the pressure-lowering effect of the epinephrine is not at least partially balanced by vasoconstriction at the optic nerve. All of this is theoretical, and I am not sure that any of it, except of course for the blurred vision, is really supported by sound experimental evidence. Nevertheless, I am rather prejudiced against any and all epinephrines, and I hardly ever use them.

Quigley: Dr. Campbell, would you like to comment on that?

Campbell: In regard to aphakia and the use of epinephrine, I think that a lot of us do steer away from it. We should remember, however, that it is a low percentage of aphakes who do get macular fluid collection with the drug, and this is reversible. So, if someone has aphakia and is a good responder to epinephrine, certainly I would go ahead and use it. If they do develop some macular edema, I will stop the medication and look for something else. In regard to the long-term efficacy in use of epinephrine, it has been used at the Massachussets Eye and Ear Infirmary, I know for over 50 years, and the general feeling has been that it does more good than harm.

Quigley: Dr. Shaffer, you probably have used epinephrine as long as or longer than anyone in your practice. Do you think epinephrine is a malignant drug for the eye or the optic nerve? Or do you think it is effective with timolol? Which is really the other question.

Shaffer: When I first came into ophthalmology, we were afraid to use epinephrine because we were afraid of precipitating angle closure before gonioscopy was standard. Beginning at about 1940, narrow angles could be recognized, and it became the best drug we had available to cut down on aqueous production, and we certainly used it right along. Certainly, as to Jim Wise's question on what does it do posteriorly, nobody has the foggiest idea. Dr. Goldman has been very suspicious of it for years, but yes, I have continued to use it and I am not very afraid of it in aphakic eyes when needed. The reason is that if a drug has a side effect the patient can recognize, that isn't very worrisome. If their vision drops, they know that something is wrong and you stop the epinephrine. With so many of these drugs, the patient doesn't know he is in trouble.

Quigley: Dr. Beckman, do you have any comment?

Beckman: I have, I guess, sort of a more casual kind of approach to it in terms of using the drugs. My feeling is that we lose a lot of vision because we try too many combinations of drugs. So, basically, to me epinephrine and timolol—which have not been shown to enhance each other very much—I sort of lump together. Pilocarpine and phospholine iodide I don't ever use together. And then there's carbonic anhydrase inhibitors; I really try never to have my patients on more than one drug in each category. I hardly ever put a patient on Timoptic and epinephrine any more than I would put them on phospholine and pilocarpine, just because one they don't work very well together at all. Two: the expense. And three: it tends to make me have too many permutations of changes while I watch the patient's vision slide down the tube.

Quigley: Dr. Simmons, you want to comment on something?

Simmons: Two thoughts. I told you what I would worry about, and I would worry about the things mentioned here and there that Jim Wise mentioned. I didn't really say what I would do. What I would do at the present time, in the absence of more firm knowledge, is as follows: I use dipivalyl epinephrine, which I find very well tolerated. I use it very frequently in combination with Timolol, both drops twice daily concurrently without using the pulse therapy, etc., since this regimen is easy for the patient. But I would be happy to change that if somebody could give me better evidence that there is really a major difference. On Jim's question, the thing that bothers me with that is that epinephrine has been used so much for so long that, well, I share his theoretical concern. I have a hunch if it were a big major effect that we should have more evidence of it by now.

Quigley: I can comment on a couple of things in terms of pharmacology. Epinephrine is a vasoconstrictor for the first hour of its action. It's a vasodilator for the next 11 hours, which is why—as every clinician who has observed a patient who takes epinephrine knows—you put your epinephrine eye drop in and the eye whitens right up. Then an hour later it turns red, which is why your patient complains to you that, "Gee, my eye whitens up, Doc, but then after the rest of the day it turns red all day." Now, one way around that, which is a little bit cheating but which works, is to say to the patient, "You know, your eye is going to be red for much of the day while you take this drop. And that is very important, because that is how the drop works; it opens up those big blood vessels so the water can get out of the eye better—so, if your eye isn't red, that is a bad sign." That is maybe a little dishonest, but it works. None of this means diddly, though, for the blood flow of the optic nerve. We must measure the blood flow of the optic nerve. The blood flow of the optic nerve has been measured with intravenous doses of metaraminol, a very severe vasconstrictor. It is published by Joel Weinstein in *Investigative Ophthalmology* recently. Blood flow in the optic nerve does not go down when you give a severe vasoconstrictor. So I don't believe we have any evidence either in the laboratory or clinically at the moment that epinephrine would be toxic to the optic nerve. I wonder, though, and I personally do use epinephrine in combination with Timolol, but I am disappointed at how infrequently I see a big additive effect.

Wise: Harry, I don't know what the reference is, but there is in fact a reference where somebody actually measured the blood flow in the optic nerve before and after topical epinephrine on the cornea, and showed that it was reduced. It was reduced quite a bit. I don't know who did it, but I do know there is such a paper in print. I don't remember who the author was.

Quigley: Flow in the choroid was measured, Jim, by Albert Alm, *Investigative Ophthalmology,* 1980. It was not measured in the optic nerve head, but we'll get together on it later.

Wise: I think it was retinal blood flow.

Quigley: Dr. Shaffer?

Shaffer: An oddity on this score—Jerry Bettman a number of years ago was studying blood flow. The only thing he could get to produce an increase in blood flow in the choroid in particular, and he thought in the optic nerve, was nicotine of all things. I don't think you can trust any of these.

Quigley: Well, good. Two other questions actually came up, and they are things I have on the list here. So, maybe we'll get to that now. Dr.Simmons mentioned that he uses dipivalyl epinephrine, and as that particular product came on the market within the last couple or 3 years, I see a tremendous initial use of dipivalyl epinephrine. Do the panel members, when they decide to use epinephrine products, choose first the cheaper and longer-standing products that are epinephrine single salts, or do you go first to dipivalyl epiniphrine, and do you think that the complication rate is actually more or less with either of those preparations? Does anybody want to take that one on first? Dr. Simmons, we already heard that you use DPE. Do you feel that it does show fewer complications?

Simmons: Yes, I think it is better tolerated than the regular epinephrine compound.

Quigley: Dr. Campbell, do you see fewer allergic responses with DPE? Do you think your clinical ''seat of the pants'' impression is that that is the case. Have you studied it?

Campbell: I have not studied it. I just have to read the literature there, and I do feel that it is tolerated a little better.

Quigley: Dr. Shaffer?

Shaffer: I don't think it works as well as epinephrine, and it costs more.

Beckman: I am delighted to hear him say that, because I have no proof of it, but I haven't been as happy with propine as I have been with the epinephrine compounds. I started off using epitrate, a bitartrate, which was many, many years ago. I was so delighted when borate came out because the borate was so much better tolerated that I have used a large amount of the borate drop over the years. I was always very happy with it. It seems like when Timoptic came along that all of a sudden everyone's latent dislike of epinephrine compounds seemed to surface, which I really never shared. Then propine came along and sort of reinforced everybody's discomforture with other epinephrine compounds. I do think some of the epinephrine compounds were sort of hard to take, but I always liked the borate compounds. Dick, what epinephrine compounds were you using before you went to propine?

Simmons: I wasn't very satisfied with them; I would very often use Glaucon, which I believe is a hydrochloride. The reason I did was that it came in a 2% solution, and there was some evidence that this was more effective. Some people thought that this provided the maximum epinephrine effect, and so I used it. But I also used the other common ones. We used to use epinephrine a lot. I would say as just an off-the-cuff impression from my point of view, I have about ⅓ or ¼ of the problems now from propine that I did from the old epinephrine compounds. Therefore, at least being in a situation that most of the panelists are in, where somebody has to travel to Baltimore, and it takes $50 to $100 for transportation to travel into town to see you, Harry, it is a big deal for an old person to travel frequently to change medical therapy. And so often the eye would be red and sore with an allergy around the skin. I think I have cut that way down. The extra cost of the propine, to me, to reduce my grief and the patient's grief and the trips and phone calls—I would go for the more expensive propine if my impression of it holds up.

Quigley: Let me ask the question another way. There are two reactions that patients have to epinephrine products. One of them is that they get a red eye, and they don't like the appearance of their eye. They might be discomforted by the sting of the drop. There are then a second group of patients whom I will refer to as the "truly allergic" patient. That is somebody who takes epinephrine, and they get a swollen eyelid and chemosis and intense tearing and watering—and that's what I call a severe allergic reaction. Has any of the panel seen patients who had that second severe allergic response to one of the previous epinephrine products, who can and have since successfully used propine for a year or more?

Simmons: You're making it tough.

Quigley: Well, no, I realize. . . But, I am asking the question for a very particular reason, because in the last 2 years I have had experiences. These are now anecdotal, and we should restudy the whole thing. But I have had more than two patients who were the second kind of truly allergic epinephrine patients who, not when they first started dipivalyl epinephrine but at sometimes shortly thereafter, redeveloped the same old really bad epinephrine allergy. Maybe there is a way out of this that I am not doing, or maybe it is that once you are allergic badly to epinephrine you are allergic badly no matter what the product is. But, I had been hoping that the second new product would be something that would beat that. OK, I didn't want to beat that to a pulp, that particular question. Dr. Campbell?

Campbell: Just a point about using the two drugs together. If one is using epinephrine in the face of narrow angles, we have many times been able to use this because there is not a large pupillary dilation associated with the use of the drug. Every now and then, however, we can see a patient who will dilate more fully when he is using the combination of epinephrine and Timoptic, and I think that in this situation: one has a patient who has a potentially closable angle, and one has got to be very careful with the two medications in this situation. Has anyone else seen that?

Quigley: Dr. Simmons?

Simmons: Yes, I sure have. I think it is an important thing, and people using contact lenses or rubbing their eyes, or people with a little irritation will rub the epithelium, and the drug will penetrate even more rapidly than usual. I think they are more predisposed to dilation than others. Thank you, Jim, you don't like what I'm saying!

Quigley: Professor Wise.

Wise: I was pulling the plug. I have seen outright angle closure from the combination.

Quigley: You have not?

Wise: I have!

Quigley: You have. I certainly have, too. OK, another question. If a patient is being told to use two different eye drops simultaneously—you have been prescribing pilocarpine, and now you say, "Ms. Jones, I want you to take epinephrine twice a day"—how do you tell them how to space the drops out? Can they take them both at the same time, or one right after the other one? Should they separate them by 3 hours? Should they have a schedule where they are totally separate in time, or does it matter? Hugh?

Beckman: This is probably going to violate just about everybody's sensibilities, but I put that patient on a combination drop which I have found to be extremely useful over the years. So that to me has been a very effective way of combining drops. It doesn't drive the patient crazy, and I really think that part of medicating people is not driving them crazy with different compounds. That one particular problem, I don't have any doubt in my mind what I would do; I would put the patient on the combination pilocarpine and epinephrine drop and have them take it four times a day.

Quigley: Dr. Campbell, what would you tell someone who is taking timolol and pilocarpine where they don't have a commercial combination preparation?

Campbell: I tell them to wait about 15 minutes between each drop if they are putting a lot of drops in at the same time. I also like to use the combination of epinephrine and pilocarpine for the reasons that Hugh has given. And finally, again, if we come back to our narrow-angle patient, this is an excellent way to avoid precipitating an attack of acute angle closure. There is simply no way that the pupil can dilate to the epinephrine if the pilo is being given at the same time.

Quigley: Dr. Simmons, do you have anything to add to this question?

Simmons: Yes, we all have pros and cons and you weigh it up and form your own balance, but the thing I don't like about the combination of epinephrine and pilo is that you need the pilocarpine four times daily, and it is really a double overdose of epinephrine, which you need twice a day at most. Therefore, I choose to separate them. I think empirically that some of the very irritated eyes and patients who complain about stinging come from those patients who are taking the epinephrine/pilo combinations four times daily. So that is the way I balance that.

Quigley: I think there is another reason why the epinephrine combination with pilocarpine drops are stinging drops. We used to call epinephrine bitartrate "fire drops"—at least, that is what the patients in our clinic called them. Most of the combinations are epinephrine bitartrate, and I am not sure why that is. I should know the pharmacology better. I believe it is because in combination you have to have a more stable epinephrine preparation with the pilocarpine at the low pH of the pilocarpine, and bitartrate is what works to do those combinations.But I agree with Hugh that once you have regulated a patient and discovered that you need both pilocarpine and epinephrine, it makes tremendous sense to have a patient who has had that determined use only one eyedrop. I believe there is a study that is going to be published soon which illustrates that fact that if you put in two drops within a minute of each other, one of them partially chases out the other one in terms of what the anterior chamber concentration is. So Dr. Campbell's admonition of 15 minutes between may be longer than what I tell people, which is 5 minutes. But at least you have to tell them that they can't put them in bing-bang right after each other for fear that one drop is going to wash the other one out—which makes it tougher to do. Another question—how many of the panel members, we'll just ask each of you, how many are using carbonic anhydrase inhibitors before laser trabeculoplasty in the majority of patients you treat?

Wise: I very often will, but I always use Neptazane and not Diamox because, as I understand it, the half-life of Diamox in the serum is 5 hours and the half-life of Neptazane in serum is 15 hours. That is, Neptazane is in fact a true twice a day medication without requiring any sort of time-release capsule. I have a lot of patients who are on a half a tablet or one tablet of neptazane twice a day. I find it is very well tolerated and will frequently allow me to control the pressure. But I don't like to go much higher than that. If I do, why then I start thinking about the laser.

Simmons: I agree with what Jim said, exactly. I have been impressed with the fact that Neptazane in small doses can have some effect. Dr. Epstein in Boston has worked on that and shown that, so you don't need the full maximum dose of Neptazane. I try it, and if it is not tolerated, however, I discontinue it.

Quigley: David Campbell?

Campbell: Nothing additional.

Quigley: Hugh?

Beckman: I think the only addition I would make to that is that I really don't use carbonic anhydrase inhibitors on anybody who is elderly, to the point where I really can't recognize immediately adverse effects. I don't like to depend on the children of patients to tell me that their mother or father is slowing up a little up. So, if I have anybody who I really feel as if I might slow them up and might not know it, I hold off on carbonic anhydrase inhibitors. So I might go directly to the laser on them. Otherwise, generally, I use Neptazane quite a lot and feel that that would be indicated before a laser trabeculoplasty.

Quigley: OK, good, so there is still some role for using pills then, the panel thinks. I am surprised; I thought we weren't going to hear that. OK. You know propranolol as an oral medicine is being sprinkled on the population for everything from high blood pressure to cardiac failure to fleas. And there are a lot of people walking around now on beta-blockers systemically. If you see a new glaucoma patient who is taking a systemic beta-blocker, is it worth adding Timolol to that patient's eye to try to control glaucoma? Dr. Shaffer, have you done that?

Shaffer: I sure keep track of what they are on. The Merck push for Timoptic really was an overkill for sure. For such a long time they refused to believe there were any side effects. There were no side effects in their study population because they used young and husky people in their study. When we began using it on our old crocks, they we suddenly had people fainting in the stores downtown. We had falls in bathrooms, and we had all kinds of problems. So Timoptic plus propranolol is certainly an overdose. Almost half of the eyedrop is said to come down into the nose, and once it gets into the nasal mucosa, it is almost exactly like a hypodermic. It is very rapidly absorbed. So, patients can get a pretty fair jolt of beta-blocker into their system. So, we always show patients how to block their tear duct when they are using timolol, whether or not they are on propranolol. I often ask them if they were told to block their tear duct. Most of them have never heard of it, so I don't think many of us are doing a good job of teaching them. If they have been told, then I ask them how they do it. Almost all of them push on their nose; they never go back and really block the tear duct. So I think this is one of the things you might keep in mind: tell patients to push back toward the back of their head, and then they will do some blocking of the ducts.

Quigley: How long do you ask them to occlude the sac?

Shaffer: A very short time. That is true, too, of your every 5 or 15 minutes between drops. Compliance is so important, and if you give them 15 minutes between, they will have forgotten to take it, I am afraid. So, I tell them to yes, wait if they can, but if they are in a hurry I would rather have them put in two within 30 seconds or so.

Quigley: Well, let me broaden the question a little bit. If anybody else would like to speak to the question about if you have a patient taking 60 mg of Inderal a day, would you give up on timolol? Would you not even prescribe it? It's $38.00 a bottle. Do you wnat them to kiss off $38.00 to find out it didn't work? You broaden the question to say there are so many side effects from topical beta-blockers that you don't use the drug. Dr. Beckman?

Beckman: I'll make a pitch for what I call "not pushing it." I think that our thinking about glaucoma has been so conservative, and perhaps properly so over the last 25 years. We really sort of like lean over backwards to just push at everything. I'm beginning to think that what we really should be thinking of is what is the maximal well-tolerated medication that you can put a patient on and have them not lose their vision? If I have somebody who is on Inderal or somebody who has a history of bradycardia or extrasystoles, I hesitate to put that patient on something that might possibly hurt him, that is, "push at it." I would at that point look for something else to use. I really look to find something that I'm reasonably content that the patient can take and continue to take without causing them a lot of extra doctoring.

Quigley: Dr. Wise?

Wise: I keep reading things where I can't quote the exact chapter and verse, but somewhere I read that the use of topical timolol in the eye was equal to something like 7 or 10 mg a day of Inderal. So, if you wanted to use timolol in the eye, you might have to cut back on the Inderal a little by mouth. There is a study which came out of England on 1/2% versus 1/4% timolol, which demonstrated that over a period of months control was just as good with 1/4% as it was with 1/2%, with of course less side effects and less expense. It has been my experience that there is no difference between the two concentrations except for the cost and the side effects, and I no longer prescribe 1/2% timolol.

Quigley: Jim, it's an important point if anyone would like to look at the study. I believe it's in the *British Journal of Ophthalmology* within the last year. In fact, I believe one of the earliest studies of the dose response curve of timolol indicated that 0.1% was near the top of the dose response curve, and 0.25% and 0.50% would therefore be expected to be similar. Nobody wants to answer my real question. Dr. Simmons, are you going to bite the bullet here?

Simmons: Well, if the patient's on propranolol, I don't believe propranolol systemically is good therapy for glaucoma, because I don't believe that it has a maximal effect on the eye and the intraocular pressure. I, therefore, in such patients—if they will tolerate it—will use timolol in the belief that the topical timolol will produce the maximal beta-blockade benefit within the eye. So, I do use them that way. I usually, on a practical note, give the patient the prescription of timolol, have them see their internist, and have him evaluate whether it is suitable to take it. In most cases this permission has been granted from the internist, and I have yet to have a serious problem from using it that way.

Quigley: I believe, just to quote a little chapter and verse, as Jim said, I believe there was a study that indicated that 80 mg of Inderal or more a day probably gets you as much pressure lowering in the eye as you are going to get. But I wouldn't stop just because the patient was on 100 mg of Inderal trying timolol additionally. Myself, personally, I would do it, and I do the same as Dr. Simmons does. I communicate with the patient's internist whenever I am adding a glaucoma medicine. You ask who the internist is and send off a day's typed or hand-written note and say you're starting the patient on a beta-blocker. Is there first degree heart block? Does this patient have bronchospasm? Is this someone who has had bradycardia in the past or mild or severe congestive failure? Please be aware of what we are doing here to your patient. I think that probably minimizes the chance of a side effect. Whether or not we actually get a pressure lowering, which as you said, I think we try it and see. Dr. Campbell mentioned about Healon the other day. Healon is not exactly one of our main pressure-lowering drugs, but it is a new thing influencing surgical therapy. Are there any other uses for Healon? Has anybody found it to be a useful or difficult drug for patients with glaucoma?

Campbell: I think, Harry, that you warned me that you were going to ask me that question, and now I still have no answer. What are you after? Surgical uses of Healon?

Quigley: Yes. Has anyone used it in filtering surgery alone, for example?

Campbell: Well, I find I am using more and more Healon for all of my anterior segment surgery. It is wonderful stuff. I think we all feel that way after we do extracapsular cataract surgery. It's indispensable for the procedure that I described to you a day or so ago for the chamber deepening and for approaches into the trabecular meshwork. Tomorrow you will hear me talk about some new approaches into the trabecular meshwork in regard to the treatment of open angle-glaucoma, and again, Healon is indispensable here to hold the chamber deep. So, we will hold off on that one.

Quigley: Dr. Simmons?

Simmons: I think that one of the things that goes through the mind of the practitioner doing trabeculectomies and other glaucoma procedures is use of Healon, such as leaving it in a bleb or in the anterior chamber to help promote the ultimate bleb success and help protect against flat chamber. I think it is worthless in that regard. I have been watching it for several years because it sounds terrific, but I think it is not usually helpful. I haven't used it frequently, because in small numbers of cases where it has been used for that purpose it has been poor.

Quigley: OK. There is—yes, David?

Campbell: I would like to just add on to that a couple of thoughts I have had about the use of Healon following filtration surgery. I think we all hoped that this was going to be the answer to our problem of flat anterior chambers and it has, disappointingly, not turned out to be so. However, it may still help us in the future, and we are going to be able to start evaluating a 2% Healon concentration, and that may do it. I would also like to ask Dick if, when he has filled the anterior chamber at the end of surgery, he also filled the bleb, because clearly what happens is that if we fill our anterior chamber, then the next morning we come in, and the chamber is flat, and the bleb is full of Healon. I recently have been filling the bleb with Healon just before I throw that last suture, and then filling the anterior chamber as well. I am still evaluating that, but I wonder if you have already tried that.

Simmons: Yes, and I have been disappointed.

Quigley: I have one or two others. You had some questions from the audience. While you are bringing those up, someone earlier had mentioned the use of echothiophate, phospholine iodide, and pilocarpine, and I certainly agree with Dr. Beckman. I certainly hope there is no one in the audience who would ever add phospholine iodide and pilocarpine together. There is a lovely study from none other than the Massachusetts Eye and Ear Infirmary that shows that there is no additive effect of echothiophate and pilocarpine. They should be used one or the other, assuming that you are actually going to use echothiophate. What does the panel tell their patients about a drug that their internist would like to give them, but it says on the FDA warning slip, "Do not use this drug in a glaucoma patient"? We are talking now about your open angle-glaucoma patients. Tricyclic antidepressant, antihistamine. Dr. Wise, what do you tell your patient about that drug?

Wise: Well, I tell them that that applies only to the type of glaucoma they don't have. It applies only to angle-closure glaucoma, and that they have a different kind, and they can take any of these medications.

Simmons: I agree with Jim. I think some of the write-ups also imply that it will make open-angle glaucoma worse. I tell them what Jim just said, that is that it doesn't apply to you because you are under therapy. What minimal effect the use of some systemic drug might have on outflow or intraocular pressure is far overshadowed by the effect of your topical therapy, so forget it.

Quigley: OK. Thank you.

APPLICATIONS OF THE PULSED NEODYMIUM:YAG LASER

DR. FRANCIS A. L'ESPERANCE, Jr.

L'Esperance: The topic today is the applications of the pulsed neodymium:YAG laser. We are going to shorten this up a little because of the presentations to follow. But I would like to show you a case. I was wondering if any of you could figure out what happened to this individual. This is a 28-year-old gentleman from a nearby laboratory. I guess we all know, at least the laser people, this fellow was what we call "bore sighting" a pulsed dye laser. A pulsed dye laser is, again, very much like the Q-switched laser; it has a 10 nanoseconds pulse length. It had a power of about 4 to 5 millijoules, and it was in the green part of the spectrum at about 500+ nanometers. When you bore sight, you are supposed to take your eye away from the part that you are sighting, and there is usually a piece of cardboard you take away. He did just the opposite, and as he took the cardboard away, the laser went off, and this is what his eye looks like the same day. The laser impact had gone completely through the foveolar region; had blown out his choroid and went directly down to the sclera. What we are seeing is blood coming from the choroidal area into the vitreous. His vision was down to counting fingers, and he had a large amount of edema around the area, but it was a perfect full-thickness macular hole. This is what he looked like about a month later. He still had counting-fingers vision, and believe it or not, he is back at work doing the same thing. I hope he is not bore sighting. This particular laboratory at this time has gone into a very extensive safety program. We have to be particularly careful as we change wavelengths that we protect our own eyes as much as we watch out for the patient's eyes. As we get into the various wavelengths that I discussed with the dye laser, for instance, and the other various wavelengths—every time you do that you have to have filters. A lot of the work that I think Marty and Hugh and people that are going to oversee a lot of these areas, the laser safety part of it—the laser safety is much for the physician as it is for the surrounding ancillary personnel and for the patient. Now that is just an interesting case that I thought you would like to see. This is what happens; we all talk about the pulsed neodymium:YAG and what could happen if it did come into the eye. Well, this is with the same amount of energy coming into the eye, except this was a collimated beam versus a beam coming into the eye at a cone angle of 16 degrees. So you can see this can be devastating.

Beckman: May I ask a question, Fran? Maybe I can get an answer from you and/or Marty. I have always routinely—when using a pulse mode laser, 1000 watts and 3 to 4 joules—used goggles in the room for doing cyclocoagulation and iridectomies. I have also always put a mirrored contact lens over the pupil. Now when we're using a really developed device such as a new YAG laser with their good delivery systems, if one is focusing on the sclera, and let's say 3.5 mm from the limbus, do you feel that it is necessary to use it to mirror off the pupil—to block off the pupil—and do you still feel that it is still necessary to wear goggles in the room?

L'Esperance: Well, I think in a situation like this, I think you get enough specular reflection, so probably you are not going to get a real tremendous amount of energy right back. I have always wondered about that. I suppose until it is proved otherwise, it is good to have all the ancillary personnel wearing some type of protective goggles for that wavelength. As we get into the visible wavelengths—the pulsed lasers have so much energy coming so fast that you can't duck. Now with the argon laser the physicists always thought, at many laboratories, that if they could see the beam they were safer than if they wore goggles where they couldn't see the beam, because they would be walking right into a beam of many watts. So they have gone back to this idea of seeing it, but with the pulsed beam I think you have to really watch out for it. And we are getting lasers that are like this. Another thing that I would like to bring up as we are going along here: it is very very easy when you are doing photocoagulation to have the little old lady who would like to have her daughter sit in with her. Now, if you are working—say you are doing an iridotomy—and you are working at 1000 or 1200 mW energy and you have a contact lens that doesn't have an antireflective coating, and you are getting a 4% reflection off of that, you are getting between 40 and 50 mW of power. With an argon beam and with somebody sitting behind you watching their mother get lased, they may coagulate the eye inadvertently, and you might be spending a long time out of your office and in another part of the municipal area. So I think it is almost one of the rules that if you have to bring the person in that you give them goggles and things for that. On the other hand, I just tell people, basically, if the patient can stand up, and if he is young and vibrant, then we just don't like other people in the photocoagulation area. We are protected, as I explain to the patient, but the patient's daughter or whomever isn't.

Simmons: Fran, there is another reason too. That is, even though they receive no reflection whatsoever, if their vision decreases or they have any macular lesion you will have a lot of explaining to do . . .

L'Esperance: Exactly. I was hoping that we would have just enough time here, because Marty has some slide to show about the pulsed neodymium:YAG and some of the other applications. Marty, could you show some of them?

Mainster: Just one quick comment so that no one is needlessly alarmed by these industrial accidents. In these accidents the victim is generally directly exposed to a laser beam of low divergence. This situation is entirely different from a clinical Nd:YAG laser photodisruptor, where the laser beam is focused by a short focal length lens and diverges rapidly posterior to the focal point. The rapid divergence of the laser beam posterior to the focal point assures low irradiances at structures posterior to the focal point. In fact, in a typical posterior capsulotomy, irradiance at the retina is orders of magnitude below maximum permissible retinal exposure levels for Nd:YAG radiation.

When you deal with experimental systems, however, it is always advisable to wear laser safety goggles for the wavelength being used. In this regard, it is important to realize that laser safety goggles that are effective for one laser wavelength may not be effective for another wavelength. What Dr. L'Esperance emphasized is also important. If you are going to have any observer in the room, whether it is a relative of the patient or a resident, they should not be standing behind you unless they are wearing laser safety goggles. For example, with an ordinary argon laser photocoagulator, the specular reflex from a treatment contact lens poses a hazard to an observer up to 1.6 m from the contact lens, even if the lens has an antireflection coating.

What I would like to do now is make some general comments about Nd:YAG lasers for those of you who are a little less familiar with their clinical applications. The most common application for Nd:YAG lasers is discission of an opacified capsule. In general, when I do a posterior capsulotomy, I make a 4 mm opening, using 7 to 15 single exposures of approximately 1 mJ. About 1 hour prior to treatment, patients receive 1% prednisolone acetate and 0.5% Timoptic, unless there is some contraindication. Patients use 1% prednisolone acetate four times a day for 48 hours after the discission. I have yet to have a problem with a pressure spike in a patient with a posterior chamber lens, but I have had two in aphakes and one in a pseudophake with an anterior chamber lens.

Quigley: Marty, could we have a dissenting opinion from the Wilmer Institute published in the *American Journal of Ophthalmology* within the last 3 or 4 months? The incidence of pressure rises in our hands, and maybe because we are using different energies—although the pressure rise we got was not dependent upon the number of deliveries or the total amount of energy—was very significant. It was well over half the patients who had a pressure rise that we would consider clinically treatable. The outflow facility dropped to half or less of what it was before the treatment. Maybe we should learn what you are doing in Boston that's right. But in our hands there are pressure rises. They should be watched for carefully, and they should be watched for for at least 3 hours.

Mainster: Well, in our standard protocol, patients spend most of the day being treated. The patient comes in in the morning, generally referred by an extracapsular surgeon in our area who does not have access to a Nd:YAG laser. We do objective preoperative intraocular pressure measurements with an Alcon tonometer, photograph the posterior capsule, and do a thorough anterior and posterior segment examination.

After careful discussion of the risks and benefits of the procedure, the patient is treated, the pressure rechecked, and the patient sent to lunch. Every patient is seen back for reevaluation 3 hours later, at which time the visual acuity and intraocular pressure are rechecked, and the capsule is photographed postoperatively. The patient is also seen for reevaluation 1 week, 1 month, 3 months, and 6 months postoperatively, in accordance with our protocol for investigational use of the Nd:YAG laser.

In general I use an energy setting between 0.7 and 1.2 mJ, although on rare occasions I have used as much as 2 mJ. As mentioned, I have had three pressure spikes in a series of approximately 70 patients, but none of those patients had a posterior chamber lens, each of them promptly responded to postoperative pilocarpine, and none of them had elevated intraocular pressure 1 week postoperatively, even though the pilocarpine was discontinued 48 hours after laser treatment. So as far as a 50% incidence of significant pressure increases postoperatively, I just do not see it with the treatment protocol that I have been using. I might add, however, that I have recently stopped using preoperative Timoptic in favor of postoperative pilocarpine, based on the results of a study by Drs. Simmons, Belcher, and Brown, which showed the effectiveness of a postoperative pilocarpine regimen in reducing the incidence of pressure elevations.

Beckman: Can I add something to this, Marty? This is a source of terrible confusion because, as everybody probably knows, Aron-Rosa reported originally 6000 cases in which she had had no pressure rises. The she subsequently reported in *Cataract* that she indeed had done a series in which she had pretreated patients with timolol and not pretreated patients with timolol. In the series in which she had not pretreated the patients with timolol, she indeed did report 25% pressure rises, and then she made the statement that if she pretreated with Timolol that she cut this down to something like 5% or 10%. Dick Keates says he doesn't have pressure rise. Harry Quigley says he does. I absolutely know I do, and will soon report almost a 30% pressure rise when one uses 3 to 4 mj to create the hole. If one cuts down, it seems that as one uses lower energy levels, one does decrease the pressure rise. But, even then, some of the rises seem to be idiosynchratic. The pressure rise seems to be of two types. One is an immediate rise, and the other is a late, delayed rise. The immediate rise can be there at an hour and then gone by 4 hours, or it can be there at 4 hours and gone by 24 hours, or it can be there at 24 hours and not have been present in the 1 to 4 hours groups. But the important thing is that once the patient has shown an immediate pressure rise they appear to be at risk for 2 weeks. I saw one patient who had a pressure rise for 40 days afterward. Generally I caution people not to use Timoptic before they perform the capsulotomy but to monitor carefully because the Timoptic may mask the immediate pressure rise, and a later rise might be missed for lack of monitoring. I was going to say, that is, the capsulotomy done by someone who has basically started off with the machine and is doing large capsulotomies. But that size capsulotomy will have a pressure rise 30% to 40% of the time. You have got to get them really small, and you have to use as little energy as possible. There is a big confusion about this and I tend to side right now with Harry. It is a big problem.

Quigley: I think we are all saying the same thing. We are just saying to watch your patient carefully, and this may occur, and so please be careful with it.

Mainster: I agree. As I said, each patient whom we treat is followed 2 to 3 hours postoperatively, and also 1 week, 1 month, 3 months, and 6 months postoperatively.

Another basic principle that is important, and one that is true not only in Nd:YAG laser therapy but also in argon or krypton laser therapy as well, is that one should never use more irradiance than necessary for a particular application.

I might also add that among patients treated with posterior capsulotomy, some of the most grateful are those who actually have good visual acuity initially but complain of glare or distortion prior to discission. When such a patient is referred to me, after talking with them to determine the seriousness of their visual problem, I still do not perform discission unless I can document first, that there is some capsular abnormality such as mild fibrosis or wrinkling, which can account for the visual deficit; second, that there is no apparent posterior segment origin for the visual problem; and third, that the visual problem can be documented, whether it be with variable contrast acuity, glare, or contrast sensitivity testing. For example, one lady had 20/25 visual acuity in an eye with a posterior chamber intraocular lens that had striae in the underlying posterior capsule, and 20/25 visual acuity in her contralateral phakic eye. She was a seamstress, complained bitterly of poor stereopsis, and had glare sensitivity in her pseudophakic eye that was 18 times normal. After a careful discussion of the risk-to-benefit ratio of the procedure, a Nd:YAG discission was performed. The acuity in the pseudophakic eye remained at the 20/25 level, but she reported a marked subjective improvement in the quality of her vision, and her glare sensitivity returned to normal. Thus there are reasons for performing Nd:YAG laser discission other than merely improving high-contrast visual acuity. Again, reliable instrumentation and careful follow-up are essential. Since my practice is directed primarily toward macular and retinal vascular diseases, I cannot speak with authority on the advantages of anterior capsulotomy prior to extracapsular cataract extraction. I do know that Dr. Aron-Rosa has reported the value of this procedure in her initial studies. At the present time, however, anterior capsulotomy does not appear to have won much favor with American extracapsular cataract surgeons.

Another application of Nd:YAG lasers which is quite useful is incising intraocular inflammatory membranes, particularly as an adjunct to retinal or anterior segment procedures. For example, a patient was referred to me who had an anterior chamber lens but was placed on HMS for postoperative inflammation. This patient developed an inflammatory pupillary membrane, with considerable debris on the PMMA lens. The patient was treated with prednisolone acetate for approximately 3 weeks, which cleared most of the debris from the lens. Then a simple discission promptly improved the patient's visual acuity.

As far as vitreous or retinal applications of Nd:YAG lasers are concerned, they still remain in the experimental or early investigational stage, except for anterior problems where noninvasive incision of an inflammatory membrane can provide visualization of essential vitreoretinal details. In general, although photodisruption of bands or membranes in the vitreous body received much early attention, treatable membranes tend to be quite rare, even in large retinal practices. In fact, one example is a patient with 20/70 visual acuity who was referred to me for a vitreous strand attached to an area of macular preretinal fibrosis. The strand was tenting the membrane upwards, and the goal of therapy would have been to incise the strand. Since it appeared to me that the vitreous strand was in the process of peeling the membrane, however, I decided not to treat the patient. Three months later, the patient's visual acuity improved to 20/30 without treatment, as the strand continued to peel the membrane. If the strand had been disrupted, the membrane would not have peeled, and acuity probably would not have improved. Thus careful preoperative vitreous examination is essential prior to any Nd:YAG laser vitreous application.

At this point, I would like to turn this session over to Dr. Simmons to talk about iris and other anterior segment applications of the Nd:YAG laser.

Simmons: The iris can be treated with the YAG, and the two major uses in the iris that we found so far is, one, iridectomy where for some reason the argon has not been useful. Particularly, the aphakic eye where argon laser iridectomy has recurrently closed, and as I mentioned the other day, going through with the YAG can make a good opening not only in the iris but the anterior vitreous. If that doesn't work, then we would turn to the miniphage technique that Dr. Wise discussed. The second use is other iris surgery such as sphincterotomy or creation of a de novo pupil in the patient with an updrawn iris. The main problem with both of these forms of surgery is a small amount of bleeding. It can be more than a small amount in a few patients, but if you have obvious vascularization of the iris, pretreatment with argon to obliterate the vessels and the YAG treatment is one technique that can be helpful.

Wise: Let me say that with regard to making pupils larger, everybody talks about burning around the pupil. But I have found a very good way to enlarge the pupil is to use the Abraham lens and just chip a linear cut across the sphincter just as if you were doing a peripheral iridectomy. I have a picture with me and will bring it along this afternoon. You can do radial sphincterotomies on a patient with a frozen pupil very nicely with a chipping technique and the argon laser with no bleeding at all.

L'Esperance: Well, I would like to thank Jim and Dick and, particularly, Marty for going through all this. I thank all the panel.

New Orleans Academy of Ophthalmology

Officers

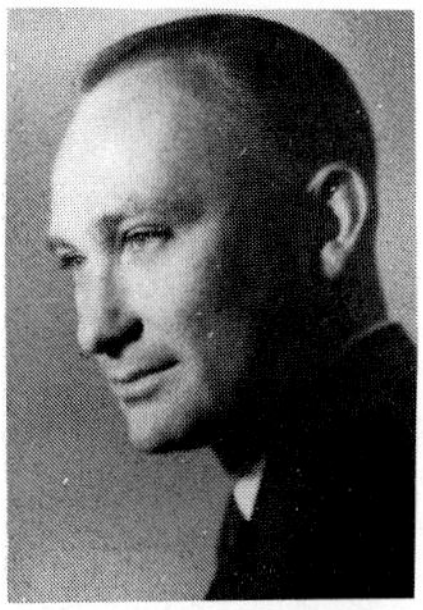

ROBERT A. SCHIMEK, M.D.
President

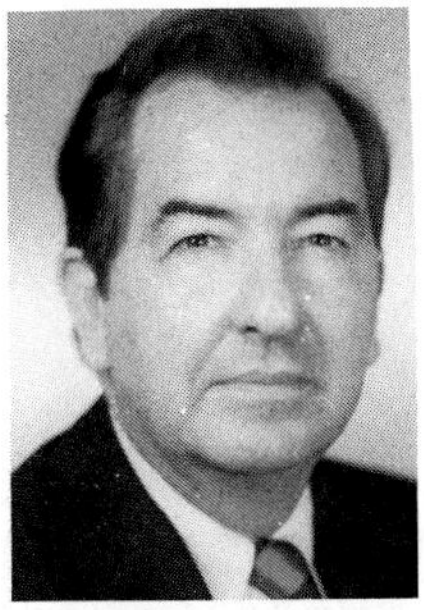

H. FRANK BOSWELL, M.D.
President-Elect

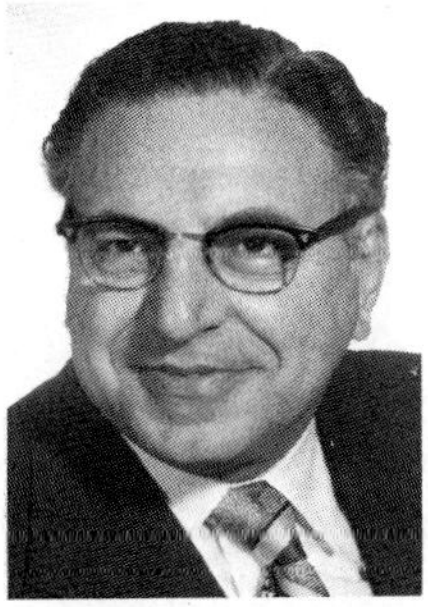

GEORGE S. ELLIS, M.D.
Vice-President

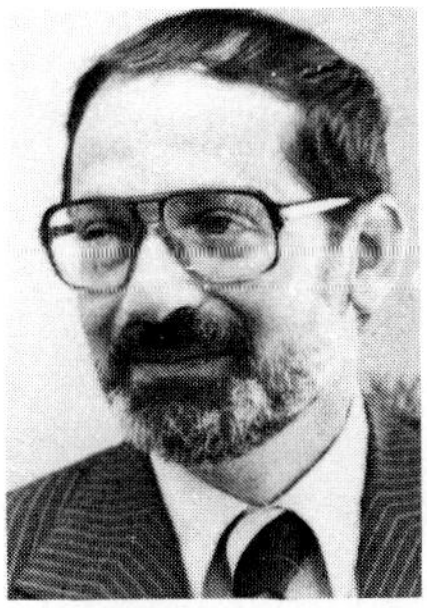

MILES H. FRIEDLANDER, M.D.
Secretary

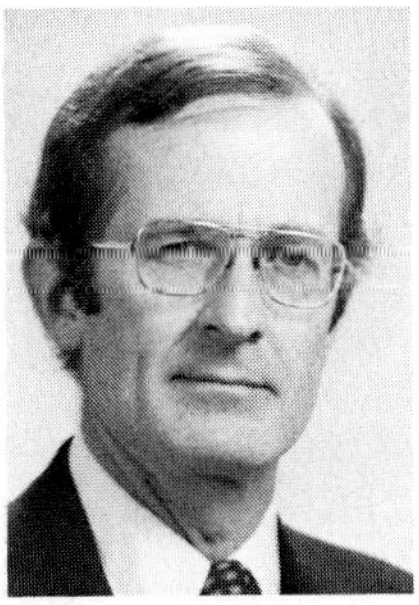

WALTER D. COCKERHAM, M.D.
Treasurer

EXECUTIVE COMMITTEE

Rodney F. Kalil, M.D.
J. William Reddoch, M.D.
Moss L. Antony, M.D.

EXECUTIVE SECRETARY

Emily Busby

ACTIVE MEMBERS
1984

NEW ORLEANS ACADEMY OF OPHTHALMOLOGY

ABERNATHY, Edward A.
ADAIR, Bonnie
ADLER, Hartwig
ALLEN, James H.
ANTONY, Moss L.
AREND, Laurence
AZAR, Robert F.
BALDONE, Joseph A.
BAXTER, Robert S.
BLAKENEY, C.C.
BOLES, William McDonald
BOSWELL, H. Frank
BOTERO, Alfredo
BOYS-SMITH, John*
BRINT, Stephen F.
BROCK, Joseph R.
CALDWELL, Delmar R.
CANGELOSI, Robert J.
CAPLAN, Dan
CAPLAN, Harry B.
CARROLL, Denis
CERISE, Don*
CLARK, Charles E.
COCKERHAM, Walter D.
COHEN, Gerald
COHEN, Sam
DABEZIES, Oliver H., Jr.
DIAMOND, James G.
DIAZ, Walter P.
DIMITRI, George J.
DOZIER, Horace B.
ELLIS, George S., Jr.
ELLIS, George, Sr.
FINKELSTEIN, Wilfred
FRANKLIN, Rudolph
FRIEDLANDER, Miles H.
GAINES, Shelly R.
GITTER, Kurt A.
GORDON, Robert A.
GRAETZ, Roger T.
GUARNIERI, Joseph
HABEEB, Albert F.W.
HAIK, George, Jr.
HAIK, George, Sr.
HAIK, Hilliard M.
HAIK, Kenneth
HANLEY, Jeanne R.
HART, N. Leon
HESSE, Richard
HORTON, Cheryl
INSLER, Michael S.
KALIL, Rodney F.
KARCIOGLU, Zeynel A.
KASTL, Peter
KAUFMAN, Herbert E.
LANDRY, Ronald
LEA, Martha Ellis
LEADER, Barry
LECKERT, Edmund L., Jr.
LONG, Daniel A.
LONG, Robert A.
McCOMISKEY, James
McDONALD, Marguerite
McKENNA, Warren P.
McNEILL, David L.
MEDLEY, Jerome T.
MORGAN, Keith S.
NAUGLE, Thomas C., Jr.
NAUGLE, Thomas C., Sr.
NELSON, Earl L.
NEWSOM, Samuel R.
NIX, Ralph R.
O'BYRNE, Alvaro
OCHSNER, Rise
PAILET, Sanford L.
PEREZ, William A.
POLLARD, Joel B.
PURYEAR, G. Porter
RACHAL, William F.
REDDOCH, J. William, Jr.
REITMAN, Howard S.
ROSENTHAL, J. William
ROSSNER, Charles W.
RUBIN, Richard L.
RUMAGE, Joseph R.
SAMSON, C.L.M.
SANDERS, C. Drew
SCHIMEK, Robert A.
SCHOEL, Robert E.
SCHOENBERGER, Martin
SIBLEY, Riley C.
SLAGLE, David F., II
SONNIER, Earl J.
STAHEL, Edward
STANBERY, Marie
STRAUSS, Howard B.
TERRELL, W. Lee
TUMAN, Walter C.
TURKISH, Lance
VAN DYK, H.J.L.
WAGNER, Nancy Jo
WOOD, Betty Jean
WOOL, Brandon*
ZIMMERMAN, Thom. J.

---

*Applications pending.

Index

D

E

S

T